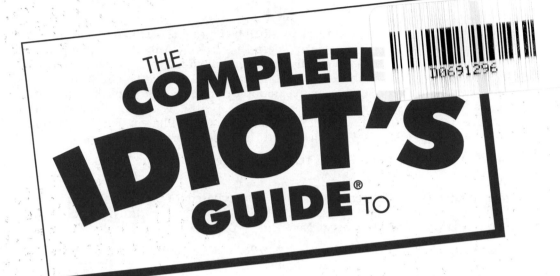

THE COMPLETE IDIOT'S GUIDE® TO

Healing
Back Pain

by Deborah S. Romaine and
Dawn E. DeWitt, M.D., M.Sc., FACP

alpha
books

A Division of Macmillan General Reference
A Pearson Education Macmillan Company
1633 Broadway, New York, NY 10019

Alpha Development Team

Publisher
Kathy Nebenhaus

Editorial Director
Gary M. Krebs

Managing Editor
Bob Shuman

Marketing Brand Manager
Felice Primeau

Acquisitions Editor
Jessica Faust

Development Editors
Phil Kitchel
Amy Zavatto

Assistant Editor
Georgette Blau

Production Team

Book Producer
Lee Ann Chearney/Amaranth

Development Editor
Lynn Northrup

Production Editor
Christy Wagner

Copy Editor
Susan Aufheimer

Cover Designer
Mike Freeland

Photo Editor
Richard H. Fox

Illustrator
Wendy Frost

Cartoonist
Jody Schaeffer

Book Designers
Scott Cook and Amy Adams of DesignLab

Indexer
Angie Bess

Layout/Proofreading
Angela Calvert
Linda Quigley

Contents at a Glance

Contents

Foreword

In my 24 years as a physician, I've seen thousands of patients with back pain. I've given hundreds of prescriptions to patients with bad backs. I've sent dozens to chiropractors, acupuncturists, massage therapists, and yoga classes. I've sent dozens more to orthopedists, radiologists, and physical therapists. And how much time was spent in my medical school class on the diagnosis and treatment of back pain? Approximately six hours out of four years!

I spent the next decade learning about backs: how to touch them, how they move, how they are injured, and how they heal. This learning came in bits, from different sources and teachers. There was no easy way to learn about this all-too-common problem, and certainly no books that adequately covered the subject.

The fact is, back pain is as poorly understood by physicians as it is widespread. Yet millions of days of productive time are lost to back pain, and billions of dollars will be spent on it. And in the end, many people will still have chronic back pain.

Deborah S. Romaine and Dr. Dawn DeWitt's remarkable book, *The Complete Idiot's Guide to Healing Back Pain*, is full of insights into the understanding and treatment of back pain. In the clear and conversational style familiar to readers of *The Complete Idiot's Guide* series, Ms. Romaine and Dr. DeWitt describe how the back works. They describe the anatomy and physiology of the back, and then give an easy-to-follow description of how we get back pain. The world of strains, sprains, and spasms is the world many of us live in daily, and this book makes that world understandable.

But understanding back pain is only the first step. This book offers the broadest approach possible to *healing* back pain. Not just medications and surgery, although these are discussed completely. *The Complete Idiot's Guide to Healing Back Pain* discusses many of the alternatives that complement a healing approach to back problems. Chiropractic, osteopathy, and hands-on therapies like massage are described, and practical tips are given to help in the decision of what treatments to seek. Acupuncture, which has been an effective tool in my own practice, is discussed from both Eastern and Western perspectives. Relaxation techniques are covered in detail, and movement therapies such as yoga and t'ai chi are included with easy directions.

This book is more than just a description of therapies, however. It's chock-full of down-to-earth wisdom on how to move, live, and cope with back pain. One chapter is even entitled "Imagine a Healthy, Pain-Free Back." Another section discusses how to go back to work and how to organize the workplace so that back pain won't recur. There are even sections describing back pain during pregnancy, during the elder years, and in children.

Reading this book, of course, will not make back pain go away. But it will be a start toward a better understanding, a better "tool chest," and a better outlook on the problem of back pain.

Enjoy!

—Glenn S. Rothfeld, M.D., M.Ac.

Glenn S. Rothfeld, M.D., M.Ac., served as a clinical fellow at Harvard University School of Medicine after his training in family medicine. He is trained in nutritional and herbal medicine and has a master's degree in acupuncture. Regional medical director for American WholeHealth, Dr. Rothfeld is also clinical assistant professor of community medicine and family health at Tufts University School of Medicine. Dr. Rothfeld is the author of four books on natural medicine, including *Natural Medicine for Back Pain*, and has written numerous articles for medical journals and health magazines.

Introduction

It's easy to rush through your day without a single thought about the back that makes your actions possible. Until, that is, your back hurts. Then nothing is easy! All you want to do is make the pain go away.

When it comes to helping back pain, a key challenge, however, is separating healing and hoax. In deciding what to include in this book, we considered a number of factors. What objective, scientific evidence supports the approach or treatment? How long have practitioners been using it? What are the known risks, short and long term? What can go wrong, and how often does it? Are you likely to feel better, worse, or no different? Sometimes the answers to these questions are incomplete at best, or even nonexistent.

New treatments tend to arrive with all the excitement and fanfare that heralds a first child. Just as sleepless nights and indescribable diapers soon notch the joy of parenting down a peg, however, these treatments quickly fade into ordinariness as the reality of their limitations takes over. After all, nothing is perfect and no treatment does everything for everyone.

Much of this book presents conventional, or allopathic, approaches to back problems because these are the approaches that are most widespread and often have been tested most rigorously. When you go to your regular doctor, you're seeking relief through one or several allopathic treatments. We also discuss different practitioners and approaches, to present a wide view of the possibilities and options.

Because the overwhelming majority of back pain isn't serious, there's often no one "right" approach for back pain (which you've probably already discovered as you've tried various remedies and treatments to help yours). Rarely, however, delay in medical care can be risky, and there are some approaches that can harm you—or at the very least, harm your checking account. Where these risks are serious and well documented, we warn you about them. Others we simply don't discuss at all because there's no evidence one way or the other. Our goal is to present information that will help you make knowledgeable decisions about keeping your back healthy and pain free. After all, you should enjoy the dawning of each new day, not dread it!

How to Use This Book

There's no right or wrong way to use this book. You can read this book cover to cover. You can take a section or chapter at a time. Or you can jump right to the parts that interest you most. Quick quizzes throughout present a lighthearted way to see what you already know...and what you don't.

We've organized the book into six parts:

Part 1, "This Back of Yours," gives you the lowdown on the structure that supports your body and your life—how it's put together, how it works, and what puts it at risk.

Part 2, "When Your Back Betrays You," discusses what can go wrong with your back and how doctors identify the problem.

Part 3, "Pain, Pain, Go Away," looks at various treatment approaches and your body's natural healing efforts.

Part 4, "Cut to the Fix," examines the surgical options for treating back problems.

Part 5, "A Healing Touch," discusses hands-on approaches to helping your back feel better.

Part 6, "Back-Healthy Living," offers guidance and suggestions about lifestyle matters that affect your back's health and well-being.

Back Tips

In each chapter, you'll find boxes with information that's interesting or helpful.

Back Talk

These boxes provide additional information, such as tidbits from history and interesting facts.

Back to Nature

These boxes offer suggestions for natural or alternative remedies.

Back Basics

These boxes give definitions for technical or medical terms.

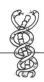

Back Care

Look in these boxes for tips and advice for taking care of your back.

Back Off!

Look in these boxes for warnings and cautions.

Acknowledgments

So many people go into making a book happen, and it's impossible to thank them all. We offer our deep gratitude to the colleagues who provided support and suggestions. We appreciate the good cheer and efficiency of the librarians who provided resources and information. We owe our families and friends, who still love us in spite of the craziness we put them through, big time. And we give thanks to (and for) Lee Ann Chearney at Amaranth, who, with patience and good humor, kept us on track.

Dawn would like to thank her colleagues who answered questions and confirmed details: Drs. Greg Gardner, Eric Kraus, Kenneth Maravilla, and Alexander Baxter. And a special thank you to Dr. Rick Deyo, who kept me focused on critically evaluating the medical evidence and repeatedly confirmed the need for good information for patients.

Special Thanks to the Technical Reviewers

The Complete Idiot's Guide® to Healing Back Pain was reviewed by several experts who double-checked the accuracy of what you'll learn here, to help us ensure that this book gives you everything you need to know about healing your back pain. Each technical editor reviewed information from the standpoint of his or her professional training (scope of care) and his or her duty of care; individual technical experts do not necessarily endorse every treatment option outlined in the text. Readers should remember to consult their primary care physicians before embarking on *any* treatment regimen for back pain—from chiropracty to surgery to beginning a fitness program. We extend special thanks to:

T. John Baumeister, D.O., assisted with Chapter 20, "Focus on Function: Osteopathy." A graduate of the Chicago College of Osteopathic Medicine, Dr. Baumeister is board certified in osteopathic family practice and in pain management and board qualified in osteopathic manipulative methods and emergency medicine. He has a special interest in osteopathic treatment of painful conditions, and practices in Redmond, Washington.

Richard A. Deyo, M.D., M.P.H., provided guidance and expertise in technical matters about back problems. Dr. Deyo received his medical degree from Pennsylvania State University College of Medicine, and completed residencies at the University of Texas (San Antonio) Health Science Center. He then completed a fellowship at the University of Washington as a Robert Wood Johnson Clinical Scholar, during which time he also received a master's degree in public health from UW. Widely published, Dr. Deyo serves on the editorial boards of several professional journals. He has a long-standing research interest in the management of back problems, and remains active in clinical teaching and practice as well as research.

Deirdre Kidder, D.C., provided invaluable assistance with chiropractic and holistic approaches to healing back pain. Dr. Kidder received her doctor of chiropractic degree from the New York Chiropractic College. She is a member of the New York Council of Chiropractors.

Sohail Mirza, M.D., provided technical assistance with the chapters in Part 4, "Cut to the Fix." After receiving his medical degree from the University of Colorado Medical School, Dr. Mirza completed his surgical residency at the University of Washington Medical Center (UWMC) in Seattle and a fellowship in spinal surgery at Harvard Medical School. Board certified in orthopedic surgery, Dr. Mirza is in practice at UWMC.

Glenn S. Rothfeld, M.D., M.Ac., offered insightful comments to Chapter 19, "Ancient Chinese Wisdom: Acupuncture," as well as graciously contributing the foreword to this book. Dr. Rothfeld was a clinical fellow at Harvard University School of Medicine after his training in family medicine. He has also been trained in nutritional and herbal medicine and has a master's degree in acupuncture.

Trademarks

All terms mentioned in this book that are known to be or are suspected of being trademarks or service marks have been appropriately capitalized. Alpha Books and Macmillan General Reference cannot attest to the accuracy of this information. Use of a term in this book should not be regarded as affecting the validity of any trademark or service mark.

Part 1
This Back of Yours

It may not be natural for man to walk upright, but it was a noble invention.
—Gorg Christoph Lichtenberg (1742–1799)

Your backbone is what separates you from other life forms on this planet. It makes it possible for you to walk, sit, stand, run, jump, and even lie down for a nap. Without it, you'd be unable to move at all on your own.

The chapters in Part 1 tell you how this intricate structure is put together and how it carries you through the activities of your day. From the bones that give it shape to the nerves and muscles that make it move, your back keeps you in motion.

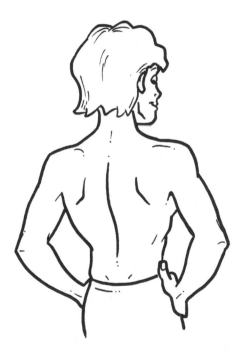

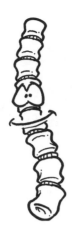

Chapter 1

The Backbone of Life

In This Chapter

➤ How posture affects back health

➤ How you treat your back: a self-quiz

➤ What stresses your back?

➤ New understandings and treatment approaches

Most of us think little about our backs when all is well. We stand, sit, bend, twist, and flex thanks to this marvel of natural engineering, all with little conscious attention on our part. But when your back hurts, you can think of little else. No other pain so completely envelopes every aspect of your being, from breathing to moving. Not even sleep offers escape from an aching back. At any given time, about 15 percent of us know this all too well—and more than 80 percent of us will experience the torment of back pain at least once during our lives.

What you want to know when you're the one experiencing back pain is how to make it go away, or at least loosen its grasp on your life for awhile. Take heart, there is hope! By taking good care of your back, you can greatly reduce the likelihood that back pain will come calling. And by giving your back a little TLC when it does bother you, you can minimize both the length and severity of your discomfort. Not all back pain is preventable, of course, and not all back pain goes away quickly. Even when you seem stuck with a bum back, there are things you can do to control the situation.

The Mixed Blessing of Upright Walking

Here we are—humankind, the most sophisticated life form inhabiting the Earth. What sets us definitively apart is not our houses, cities, cars, and other trappings of modern living, but a characteristic we can trace to the beginning of human existence—an erect posture. (And opposable thumbs, but that's another story.) Among all the creatures that populate our world, only human beings walk exclusively upright. While this certainly makes it easier to reach for that bag of cookies stashed on the cupboard's top shelf, it doesn't always bode well for back health.

Back Talk

Every year in America, back pain accounts for more than 14 million visits to the doctor, 100 million lost days of work, and $30 to $60 billion in related costs. Back pain is the second most common symptomatic reason people go to the doctor (pregnancy care, checkups, well-baby visits are more common), and the second leading reason for missing work. While people in other countries seem to experience just as much back pain as we do, they seek less medical attention and spend less money trying to make it better. America's back surgery rate is five times that of Great Britain's.

One theory holds that upright posture would not have survived the strenuous *survival of the fittest* process of evolution were it not the most efficient means of movement. That would certainly be the case if we still hunted and gathered our food in the fields and woods instead of at the grocery store. In such an existence, we would spend most of our waking hours running and walking, activities that keep the back in good working condition. But our modern lifestyle turns that formula upside down—we spend far more time standing and sitting. This puts incredible pressure on the complex structures of the spine and back, with your lower back supporting most of your weight.

Walking on all fours, according to other theories, relieves this pressure. The burden of balance goes to the legs rather than the back, easing the load the back bears. In this posture, there is no pressure on the sensitive structures that form the spine. Walking on all fours is not likely to help humans today, since our bodies are designed to walk upright. (Though walking on all fours

Back Basics

Survival of the fittest describes the way traits that help a species survive are passed on to future generations.

does little to help the poor daschund, whose long body and short legs mean the little dog's entire body weight hangs from its spine.)

Following a regular yoga practice is just one way we humans can ease the demands of our upright frame. Developed over centuries, many of the poses were created from careful observance of the natural world: from the tranquil power of standing in mountain pose or the peaceful balance of tree pose to the graceful stretch of downward facing dog pose. For more about how yoga can help your back, see Chapter 5, "Posture Perfect," or pick up a copy of *The Complete Idiot's Guide to Yoga* (Alpha Books, 1998).

Bad Backs Keep Good Company

Back problems can affect anyone. Indeed, 8 out of every 10 of us will experience at least one episode of back pain in our lifetimes. Back pain doesn't care how famous you are (or aren't), how much money you have, or what you do for a living. From athletes to zookeepers, no one is immune.

Athletes are often in the news for various injuries. Back pain has sidelined many of America's star athletes such as hockey legend Wayne Gretsky and basketball great Larry Bird. Some have even changed direction and careers, such as first baseman Tony Clark, who was a standout college basketball player until back problems forced him to switch from the court to the diamond. Athletes, whether of the professional or "weekend warrior" persuasion, push the limits of tolerance in many areas. Their backs take unusual punishment from extremes in both movement and blows. But more often than not, there is no clear injury or action that causes back pain. It just shows up one day.

Back Talk

John F. Kennedy, the popular thirty-fifth president of the United States, experienced nearly incapacitating back pain for most of his adult life. Born with a number of physical ailments that resulted in back problems, Kennedy underwent several surgeries that did little to relieve his pain. Outwardly the picture of healthy youthfulness, by 1954 Kennedy could walk without crutches for only very short distances—though none but his closest acquaintances knew.

Are You Good to Your Back? A Self-Quiz

If you're among the fortunate few whose back seldom pains you, you're probably not even aware of the amazing structure that keeps you upright. But if twinges and aches are familiar reminders that your back's back there, you know how easy it is to just "do something" that turns your day upside down. How do you treat your back? Take this quick quiz to see. Circle the letter that best describes how you would respond to each situation.

1. There's a box at the front door when you get home. To pick it up, you...

    a) Shift the two bags of groceries you're carrying into one arm, then swoop down with your free hand to scoop the box up.

    b) Anchor one bag of groceries in each arm, squat down, and pinch the box between the two bags.

    c) Bend over, put the bags of groceries down, and pick up the box.

    d) Take the groceries in the house, come back out, squat down, take the box in both hands, and stand up.

2. The copy machine is out of paper, and there's no more on the shelf. You have to get a case of paper that weighs about 60 pounds from the storeroom. To get it back to the copy machine, you...

    a) Bend down, pick it up, and shuffle as fast as you can so you don't drop it before you get there.

    b) Pull the box to the edge of the shelf, let it drop onto the floor, then take out one ream of paper and take that back to the copy machine. Someone else can deal with the rest of it.

    c) Stop by the utility room on your way to the storeroom to pick up a hand cart. You pull the case of paper onto the cart, then wheel it back to the copy machine.

    d) Ask a coworker to give you a hand. Together, you get a hand cart, lift the case of paper onto the cart, and wheel the cart back to the copy machine.

3. When you work at a desk, you sit...

    a) In whatever chair happens to be available.

    b) In a chair with wheels, so you can prop your feet up on the legs.

    c) In an old but comfortable steno chair.

    d) In a fully adjustable, ergonomically designed chair fitted especially for you.

4. When you get out of bed in the morning, you feel...

    a) Like you were involved in every tackle on *Monday Night Football*.

    b) A little stiff, but nothing a hot shower won't fix.

    c) You don't really think about it.

    d) Refreshed and ready to start a new day.

5. You're standing in line at the library with an armload of books to check out. You…

   a) Hold the books in a stack at waist level, standing with your knees locked and your feet about shoulder's width apart.

   b) Rest the books first against one hip and then the other, shifting your weight from one leg to the other as you change position.

   c) Stack the books on the floor and shove them forward with your foot as the line moves.

   d) Place the books on the counter, then step back into line to finish waiting your turn.

6. It's time to get that box of holiday decorations down from the top shelf in the closet. You…

   a) Stretch up to scrape the box with your fingertips until it reaches the edge of the shelf, then catch it as it falls.

   b) Stack enough books to let you reach the box, then pull it down and jump to the floor before the stack topples over.

   c) Stand on a chair, pull the box off the shelf, step off the chair holding the box, then bend over and put the box on the floor.

   d) Call a spouse, partner, or friend to give you a hand. Using a stepladder, you stand so the box is at least level with your chest. Grabbing the box with both hands, you pull it toward you. When it's completely off the shelf, you hold the box tight against your chest, then pass it to your waiting helper.

7. Your credit card has somehow ended up under the sofa, where you can see but not quite reach it. You…

   a) Bend down, put your hands under the bottom edge of the sofa, and try to move it enough to let you reach the card.

   b) Pull all the cushions off and try to squeeze your arm through the same opening the card went through.

   c) Poke under the sofa with a yardstick or broom handle to see if you can snag the card and pull it to where you can reach it.

   d) Muster enough help to safely move the sofa to retrieve your card (and do a little cleaning while you're there).

Tally the number of As, Bs, Cs, and Ds you marked. If you scored mostly As and Bs, your habits are likely to bring you back problems. If you scored mostly Cs, your back thanks you. And if you marked five or more Ds, give yourself a pat on the back. You're treating your back with care!

Your Stressed Back

It's probably fair to say that life through the centuries has never been without its physical stresses. For primitive cultures, survival itself was a struggle, with nearly all the elements of the environment more enemy than friend. An aching back was merely an annoyance, no doubt. There were more serious matters to worry about, not the least of which were the hazards of the hunt during the day and the predatory animals that lurked in the darkness of night. A minor mishap such as a sprained ankle could doom an individual's existence; more severe injuries would almost certainly end it. And of course, life spans were much shorter then, with the average adult living only to age 30 or so well into the sixteenth century. (Today, by comparison, the average American will live to age 75, bad backs notwithstanding. Indeed, according to the MacArthur Foundation study of aging, the increases in the human life span in the twentieth century are so significant that of all the humans throughout the history of humankind who've lived to be age 65, fully half of them are alive *today*!)

In most parts of our twenty-first-century world, few people hunt to eat. By comparison with our predecessors, our lives are quite cushy. We walk for exercise, not necessarily transportation. Mechanical devices assist in nearly all heavy lifting tasks. In fact, more Americans sit all day than ever before in history. So why do we have more back problems? Because we sit so much. Believe it or not, all that running through the forests in search of the day's meal was actually healthy for the human back! It kept muscles strong and limber, and the nearly continual movement kept pressure on the spine at a minimum. When in motion, your back's muscles, bones, and ligaments work in harmony. When your back is in balance, your body is in balance.

Of course, there are other reasons for back problems. Our longer life span means that some people live long enough to develop back problems that are related to the natural deteriorations of bone and connective tissue related to the aging process. Osteoporosis, a decrease in bone density with age that is common in many American women, is a good example of such a condition. Modern living also involves significant lifting. Primitive humans hefted deer from the hunt and harvested grain by hand, and we modern humans, despite all our advanced machines, still have to do repetitive lifting. It's no wonder we suffer occasional back problems! Luckily, primitive and agricultural humans were rarely chronically disabled by back pain and the same remains true for us.

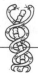

Back Care

Prolonged sitting alters the natural curvature of your spine, stressing the muscles and ligaments in your back. Stand and move around or stretch for 5 or 10 minutes every half-hour or so to relieve this stress and help your back feel better.

Postures Nature Never Intended

The next time you're getting ready for a bath or shower, stand sideways and take a look at your back. You'll notice a prominent inward curve at your waist. When you sit, that curve nearly disappears, changing the relationships among the muscles, bones, ligaments, and nerves. And we sit a lot. Even if your job requires standing, walking, and lifting, odds are you still spend more time in a chair than in all other positions combined (except lying in bed).

Obviously nature intended for humans to sit. Just not so much for so long in so many different ways! Many of us sit in our cars to get to work, sit at a desk all day, sit in our cars to get home again, and sit on the sofa to relax. Even if your job is physically demanding, odds are you spend more time sitting than doing anything else. And if you're not sitting, you're standing—a posture that, even though it maintains your back's natural curves (provided you're wearing flat-heeled shoes), is equally challenging for your back. Factor in lifting or repetitive movements, and you're a backache waiting to happen.

Of course, you can't just stop living because your back *might* hurt at some point. The key is to add activities to your life that keep your back healthy and strong so it can resist the challenges it faces.

The Body/Mind Connection

Would it surprise you to learn that pain is as much about how you perceive it as how it feels? Your perception of pain generally determines how much that pain limits your usual activities. Pain is highly subjective. What you might find tolerable could well drive someone else nuts, or vice versa. This is not to say that you can wish away back pain if you just think about it hard enough or that back pain is all in your head. But you can change the way you feel about pain, which in turn changes how that pain affects your life. We talk more about this in later chapters.

Natural Alternatives to Heal Back Pain

Therapy	Healing Back Benefit
Yoga	Yoga's gentle stretching and strengthening exercises increase range of motion, build flexibility, muscle tone and muscle strength, and calm and center the mind.
T'ai chi and QiGong	These ancient Chinese practices are believed to harness and channel life force energy for healing benefit. The slow movements and poses center the mind and body and have therapeutic value for stress reduction and chronic pain conditions, such as back pain.
Meditation	Seated meditation promotes good posture (and the meditator's conscious awareness of what good posture is!). Breathing exercises can strengthen abdominal muscles and the diaphragm muscle. Concentration promotes relaxation and stress reduction, which lessens the perception of pain.

continues

9

Natural Alternatives to Heal Back Pain (continued)

Therapy	Healing Back Benefit
Guided imagery	The connection between the mind and body is a powerful one. Directing thought to address a specific problem, such as healing back pain, can have positive results.

Back-Breaking Habits

How did you do on the earlier back quiz? Many of our back problems are those we bring on ourselves, not through intent but as a result of the everyday activities we perform and even the shoes we wear. Over time, the bad habits that form our daily routines will break down even the strongest backs. It's usually the constant assault of little things that add up to major problems. After all, pain is often a message from your body that something's not right. To end the pain, you have to right the wrong.

Back Off!

If you feel pain in the small of your back, particularly on just one side, and have pain when you urinate or a fever over 100°, see your doctor. This kind of pain can indicate a kidney infection.

Back Basics

An **anti-inflammatory** medication works to reduce the swelling or inflammation at the site of an injury. An **analgesic** is a drug that relieves pain. Many anti-inflammatory drugs also work as analgesics.

When Back Pain Rules (and Ruins) Your Life

When we hurt, we want to know why. The truth is, doctors can't determine a definitive cause for 85 percent of all back pain complaints. Nonetheless, most people see significant improvement within two weeks of the onset of pain and their back pain entirely disappears within six weeks. For some people, unfortunately, the pain stays. If you're among them, you have our sympathy. We know that for some of you, your pain has come to define your life and your activities.

While we'd like nothing more than to tell you this book holds the magic answers you've been seeking, we can't. There aren't any. There is just a process, a long one for some people, of searching for relief. For all the marvels of modern medicine that have emerged in the last 20 years, we still can't fix everything. What we *can* offer you are alternatives and approaches for the relief of back pain that you may not have considered or already tried.

Temporary Setback

Maybe it was that drive from the eleventh green, when your foot slipped just as your club connected. The ball and your back both took it rough, with a sharp jab just below the right side of your rib cage in the back, cutting short what would've been a textbook-perfect follow-through. Even breathing hurts. But as bad as your back hurts in the first few hours, your injury is not likely serious and odds are good that you'll be back in good form within a few weeks.

The twisting, sudden movements common in many activities from sports to household chores often cause strains and pulls that are temporary setbacks. Most such injuries heal in two to six weeks whether you seek medical treatment or not. An over-the-counter *anti-inflammatory* medication such as ibuprofen or an *analgesic* such as acetaminophen may help you feel better, but time is the true healer.

No End in Sight

Are you among the 1 to 2 percent of Americans who have disabling back problems? Not all back problems are curable, and when it happens to you, it can change your life. In such situations, the best thing you can do is take a realistic appraisal of your circumstances. What *can* you do and still tolerate your back's response? Where are your limits, and what things do you do that stretch them? What happens? Sometimes it's helpful to keep a daily journal for a few weeks, to record how you actually feel during certain activities. You might be surprised that you've become accustomed to limitations imposed by your perceptions, not by the reality of your condition. After you've documented your aches and pains, you might see ways to work around problem areas and to restore at least some aspects of your life to normal.

And if you complete this journaling exercise and conclude that all you can do is sit around, read on. While bed rest and inactivity were once the mainstays of treatment for back problems, this is no longer true. Numerous studies demonstrate that activity and exercise (in moderation and usually under the guidance of a physical trainer and your health care provider, of course) are the weapons for winning the war against back pain.

There's Always Hope

If you've lived with back pain for a long time, you might feel there's little hope for improvement. At first glance, statistics support this belief. After one year of back injury disability, according to studies conducted for the insurance industry, your odds of returning to work are one in four. After two years, those odds drop to nil. There are many reasons for this, some of which have little relationship to the back injury (more on this in later chapters). With nearly 50,000 people experiencing disabling back injuries every year, this is a serious situation.

New understandings about the workings of the back coupled with studies of the effectiveness of various treatments hold promise for improving these odds. Herniated, or "slipped," disks bear the

Back Basics

Computerized tomography, or **CT scan**, and magnetic resonance imaging, or **MRI**, are high-tech procedures that allow doctors to see what's going on inside your spine without surgery. These tests are sometimes useful in diagnosing the cause of certain kinds of back pain.

blame for much back pain, for example, yet sophisticated new technologies like *CT scans* and *MRIs* show that damaged disks are at least as common in people with no complaints of back pain as they are in people experiencing incapacitating back pain. While so far no miracle cures have come of these studies, they nonetheless give physicians new guidance in that famed edict from the famous ancient Greek physician Hippocrates: "Above all, do no harm."

Back Basics

Vertebrae are the bones of the spine. **Intervertebral disks** are the gel-filled tissue cushions that separate the vertebrae from one another. When a disk **herniates**, the outer tissue tears and allows some of the soft internal material to escape, reducing the disk's ability to cushion the vertebrae and sometimes placing pressure on nerves.

New Understanding

The Belgian physician Andreas Vesalius (1514–1564) first identified and published drawings of the *vertebrae* and *intervertebral disks* in 1543. It took nearly another 300 years for scientists to understand the relationship between them. In 1934 a pair of Boston surgeons removed a swelling in the disk of a patient's spine and cured the patient's leg pain—the first surgery to remove a *herniated disk*. This helped identify one source for back and leg pain. In the years since, doctors have refined this knowledge into a greater understanding of the intricate relationships among the back's bones, muscles, tendons, ligaments, and nerves. They've learned that not all herniated disks cause pain, and that surgery helps only 5 to 10 percent of those that do.

New Treatment Approaches

Just 10 years ago, the treatment of choice for back pain was complete bed rest until the pain went away. The logic behind this approach was that lying flat on your back relieved stress on your spine and back, allowing healing to take place. What actually happened, researchers discovered after years of studies, was that the longer you stayed in bed, the more atrophied, or withered away, your muscles became. Maybe stretched out in your bed you didn't feel any pain, but as soon as you got up and started moving around, your back pain flared up. Studies show that, in fact, the opposite approach is far more likely to ease both the pain and the problem causing it. Doctors now recommend returning to normal activity as quickly as possible, and people start feeling better faster.

Other technologies have entered the treatment picture, too. Ultrasound treatment performed by a qualified health care professional sends high-frequency sound waves into damaged soft tissues like muscles and tendons to speed healing. New anti-inflammatory drugs reduce swelling and pain with few side effects, enhancing the body's natural healing efforts. Therapeutic massage and physical therapy are also helpful. Some people get relief from chiropractic adjustments or acupuncture treatments.

Just for You

Throughout this book, we'll be "rounding up the usual suspects"—the sources of back pain most likely to be giving you trouble—and providing insight and strategies for healing your back and reducing pain. Do you see yourself in any of the people in the following list?

➤ You deliver or process thousands of letters and packages each year at work for the United States Post Office or for a major courier service, such as Airborne Express, FedEx, or UPS.

➤ As a nurse or an allied health care provider—a health professional who has special training in supportive health care tasks, such as a physical therapist, massage therapist, or medical assistant—you're often called upon to lift or assist patients and sometimes to handle heavy medical equipment.

➤ You drive a truck for a living, spending most of your waking hours sitting behind the wheel.

➤ You don't drive a truck for a living, but you spend at least an hour in the car per day commuting to the office or on mass transportation in the big cities just getting where you're going.

➤ Your office job requires handling, sorting, and filing documents, files, and reports every day.

➤ You're seven months pregnant and still trying to do everything you always do anyway! Hey, your world doesn't slow down while you're having a baby…that is, of course, unless *you* slow it down!

➤ You've got a toddler to tote.

➤ You wait in line.

➤ You've got an aging parent to assist in daily activities such as dressing and bathing.

➤ You're a computer programmer who's spending every waking moment sitting at the computer working on changing code to solve that pesky Y2K conundrum. Not only does your back hurt, but you've got a headache, too!

➤ After a hard day's work hefting, toting, commuting, and sitting at a desk, all you want to do is collapse in front of the TV for the evening.

It seems that no matter who you are or what you do every day, our twenty-first-century world presents interesting challenges for healing back pain. We may have richly diverse lives and interests, but when it comes down to it, Americans share a struggle to control and manage back pain—and the many lifestyle circumstances that contribute to it. Perhaps we should put healing back pain on the national agenda!

The Least You Need to Know

➤ Most back pain improves within two to six weeks of the initial injury, with or without medical treatment.

➤ The postures of modern times—sitting and standing—account for the majority of back problems.

➤ Gentle exercise and activity do the most to help heal back injuries.

➤ Though you may not be able to completely eliminate your back pain, you can take charge of how it affects your life.

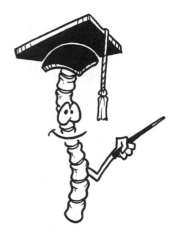

Chapter 2

Back School

In This Chapter

➤ All about bones, muscles, ligaments, and tendons

➤ Drawings that show what your spine looks like

➤ Your spinal cord and major nerves

➤ The five sections of your spine

Remember that saying, "Knowledge is power!" Understanding how your back is constructed and how and why it all works will help you understand the possible causes of back pain, the healing process, and treatment options. You wouldn't go under the hood to try to fix your car yourself without first reading a manual or taking an auto repair workshop, would you? Well, the same logic applies here. While we're not suggesting you open up your back to take a look around, we do think learning more about your back will give you a better understanding of how it works. So, let's go back to school—back school, that is—to learn what a healthy back is made of, and how to keep it strong and pain free.

Giving your back its structure is 33 bones, 23 cartilage disks, 31 pairs of spinal nerves, and dozens of muscles. Ligaments rope the whole contraption together so it both supports your body and encases your spinal cord. The knobby protrusions you feel when you run your fingers down your spine are bone spikes that offer attachment points for your back muscles. To the front, facing your chest and abdominal cavities, your spine presents a smoother surface that serves as the "back wall" for your organ systems.

Not surprisingly, this complex architecture doesn't always come together quite right. About 8 out of every 10 of us have some variation from the ideal in our backs. While most of these differences are minor, occasionally there are significant anomalies, as was the case with former U.S. president John F. Kennedy. Born with what one of his doctors summarized as "the left side of his body smaller than the right," Kennedy suffered from back problems and pain, sometimes severe enough to confine him to a wheelchair or bed, all his life. Fortunately, relatively few backs enter the world in such shape, and most function as nature intended despite minor design flaws.

Back Basics

Vertebrae are the irregularly shaped bones that form your spine; if you're talking about just one, it's a **verte-bra**. The term comes from the Latin word *vertere*, meaning "to turn." **Facet joints** are the small, flat, circular bone surfaces that connect the vertebrae into a column. The term comes from the Latin word *facere*, which means "to form."

Getting Down to Bare Bones: Your Vertebral Column

The 33 bones that form your spine are called *vertebrae*. Five are fused together to form the sacrum, and another four are fused to form the coccyx. When you're born, these bones are all separate; they form into their prospective fused structures by early adulthood. Fingerlike projections called *spinous processes* extend from the back of each vertebra, giving your back its familiar bumpy feel.

Structures called *facet joints* allow the vertebrae to interlock for stability and flexibility. Facet joints have small, flat, circular surfaces separated by a thin film of a substance called *synovial fluid*. Functioning as a lubricant, this fluid lets the bone surfaces glide over one another so your spine can twist and bend. Because they connect the vertebrae, facet joints also keep the bones of your back from separating when you move. Most of us can bend forward far enough to see the upside-down world behind us from between our legs, but can flex backward only about 10 or 20 degrees.

Back Talk

How many vertebrae do you think make up the back and long neck of the giraffe? Despite being able to graze treetops we can barely see, this graceful creature has the same number of bones in its back as do we much shorter humans—33.

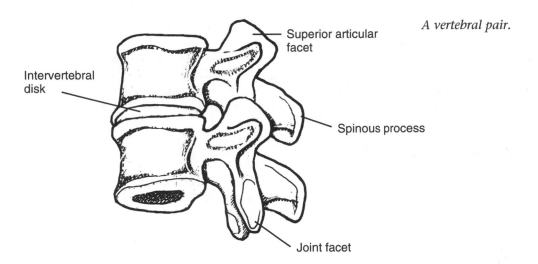

A vertebral pair.

Superior articular facet

Intervertebral disk

Spinous process

Joint facet

Cushioning the Shock: Intervertebral Disks

You wouldn't think walking is such a shock to your back. After all, you usually don't feel a thing in your back just from putting one foot in front of the other. That's because nature gave you built-in shock absorbers—your intervertebral disks. Conveniently wedged in between each vertebra, these keep the bones in your back from crunching into each other with your every move.

Flat and more or less round, each disk has an outer surface of cartilage and an inner core filled with a jelly-like goo about the consistency of the lubricating gel that's a familiar item in your doctor's exam room. Like a water-filled balloon, the disk changes shape in response to pressure your spine puts on it, such as when you sit, walk, jump, or even sneeze. Unlike a water balloon, however, your intervertebral disks are amazingly durable and can take quite a lot of wear and tear before they start to show signs of damage.

Back Talk

There really is no such thing as a "slipped disk." It's pretty much impossible for a disk to slip, since several ligaments anchor it in place. A damaged disk often bulges out from between the vertebrae, however, giving the impression that it has slipped out of place. By itself, a bulging disk doesn't identify the cause of your pain, or even signal a problem. Even normal disks can protrude somewhat.

Contrary to popular belief, a damaged disk doesn't slip. It *herniates* (bulges at a weak place in the disk's outer surface) or ruptures (leaks its inner core of jelly-like fluid through a crack in the outer surface). Either situation reduces the disk's ability to keep the vertebrae on either side of it from clanking into each other with your every move. A herniated disk may push against sensitive nerves or even your spinal cord. Once damaged, a disk cannot fully restore itself. Fortunately, most heal with time and noninvasive treatment (more on this in later chapters).

Holding It All Together

It takes more than rubber bands and baling wire to hold together a structure as complex as the human back. The ties that bind must also flex and stretch. Ligaments, tendons, and muscles tether and wrap your spine, making it possible for you to stand at attention or shake, shimmy, and roll.

Ligaments

Ligaments are tough, fibrous cords of connective tissue that band bones together. In your back, two long, thick ligaments run the length of your spine on either side, linking and aligning the vertebrae into a vertical column. Numerous smaller ligaments intertwine among the vertebrae, anchoring themselves to the spinous processes to form a fibrous web that further restricts each bone's movement. Other ligaments tie the bones of the spine to the ribs and to the pelvis. It's difficult, though certainly not impossible, to damage the ligaments in your back. Other structures, especially muscles, are more likely to give in a potential injury situation.

Back Basics

Ligament comes from the Latin word *ligare*, meaning "to tie." Ligaments connect bones to each other. **Tendon** comes from the Latin word *tendere*, meaning "to stretch." Tendons connect muscles to bones.

Tendons

Similar in structure to ligaments, *tendons* connect muscles to bones. Tendons hold steady as your muscles relax and contract, providing the tension necessary to allow movement. Unlike ligaments, tendons have a supply of nerves that respond to injury by sending pain signals flashing to your brain.

Back Muscles

More than 600 muscles move your body, ranging in size from the barely visible stapedius inside your inner ear to the prominent gluteus maximus that makes it possible for you to move your leg to walk and run (and gives you a nice natural cushion for sitting). About 20 percent of them are in your back. When you have a backache, however, only one muscle matters—the one that hurts.

As often as not, that muscle is the *latissimus dorsus*, a broad, thick band that wraps across your back from the side of your rib cage to the base of your spine. You have a matched pair, one on each side (together they're called the *latissimus dorsi*). These workhorse muscles extend and contract to let you bend and stretch from the waist. In tandem, your latissimus dorsi make it possible for you to stand, sit, walk, and run. Under ordinary circumstances you'll never even notice these muscles at work. Twist or lift wrong, however, and you'll get a sudden and rather rude introduction. Other muscles in your back are also susceptible to injury, particularly from sudden twisting and lifting.

Back Care

A back that's in good physical shape is less likely to hurt than one that doesn't know the meaning of exercise. Walking, yoga, aerobics, and swimming are all excellent activities for the back, as well as overall health.

What Back Muscles Do

Muscle	Function
Deltoids	Each deltoid muscle covers the shoulder joint and controls movement and rotation of the arm.
Erector spinae	Also called the sacrospinalis, this muscle deep in your back draws the ribs down and extends and flexes the vertebrae and head.
Gluteus maximus	This muscle originates in the sacrum and controls thigh extension.
Infraspinatus	This muscle covers the shoulder blade and pulls the arm in toward the body.
Latissimus dorsi	This large muscle draws the shoulder back and down, helps the arm move toward the body, and assists in pulling the body up when climbing.
Rhomboideus major and minor	This pair of muscles located between the shoulder blades helps with pulling.
Teres major and minor	This muscle pair, located beneath the shoulder blade, moves and rotates the arm down and back.
Trapezius	Running from the shoulder blade to the base of the skull, this muscle braces the shoulder and pulls the head back.

The muscles that move your back, like skeletal muscles throughout your body, are called *striated muscles*—under a microscope, their cells appear striped. They are also called voluntary muscles, since you can consciously choose to make them move. (Unlike the muscles of your intestines, for example, which are involuntary—no matter how hard you concentrate, you won't get them to flinch. Involuntary muscles take their marching orders from a part of your brain your conscious awareness never visits.)

The back muscles.

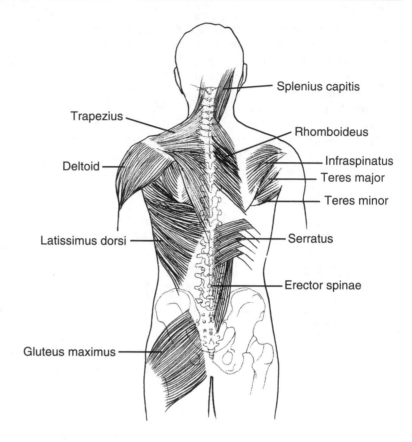

Splenius capitis

Trapezius

Rhomboideus

Deltoid

Infraspinatus

Teres major

Teres minor

Latissimus dorsi

Serratus

Erector spinae

Gluteus maximus

Minute electrical impulses cause striated muscle cells to contract, which they do in unison—only in numbers is there strength. When each electrical impulse ends, the cells relax. Of course, you don't really call out the cadence for these muscles, either. The entire communication process between your brain and your voluntary muscles moves at nearly the speed of light, and can walk you around the block before your conscious instructions could get a single foot off the ground.

Abdominal Muscles

The human body is a marvel of balance and symmetry. Making it possible for the muscles of your back to do their jobs are the muscles of your front side, the abdominal muscles. Amazing abs give you more than just a pleasing physique. As well as holding in the contents of your abdomen, your abdominal muscles counter the actions of the muscles in your back. When you bend over, the muscles in your back relax and stretch and your abdominal muscles contract or tighten. When you straighten up, the reverse happens—your back muscles contract, and your abdominal muscles relax. Weak abdominal muscles force your back muscles to do more of the work in movements such as straightening and lifting. Your abdominal muscles are sometimes called "flexor muscles," and your back muscles "extensor muscles."

What Chest and Abdominal Muscles Do

Muscle	Function
Pectoralis major	This large chest muscle pulls and rotates the arm inward.
Pectoralis minor	Connecting the chest to the collarbone, this muscle pulls the shoulder downward.
Rectus abdominis	These muscles, which flank the belly button, hold the abdomen tight.
External oblique	This muscle runs diagonally across the belly like a band to hold the abdomen tight and keep its contents in place.
Internal oblique	This muscle runs beneath the external oblique at a slightly different angle to further support the abdomen.
Serratus anterior	Wrapping around the side of the ribs, this muscle draws the shoulder blade forward and helps raise the arm. It also aids in pushing.
Sartorius	Running from your pelvis across the thigh, this muscle pulls the thigh up and helps rotate it outward.

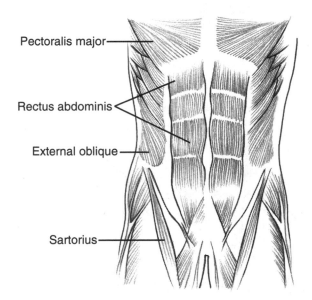

Pectoralis major

Rectus abdominis

External oblique

Sartorius

The chest and abdominal muscles.

The "Body-Wide Web": Your Spinal Cord

Ah, yet another body part you know nothing about unless something happens to interrupt its work: your spinal cord. This bundled cable that extends about 18 inches downward from your brain is teeming with nerve cells—10 billion electrified, microscopic particles, give or take a few million. Your spinal cord and brain together are

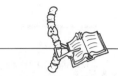

Back Basics

The **cauda equina** is so-named because this branching nerve structure resembles the tail of a horse. The term is Latin for, you guessed it, "horse's tail."

called your *central nervous system*. All messages from your brain to your body travel along this neuro-superhighway until they reach the branching nerve structures that will take them to their targets.

Major nerve channels branch off from your spinal cord at each of the five sections of your spine. Your spinal cord branches out at your lumbar spine into a configuration called the *cauda equina*, which continues to the end of your spine. About the diameter of your index finger, your spinal cord is the largest and most important nerve bundle in your body.

The spinal cord and major nerves.

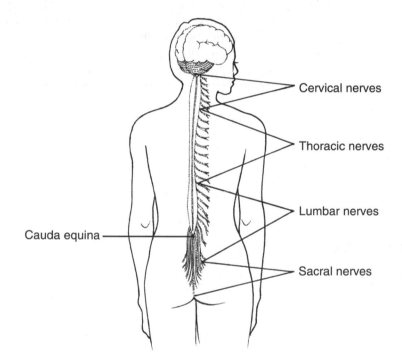

Cervical nerves

Thoracic nerves

Lumbar nerves

Cauda equina

Sacral nerves

Byways and Side Roads: Major Nerves

Signals from your brain travel along your spinal cord until they reach the nerve bundles that say "turn here." A message telling your hand to get off that hot stove, for example, exits your spinal cord at the thoracic nerve trunk intersection at about shoulder level. This nerve path then routes the electronic impulses on down the peripheral (sort of the country roads of your nervous system) nerves to your fingers—which jump off the stove in response to the most powerful message of all, pain. Key nerve intersections are:

➤ The cervical nerves, serving the head and neck

➤ The thoracic nerves, serving the chest and abdomen

➤ The lumbar nerves, serving the trunk and legs

➤ The sacral nerves, serving the lower extremities

These major nerve routes are important because they branch directly from your spinal cord. Any injury to your back, such as a bulging disk, may show up as pain in an area served by the affected major nerve route. For example, sciatica, an inflammation of the sciatic nerve running down the back of your leg, is a prime symptom of a disk problem in your lumbar spine.

Divide and Conquer: Your Back's Five Sections

Your back has too many parts to remember! How do you keep all of this straight? Well, for easy reference, the back's structure is divided into five sections. Knowing which part of your back you're talking about is as easy as cervical, thoracic, lumbar, sacrum, and coccyx (you don't have to spell them, just remember them). In general, each is marked by a change in the direction of your spine's curves.

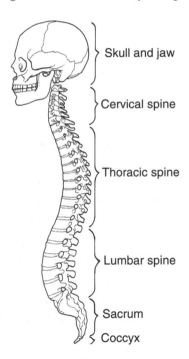

The head and spine.

Skull and jaw

Cervical spine

Thoracic spine

Lumbar spine

Sacrum

Coccyx

Your Neck: The Cervical Spine

The first seven vertebrae under your skull are called the cervical spine, and they form your neck. Doctors often refer to these bones as C1, C2, C3, C4, C5, C6, and C7—not especially inspired, though unmistakably clear. Their main job is to hold your head upright and steady. The top or first cervical vertebra, also called the atlas, has a special surface that allows it to "dock" with the occipital bone of your skull, locking your head and spine together. Movement between the atlas and the second vertebra, the axis, is what allows your head to turn from side to side and to tip back and forth. Your cervical spine curves inward.

Back Off!

Diving into shallow water is a common cause of cervical spine fractures, which can result in paralysis from the neck down if the impact damages the spinal cord as well. If you don't know how deep the water is, save your neck—*don't dive.*

Rib Racks: The Thoracic Spine

The next 12 vertebrae are the thoracic vertebrae, and are numbered T1 through T12. They each anchor a pair of ribs, providing support for your chest. This provides the structure that makes it possible for that vital function, breathing, to take place. Your ribs move up and down as you breathe in and out, allowing your lungs to expand and contract. (Bet you didn't know your back helps you breathe!) Your thoracic spine curves outward.

Back Talk

The so-called "dowager's hump" sometimes seen in elderly women is, in fact, evidence of multiple fractures that cause the cervical and thoracic vertebrae to crumple and their shape changes from nice square boxes to wedge-like, resulting in a curved "leaning tower" effect. Osteoporosis, a condition in which the bones lose calcium and other minerals, causes this disfiguration. We'll talk more about this in the next chapter.

Bend and Stretch: The Lumbar Spine

Moving on down your back, the next five vertebrae form your lumbar spine. This is where you likely put your hands when you complain, "Oh, my aching back!" Your doctor calls these vertebrae L1 through L5, though you may have more expressive names for them when they cause you pain. Your lumbar spine bears the brunt of lifting efforts, and more than 80 percent of those who injure their backs do so while lifting. Its most vulnerable point is the joint between the last lumbar vertebra and the next section of the spine, the sacrum. Your lumbar spine curves inward.

Nothing Sacred: The Sacrum

Your sacrum looks like someone took a hammer to several vertebrae and flattened them into a spade-like, triangular configuration. The sacrum's five vertebrae, which fuse together into a single bony structure in early adulthood, form the back of your pelvis. This is the only part of your spine that looks different depending on whether you're a man or a woman. A woman's sacrum is broader and straighter than a man's sacrum, which is narrow and has a distinct outward curve.

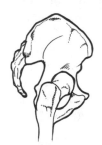

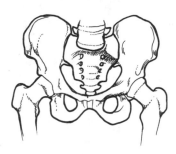

The sacrum and the pelvic structure from side and front views.

Tail End: The Coccyx

Bringing up the rear is your coccyx, the four fused bones that form your tailbone. To some ancient and anonymous anatomist, this structure looked like the beak of a cuckoo bird. So he named it *kokkyx*, Greek for "cuckoo." (We think it looks more like a crooked finger, but the Greek version of that probably wouldn't sound any better.) Translating this word, which is pronounced *kock-six*, into English made it no less peculiar. Rumor has it that if humans had tails, they would start here. Since we don't, this bone configuration is simply the end of the line for your spine. Falling on your tush is a common (and painful!) way to fracture your coccyx.

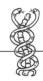

Back Care

While lifting is one risk factor for back pain, people who sit a lot are also at high risk. Prolonged sitting places unnatural tension on the structures of your spine. You can easily relieve this tension and reduce your risk of back problems by standing and walking for a few minutes every hour.

Back to Nature

Your body develops most of your bone mass and strength when you're young. The calcium you feed your body during this time is crucial for good bone density. Dairy products are a common and easy source of calcium, as are tuna, nuts, broccoli, spinach, collard greens, and sardines.

The Backbone's Connected to the...

When it comes right down to it, your back affects almost every other part of your body. Without a strong spine, you couldn't stand, sit, walk, run, twist, jump, or even breathe. Your spine supports your skull, which houses your brain. It shelters your spinal cord, along which your brain sends the millions of signals your body needs to function. It shields vital organ systems from injury, and provides the structure your lungs need to expand and contract. And your spine is the center of your skeleton, providing a place for your arms to hang and your legs to attach. Your backbone really is connected to everything!

A strong spine is central to the proper functioning of the human frame at rest and in motion.

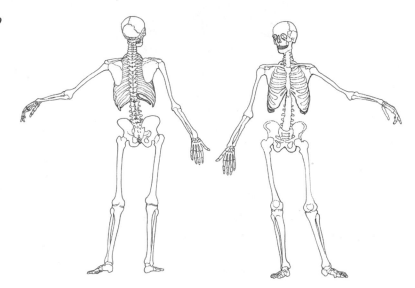

The Least You Need to Know

➤ While few backs are perfect, most work as nature intended.

➤ Your back is a complex structure where bones, ligaments, tendons, muscles, and nerves all have important roles in maintaining back health.

➤ Your spinal cord is the most important nerve structure, besides your brain, in your body.

➤ The best thing you can do for your back is keep it in shape.

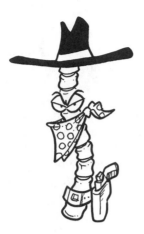

Chapter 3

Why Backs Go Bad

In This Chapter

➤ Extra height and weight are extra trouble

➤ The importance of calcium in your diet

➤ How does your job treat your back? A self-quiz

➤ What happens to your back as you age

Scientists speculate that humans are coming close to the maximum height their backs can support. Our prehistoric ancestors weren't exactly giants. Archaeological discoveries tell us they measured in at a mere $3^1/_2$ feet, about the size of a typical kindergartner today. While those twice that height crowd the ranks of professional basketball, the average man tops out at 5-feet 10-inches. The average woman is about six inches shorter, 5-feet 4-inches.

The spine of a creature that walks on all fours curves slightly upward in a single arc that runs the full length of the back. While this spine design might alleviate some kinds of back problems, it has its drawbacks. Your favorite recliner would be useless, for example, and you couldn't reach the ice cream in the back of the freezer. All in all, the spine design we have isn't so bad!

Who's at Risk and Why

Any back can have problems, since much back pain seems to be the result of simply being human. However, extremes in height and weight can stress your back.

The Tall and Short of It

As height inches upward, it puts more strain on the structures of the back. Among professional basketball players, back problems are second only to ankle injuries in shortening careers—Larry Bird, Charles Barkley, Mike Gminski, Mark Eaton, and Moses Malone are but a handful of court stars sidelined by bad backs. Other tall athletes suffer similar problems. While pitching sensation Randy Johnson's 6-foot 10-inch frame makes him the tallest player in major league baseball, it also has cost him playing time throughout his career. And hockey's big man on the ice, 6-foot 4-inch Mario Lemieux, towered over teammates and opponents alike until persistent back injuries forced his retirement.

All that height requires substance to support it. Taller people have more muscle mass and bigger bones—and more weight. Malone, Johnson, Lemieux, and their tall colleagues weigh in at around 220 pounds. This puts tremendous pressure on the vertebrae and back, especially during bending and straightening. So you're not a great athlete, just tall enough to wash the roof of your 4×4 without a stepstool? Your height still puts you at greater risk for back problems.

Back Care

Women who wear high heels could be setting themselves up for a variety of musculoskeletal problems, from low back pain to osteoarthritis of the knees and foot trouble. Lower heels—ideally no higher than one inch—may not be fashion chic, but they're a good health pick.

Back Talk

According to *Prevention Magazine's Giant Book of Health Facts*, although tall people grab attention wherever they go, short people are more common. Only about 3 percent of American men are taller than 6-feet 4-inches, while more than 15 percent are shorter than 5-feet 6-inches.

What if you're short—say, under five feet tall? While your lack of height doesn't give you immunity, smaller adults do seem less prone to back problems. Use care when stretching, reaching, and twisting, though, to minimize your risks of injury. These actions can make any back twinge.

Weighing In

So you'd walk more, if only you could bend down far enough to tie your shoelaces? Better invest in a pair of slip-ons and start hoofing it before your burgeoning "love handles" carry you right into bad-back country. Extra weight, no matter what your height, places additional stress on muscles, bones, and especially joints. Over time, this stress can strain muscles and ligaments, and become *osteoarthritis*. Not only does walking help your overall fitness level (including weight management), but it keeps your back in motion. This makes your back less prone to injury.

You produce about one pound of pressure for every pound you weigh each time your foot hits the ground. Your body feels the impact of this pressure from the soles of your feet to the base of your skull. As you learned in Chapter 2, "Back School," your body's primary shock absorbers are the intervertebral disks separating the bones in your spine. Unlike bad shocks in your car, however, the cushiony disks in your spine are yours for keeps. If they go bad, there's no way to replace them. This is not to say that you're a frail little thing, certain to break under pressure. To the contrary, intermittent pressure (from walking and other exercise) helps keep your disks and spine healthy.

One way to think of it is that athletes train for anything they do. We'd never encourage someone to run a marathon without training or do gymnastics without coaching. It's harder to keep our backs "in training" because they're harder to isolate as an area, and because we use them so much on a daily basis. Think about how to keep your back strong, though also expect, just as an athlete does, that you'll have the usual sprains and strains of life. This doesn't mean you should approach every move (for example, a new gymnastic routine) with fear and trepidation. Just use common sense and try to enjoy life anyway.

Gender Inequality

How likely you are to have back problems, and what kind, may depend in part on whether you're a man or a woman. According to the American Academy of Orthopedic Surgeons (AAOS), before age 45, men are more than twice as likely to hurt their backs than are women. After age 65, the balance shifts the other way as osteoporosis and compression fractures of the vertebrae become a major concern for women. Both men and women are at greatest risk of back injury between the ages

Back Basics

Osteoarthritis is a "wear and tear" irritation and inflammation of the joints, usually those that are weight-bearing such as knees, hips, and backs. Osteoarthritis can cause joints to deteriorate to a point where movement becomes limited and painful.

Back Basics

A **congenital** condition is one you're born with, and can be random (without an identifiable cause), inherited (linked to your genes), or environmental (caused by viruses, for example). **Spina bifida**, a rare congenital condition affecting the spine, occurs when an abnormal gap forms between the vertebrae in a developing unborn child, leaving part of the spinal cord outside the spine at birth.

of 25 and 55. Of course, most people who have back pain don't have a specific injury. Most of the time, no one really knows why your back hurts.

When You're Born with Back Problems

Congenital back problems, which account for a very small percentage of adult back pain, can range from random deformities in which bone and muscle structures fail to form correctly, such as those suffered by John F. Kennedy, to conditions such as *spina bifida* that appear to be caused by a combination of hereditary and environmental factors. To what extent such problems limit activity depends on their severity as well as the determination of the individual. Kennedy, for example, was a standout athlete, soldier, and politician despite nearly constant back pain.

Back Talk

Spina bifida ranges in severity from a small dimple in the skin above the problem area to complete paralysis below the exposure. Treatment usually includes surgery to enclose the spinal cord within the vertebrae, followed by physical therapy to restore mobility.

While the likelihood of spina bifida is not linked to any single factor, there are several circumstances that appear connected, including high body temperature and folate levels during pregnancy. Doctors recommend that in the first trimester of pregnancy when the unborn child's nervous system is developing, women avoid hot tubs and heavy exercise, and take a folate (vitamin B complex) supplement.

Corrective Treatments

Advances in medical technology are changing the face of disability. Twenty years ago, a child born with spina bifida or other serious back defects was likely to face lifelong limitations. For children born today, early diagnosis and treatment or surgery followed by physical therapy can sometimes restore a problem back to a near-normal condition early in life. With proper care, a back so reborn can carry a body through a full and active life.

Hurdles and Challenges

If you have a congenital back problem that gives you symptoms, such as scoliosis, it's important to take the best possible care of your back to prevent further problems. And as this book describes, there are many ways to manage back problems to keep them from ruling (and ruining) your life.

I've Been Working on the Railroad...

Not many people drive spikes into rails for a living these days. But no doubt about it, there are plenty of jobs that are flat-out back breakers. Physical work that involves heavy lifting and frequent twisting is the most likely to create back problems. Logging, construction, commercial fishing, fire fighting, landscaping, and longshoring are but a handful of occupations that can seriously stress your back.

Other jobs carry less obvious risks. Nursing assistants post the highest rate in the United States of on-the-job back injuries, followed by child-care workers. Even people with sedentary jobs—those where it's mostly your fingers that do any walking—can find their backs aching at the end of the day. Standing and especially sitting for prolonged periods of time force your back into curves nature didn't design. Supreme Court Chief Justice William Rehnquist struggles with back pain. The Chief Justice sometimes designs the length of court sessions to coincide with the length of time he can sit; often, he has to stand up.

So should you give up your job to save your back? Good heavens, no! You could bend down to pluck a yogurt container from the bottom shelf of your refrigerator and get a pain in your back in the process. You wouldn't throw out your fridge, though! Looking at the various ways what you do for a living can affect your back is *not* about blame. It's about identifying potential risks and doing your best to minimize them (which could be as simple as taking a two-minute stretch break every half-hour). Yes, some people will suffer serious back injuries at work—just as some people will cut fingers and break bones. But most of us will just have the ordinary, albeit uncomfortable, variety of aches and pains. Indeed, current research indicates that continuing regular activities, including work, is the best course of action for most back pain.

Back Care

Does your job require you to sit or stand in the same place for long periods of time? Give your back a break by standing, stretching, and walking around for a few minutes every hour. You'll feel more alert, too.

Is Your Job Good to Your Back? A Self-Quiz

While there are many reasons your back could hurt, what you spend the most time doing can have considerable influence. Sometimes the jobs we think of as "back busters" are in fact better than those we view as low risk. Look at the following list of pairs of jobs, occupations, and tasks. Can you pick out which in each pair is the more risky for your back?

1. (a) Computer programmer or (b) warehouse stocker?

2. (a) Veterinarian or (b) long-haul truck driver?

3. (a) Firefighter or (b) nursing assistant?

4. (a) Assembly worker in an electronics plant or (b) assembly worker in an automotive plant?

5. (a) Airline pilot or (b) school bus driver?

6. (a) Pharmacist or (b) punch press operator?

7. (a) Professional athlete or (b) couch potato?

8. (a) Elementary school teacher or (b) tax accountant?

9. (a) Store clerk or (b) mail carrier?

10. (a) Librarian or (b) ballet dancer?

Back Talk

What puts more pressure on your back—bending forward at the waist or a good belly laugh? Both exert the same pressure on your spine, about 265 pounds. Laughing, however, is certainly more fun.

Here are the answers. How well did you do?

1. While computer programmers risk stiff shoulders and sore necks from scrunching in front of a computer screen all day, warehouse stockers spend a lot of time lifting and twisting—two of the most common activities that result in back strain. Answer: (b).

2. Animal bites can be nasty, and its certainly no treat trying to wrestle a St. Bernard onto an exam table. But at least the vet gets to move around, and hopefully summons help when hoisting squirming pets. The long-haul trucker sits in one position for several hours at a time, which is a major stress for your back. Answer: (b).

3. Firefighters generally have very fit backs and are less likely to experience back pain than are nursing assistants. The latter occupation requires much lifting, twisting, pulling, and supporting of human bodies that can't help or react unpredictably because of disabilities. Answer: (b).

4. If you made it through school by always guessing (b) on multiple-choice tests, your luck just ran out. An assembly worker in an automotive plant typically works on large items that come down the line, moving around to handle the necessary tasks. The assembly worker in an electronics plant is more likely to

stand or sit in one place for long periods of time, maybe even hunched over to work on small objects in confined spaces. A good backrub would be a much-appreciated fringe benefit, for sure. Answer: (a).

5. Hmmm. At first glance, these occupations seem quite similar—a lot of sitting in enclosed places, noisy kids in the background. But the cockpit of a plane is designed to place controls and gauges within easy reach. Pilot seats are contoured and have armrests. And the pilot can usually stand to stretch every now and again. The ergonomics of a school bus, on the other hand, are far less sophisticated. The driver sits on a seat seemingly designed by Sparticus—just enough to get the job done, no more. Though a school bus driver may spend fewer hours at a time in this "cockpit," they're harder hours for the back. Answer: (b).

6. Both occupations require a substantial amount of standing. A punch press operator is more likely to move around, however, keeping the back in motion. A pharmacist may stand in the same place for long periods of time, moving little except his or her hands. Answer: (a).

7. No, this is not a trick question. Most people view the stresses an athlete's body faces in practice and competition as extraordinarily challenging—and they are. But an athlete is in top shape. A couch potato isn't. A couch potato could get hurt sneezing, particularly if he or she is attempting to change positions at the same time. Nothing does more to keep your back in good shape than regular exercise. Answer: (b).

8. From May through March, the nod could go to the teacher—especially if those kids are young and active. During tax season, though, the accountant may appear to have become one with the chair—definitely not a good thing for the back. While teachers spend a lot of time on their feet, they move around quite a bit, which helps keep their backs from tightening up. An accountant going through shoeboxes of records doesn't move much at all. Answer: (b).

9. Some store clerks do a lot of standing in one place (cashiering) or lifting (stocking shelves), which definitely presents risks for the back. Mail carriers who walk a route carrying a mailbag come home at the end of the day with at least a sore shoulder. And while vaulting fences to escape the fangs of "Oh, he won't bite!" qualifies as movement, it's not likely to make the back feel good. Answer: (b).

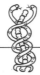

Back Care

"Drink your milk," we counsel our children. Their growing bones need the calcium and other nutrients milk provides. But did you know you need *more* calcium after age 45 than when you were 10? An adult needs 1,000 to 1,200 milligrams of calcium each day, equal to three servings of dairy products or a couple extra-strength TUMS. You also need 400 units of vitamin D, which you might want to get from a supplement, especially if you're over age 65.

10. The body of a ballet dancer is as fine-tuned as any athlete's. The swoops and leaps and even lifts of the dance demand a strong back—and the dancer has it. Librarians don't often get such a demanding workout, though they do spend a good deal of time lifting and twisting. Carrying an armful of books from the desk to the shelves doesn't seem like such a big deal until halfway there, when suddenly it feels like a ton of bricks. Answer: (a).

Back to Nature

There's more to good posture than looking good. Sitting up straight and standing tall help your spine retain its natural curves. Good posture also aids other body systems by giving your internal organs the room they need to work properly. Good posture also makes it easier to breathe fully and deeply.

Back Off!

Are you taking a diuretic (water pill) for your blood pressure or other reason? Then don't take calcium supplements without first talking it over with your doctor. Taking calcium supplements at the same time you're taking a diuretic can put you at increased risk for kidney or bladder stones. Take calcium with meals, and drink eight glasses of water a day.

Back Health Across the Life Span

Your body goes through a number of changes as you grow older. You can easily accommodate some, like gray hair. Others create more of a challenge. With increasing age comes a decreasing ability to absorb and use calcium. Yet calcium remains an important nutrient for your cells to carry out the various activities that keep you alive and kicking. When your cells can't get the calcium they need from the foods you eat, your bones suddenly look like the First Elemental Bank of Calcium. Your body draws out calcium your bones store and uses it for other cell functions.

By about age 40, the typical American starts losing one-half percent of his or her bone mass each year. If you don't prevent or replace this loss in some way, it doesn't take a crystal ball to see that back problems are most certainly in your future.

Brittle Bones: Osteoporosis

As we age, most of us realize we'd better start taking better care of our bodies. We switch to diets lower in saturated fats, the first step of which is often to drop dairy products. And boom! There goes your main calcium supply. If you don't do something to get your calcium intake back up to par, the next crack you hear may be a breaking bone. Osteoporosis, sometimes called "brittle bone disease," is a leading cause of spontaneous fractures in the spine and other bones.

Don't feel you're safe from osteoporosis just because you're a man. While a man's thicker, denser bones can delay the effects, the older a man is, the more likely he is to have osteoporosis. Osteoporosis strikes women more frequently and more severely than it strikes men. Women have smaller, lighter bones to start with, and the natural protection against bone loss they enjoy for the first half of their adult lives—estrogen—disappears after menopause.

Back Talk

Men with alcoholism are more likely to get osteoporosis than their nondrinking counter-parts. Excessive alcohol consumption (more than two alcoholic drinks a day) interferes with your body's ability to absorb and metabolize nutrients, depleting your bones of vital calcium and other minerals.

While there are treatments for osteoporosis, by far the best approach is pre-menopausal prevention. For women past menopause, estrogen replacement therapy has the added benefit of slowing calcium loss. Regular weight-bearing exercise, which is also good for the rest of your body, helps your bones keep their calcium and even rebuild to become stronger and more dense. Medications can help restore some, but not all, of the lost calcium and bone mass in moderate and severe osteoporosis.

Dietary Sources of Calcium

Dairy products are by far the most abundant natural source of calcium. Many items, such as yogurt, cheese, milk, and even ice cream, are available in low-fat or no-fat varieties. For people who can't tolerate or don't like dairy products, there are many other sources of calcium, from over-the-counter supplements you can buy at your drug store to foods such as certain vegetables, fish, nuts, and soybean products. A single stalk of cooked broccoli, for example, contains as much calcium as an ounce of cheddar cheese (about 200 milligrams). A cup of cooked spinach (300 milli-grams) or collards (350 milligrams) has more (and far less fat).

Back Care

If you're taking a calcium supple-ment, be sure you're also getting enough vitamin D. While your body has to have this essential substance to use calcium and other minerals, it doesn't need much. The sun's ultraviolet rays cause a chemical reaction in your skin that produces vitamin D, so get a little sun. Daily multivitamins and animal-based foods that are high in calcium are also naturally high in vitamin D.

Natural Sources of Calcium	
Dairy products	Choose low-fat hard cheeses, yogurt, milk, and cottage cheese
Vegetables	Collards, turnip greens, broccoli, kale, okra, beans (white or pinto), chickpeas, and spinach
Grains	Many breads and breakfast cereals are fortified with calcium and other nutrients
Fruits	Figs and calcium-fortified orange juice
Fish	Salmon, mackerel, sardines, and tuna
Other foods	Soybeans and soybean products such as tofu, sunflower seeds, and peanuts

Calcium Supplements

With 100 or more calcium supplements on the market, how do you know which is right for you? Are there any real differences between all these products?

Calcium comes from different sources. Calcium carbonate, for example, is often prepared from chalk (you knew there was a good reason those chewable tablets taste so, well, chalky!). Oyster shell calcium carbonate comes from limestone quarries, drawing its calcium from the fossilized shells that are abundant in such quarries. So does dolomite, another form of calcium.

More expensive doesn't necessarily mean better when it comes to choosing a calcium supplement, advise the experts. Calcium carbonate and calcium citrate are often the least costly—and most easily absorbed. If you're drawn to "natural" formulations, beware that many oyster shell and dolomite supplements may contain higher levels of aluminum and lead—heavy metals that can be poisonous. Read and compare labels!

Yes, Violet, You Really Are Shrinking!

If that closet shelf seems like it's harder to reach now than it was 10 years ago, it's no delusion. You really are shrinking! Most adults in their 70s are at least an inch or two shorter than they were in their 30s. Osteoporosis and the natural degeneration of disk material causes your spine to flatten somewhat, moving the vertebrae closer together.

With severe osteoporosis you could shrink by 10 to 15 percent, meaning that if you measured 5-feet 10-inches in your prime, by the time you're in your 80s you could be once again looking at that five-foot mark. Since women are more likely to have osteoporosis, they tend to lose more height.

Back Talk

Always wanted to be tall? Head for space! Without gravity to contain their spines, astronauts "grow" four to six inches in the weightlessness of space. Of course, they lose the extra inches after a few days back on Earth.

Get It Off Your Back!

What do you carry on your back? A purse? A backpack or book bag? Just for fun, put it on the scale. Surprise! Often the items you're packing on your back weigh more than a small child. Now empty the contents. How much of what's in there do you really need? How much can you do without? Lighten your load as much as possible, and your back'll love you.

If you must carry heavy items, such as books, invest in a well-made backpack. It should have sturdy seams and adjustable straps. When you carry the pack, put both straps over your shoulders. Carrying a loaded backpack slung over one shoulder is an invitation to disaster. Not only is your load (and your body) unbalanced, but you're also putting a lot of strain on structures not intended to bear such burdens. Your shoulders should carry the bulk of the weight—a bag that hangs too low or too high puts pressure on your lower back.

Do you carry a wallet in your back pants pocket? If so, take it out right now and look at it. Is it more than half an inch thick? That's what you're sitting on every time you take a seat, and it's throwing your spine a curve. If you really need everything that's crammed into your wallet, look for other ways to carry it. Perhaps a briefcase might work better. Or consider carrying your wallet in an inside jacket pocket. Just get that lump off your hip!

Back Off!

Doctors are seeing more young people with back problems as a result of carrying heavy backpacks and book bags. Chiropractors and pediatricians recommend that children carry a backpack that weighs no more than 10 to 20 percent as much as they do. One trendy item on the market that might help is a book bag on wheels that a child can pull instead of wear.

The Least You Need to Know

➤ While it might be handy to be tall, it's also a challenge for your back. If you're over six feet, you're at extra risk for back problems.

➤ Regular exercise is the best way to keep your back in good shape. Exercise tones and strengthens muscles, builds strong bone tissue, and helps keep your weight under control.

➤ Getting enough calcium and controlling your weight can help prevent long-term back problems.

➤ Items you carry on your back—purses, book bags, backpacks—may be weighing you down more than you realize. And sitting on a billfold that's more than a half-inch thick throws your back a curve it could do without.

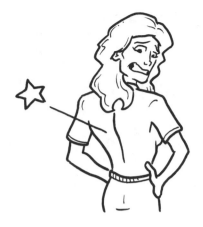

Chapter 4

Oh, Your Aching Back

In This Chapter

➤ The subjective nature of pain

➤ New understandings about how pain works

➤ Other problems that can cause back pain

➤ When to see a health care professional

If you can't touch it, see it, hear it, smell it, taste it, or measure it, how do you know it's real? Even the air you breathe is easier to quantify than the pain in your back. Your pain is real because you can feel it. But just you, no one else. This is both the characteristic and the dilemma of pain. What researchers know about pain comes largely through the experiences people report.

The Physiology of Pain

Studies in *physiology* show that pain usually originates as a series of chemical and electrical signals that travel along the *neuron* pathways of your body—your nerves—to your brain. Say, for example, you cut your finger. The damaged nerves in your fingertip send a message along a *sensory nerve* to your spinal cord. When it receives the message, your spinal cord does two things simultaneously. It sends a signal back through a *motor nerve* instructing the muscles of your arm, hand, and finger to contract and pull away from the knife. It sends another signal to your brain, which your brain translates into the universal language of pain. All this happens in just a fraction of a nanosecond.

While the physiology of pain seems fairly straightforward, there is much about pain that we don't yet understand. Why, for example, do people who have had an arm or leg amputated continue to feel pain in the limb even though it's not there anymore? How can one person whose back MRI (see Chapter 9, "What the Tests Tell") shows such extensive damage that walking should be impossible feel not the slightest discomfort; yet another person whose pain interferes with all aspects of life has no evidence of any physical cause?

Back Basics

From the Greek root words *physio*, meaning "natural," and *ology*, meaning "study," **physiology** is the study of how the human body works. A **neuron** is a nerve cell. Like the two directions of a highway, **sensory nerves** carry signals of sensation to the brain, and **motor nerves** carry signals of action away from the brain.

Back Off!

Thinking of rubbing a little topical pain reliever (like Ben-Gay) over those aching back muscles? Lay off the heating pad if you do! Topical pain relievers increase circulation near the skin's surface. Adding heat to the mix could result in serious skin damage.

Is Your Brain "Hardwired" for Pain?

What if somewhere deep in your brain, there's a "pain switch" that certain events, such as injuries, trigger? The idea might not be as far-fetched as it sounds. Neurosurgeons have discovered that stimulating certain areas of brain cells in some people can falsely re-create specific pain symptoms (which they learned by accident, not through intentional torture). If the brain itself is programmed to present an experience of pain in a particular way, then all we need to do is figure out how to turn off the switch.

Easier said than done, unfortunately. Your brain is a marvelous and mysterious organ, and there is much scientists still don't know about how it works. New medications that seem to attack pain by shutting down the "pain switch" could be the next revolution in treatment for chronic pain. As promising as such discoveries are, it will be some time before doctors can use them in practical ways. In the here and now, you're not likely to have brain surgery for your back pain.

Busy Messengers: Neurotransmitters

If nerves are the highways and byways of communication within your body, neurotransmitters are the cars that zip along them. These microscopic messengers are actually chemicals that transfer electronic signals from nerve cells to each other and to other cells such as muscle cells. Serotonin is perhaps the most familiar neurotransmitter; it affects conscious processes such as thinking and concentration.

Also in the neurotransmitter family are protein molecules called neuropeptides. Somewhat larger than other neurotransmitters though still microscopic, neuropeptides appear to be a biochemical link between emotions and the brain. Researchers believe neuropeptides affect emotion, learning, stress response, and memory. Neuropeptides called endorphins affect your brain's perception of pain.

Pain and Social Expectations

We don't usually think of pain as a social event. We usually keep how much we hurt to ourselves, perhaps as a leftover protective mechanism to hide our vulnerability. But back pain has become somewhat of a community affair.

Now don't throw this book across the room—you might break something, or throw out your back. We're not saying you have back pain just 'cause everyone else does. We just want to point out a few interesting facts. Can you pick out which of the following statements are true?

1. The more severe your pain, the more likely you are to have a long-term disability. True or false?

2. The longer you're off work, the less likely it is that you will return. True or false?

3. The nature of your problem (sprain, herniated disk) determines how long you'll be out of action. True or false?

4. The United States has the highest rate of back surgery in the world. True or false?

5. Job satisfaction is the most significant predictor that back pain will become disabling. True or false?

6. If we could teach everyone how to lift properly, most back pain would be a thing of the past. True or false?

7. When your back hurts, get in to see the doctor right away to get the problem "fixed" before it gets worse. True or false?

Did you come up with four false and three true answers? Let's see how well you separated fact from fiction.

1. *False.* When it comes to back problems, there is little relationship between the severity of pain and the seriousness of the condition that causes it. Pain that incapacitates you when it first hits could be completely gone in just a few weeks.

2. *True.* About 85 percent of those with back problems severe enough to stay away from work return within six weeks. Fewer than half those who miss six months of work will go back. And less than 1 percent of those who are off for two years ever return to work.

3. *False.* A sprain could be a bother for months, while a herniated disk might heal in six weeks or so. Your attitude is far more likely to influence the length of time your back problem puts your regular life on hold.

4. *True.* American surgeons operate on backs twice as often as their Canadian counterparts, and nearly five times more often than surgeons in Great Britain.

Back Off!

If your back pain could be due to a fracture related to an acute injury (such as a fall or car accident), get medical attention immediately. A broken bone in your back can bruise or cut your spinal cord, putting you at risk for paralysis. Osteoporosis-related compression fractures rarely put your spinal cord at risk.

5. *True.* Numerous studies in the United States as well as in other countries support this premise.

6. *False.* While about 80 percent of back sprains occur while lifting, such injuries are only part of the big picture when it comes to back problems. Many back problems develop as a result of aging and normal deterioration.

7. *False.* Unless you have reason to suspect that you have a fracture, tumor, or other rare problem, less is more when it comes to most back pain. Your doctor is likely to recommend the same things you can do on your own—ice or heat, anti-inflammatory or pain-relieving medication, and patience. For most back pain, the best "fix" is time.

Back Talk

The beliefs of French philosopher Rene Descartes (1596–1650) shaped medicine's approach to understanding and treating pain for several centuries. Blending the religious influences of his day with his understanding of human anatomy, Descartes determined that pain was a function of the body, not of the mind or the soul. If only humans had souls and minds, Descartes reasoned, yet animals could also feel pain, then pain must be a purely physical event.

Back Basics

Acute pain comes on suddenly, is often severe, and improves quickly. The word "acute" comes from the Latin *acutus,* meaning "sharp."

The Pain in Your Back

Back pain can come on sharply and suddenly, freezing you in your tracks. Or it can develop slowly, over time, until one day you notice that you hurt. Pain can drop in for a short stay, or become like a relative who stays for an extended visit.

Not So Cute

You're late for the sales meeting. Papers and notebooks fill your arms as you rush down the hallway to the conference room. Your pencil flies out of your hand and rolls across the floor. You reach down to pick it up and wham!—a sharp, stabbing pain freezes you in an unflattering position. You can barely breathe, and your life flashes before your eyes. This is what doctors call *acute* pain. And it's not exactly a pretty picture!

Acute back pain can start without apparent reason or may result from a strain or sprain, or even a fracture. The injury can be slight or significant. The amount of pain you feel is not always a helpful way to distinguish between the two. Heat or ice, rest, and analgesic or anti-inflammatory drugs such as aspirin or ibuprofen can help you feel better more quickly.

When your back suddenly gives you pain, take prompt action to keep the situation from getting worse. During the first 24 hours, use ice to soothe irritated or strained muscles and reduce swelling. After 24 hours, switch to heat to help your sore muscles relax and feel better. Your doctor may suggest an anti-inflammatory medication to keep you comfortable while your back heals.

Don't rest too long, or you'll do more harm than good. Doctors sometimes recommend two or three days of restricted activity, and seldom suggest complete bed rest for strains, sprains, and other muscle-related injuries. For one thing, lying in bed doesn't put your back in the best position. (Lying on your side is usually best; on your back is definitely not good, and neither is on your stomach.) You usually fall asleep, which means you're not moving at all. Your muscles get stiff, and other muscles will begin to ache. Try to get up and move around, however slowly, every few hours. Even though your back hurts, a little bit of movement is the best way to keep the healing process moving along.

Of course, follow any specific instructions your doctor gives you. As common as back problems are, every back injury is unique, so only you and your doctor know your particular circumstances. If you're taking prescription or over-the-counter medications for any other purpose, check with your doctor or pharmacist before adding any pain relievers or anti-inflammatory drugs.

Back to Nature

Some people find standing in a warm shower or sitting in a hot tub helps relieve the pain of a back injury. Limit your time in the water to no more than 20 minutes. Try to stretch and move around to help loosen stiff muscles. If you've been taking medication that makes you sleepy, don't relax in the tub or spa unless someone can check on you frequently.

Back Off!

DO NOT take aspirin for your back pain if you're taking a blood thinner (anticoagulant). And don't combine over-the-counter analgesics and anti-inflammatory drugs with each other or with prescription medications unless your pharmacist or doctor instructs you to do so.

Still Hurting

If your pain lasts longer than a week but less than three months, your doctor calls it "subacute." Even if you're still not feeling that great, the initial injury has started to heal. By this time the sharp pain is usually gone (except for those nasty reminder twinges when you bend or twist wrong), though you may have aching and soreness. Sometimes secondary problems, such as muscle spasms in the injured area, develop as the initial pain begins to wane. Your doctor might prescribe medication to help your muscles relax. This is also a time when physical therapy or therapeutic massage might help (more on these in Chapter 21, "Hands-On Healing: Therapeutic Massage and Physical Therapy"). Chiropractic care and acupuncture provide pain relief for some people, too (more in Chapters 18, "A Hands-On Approach: Chiropractic," and 19, "Ancient Chinese Wisdom: Acupuncture").

When your pain lingers longer than a Wisconsin winter, it's enough to make you want to scream. While you might call this a pain in the wahtusi, doctors call it *chronic*. Sorry, but you're now among the minority whose back pain has become more than a limited episode. Unfortunately, it's not uncommon for back pain to ebb and flow. You can go along for a few months with just little stuff to grumble about, then your pain surges back with a vengeance.

Back Basics

Chronic pain is pain that's been going on for a while, though it may still be intense. The word "chronic" comes from the Greek *chronos*, which means "time or duration."

We humans have inquiring (some would say nosy) minds. We like to know why and how things happen. You want to know why your back hurts, and how you can make the pain go away. As often as not, however, your inquiring mind is going to be disappointed. "We don't know for sure" is the most common answer. Sometimes extensive testing reveals a problem that's not causing any symptoms, yet fails to identify the source of debilitating pain. The truth is, more than half of the time neither you nor your health care provider will know for sure what caused your back pain.

My Pain's Worse Than Your Pain

Pain operates under its own theory of relativity (sorry, Albert). How much does your back hurt? Well, it depends…on what's causing your pain, what you're doing, who you're with, where you are, what your mood is, and even what time of day it is. Pain is relative to your unique circumstances. Your sprain may well be more painful than your neighbor's…or less. Having the same problem doesn't mean we'll have the same level of pain, or that our experience of our pain will be the same.

Is It Really All in Your Head?

The Greek philosopher Aristotle (384–322 B.C.) believed that the mind and the body were two functions of the same structure. One influenced the other to the point where distinguishing between them was useless. Not many of his counterparts or followers shared this belief, however, and through the ages the mind and the body became viewed as separate structures. And pain was a feature of the physical body.

Then came the World War II and a landmark study of battlefield injuries. Wounded soldiers didn't seem to need medications to control their pain despite serious and even life-threatening injuries. Were these warriors exceptionally brave, or was there something else that accounted for their stoicism? As it turns out, Aristotle was on the right track. Emotions often affect the body and its functions. Military surgeons speculated that their courageous patients felt little pain despite serious wounds because they were so relieved and overjoyed about just being alive.

It's not just soldiers in battle who can put mind over matter. Every game day, the body of a professional football player takes a pounding that brings tears to the eyes of even the most seasoned couch potato. Yet down after down, the player trots back to the line of scrimmage. Professional ballet dancers have been known to perform with stress fractures. Determination, it seems, can overcome pain that would melt the rest of us.

So what's your problem, you who's crashed there on the sofa with a heating pad behind your back and a bottle of ibuprofen in your hand? Are you just wimping out? Heavens, no! While courage under fire is admirable, when your aching back tells you to back off, you'd better pay attention. There's a price, sometimes a steep one, for ignoring your body's cries of pain. Just look at the faces during post-game dressing room interviews.

When your back hurts, do what you know will help it feel better. Then consider adding a dab of attitude adjustment to your treatment regimen. Concentrate on what *doesn't* hurt, for example. Tell yourself—out loud, even—that *you* are in control. You may not be able to end the pain, but you can change how you feel about it (and maybe cut it back to a dull roar). You might be surprised at what a difference it makes.

The Reality of Perception

Your back hurts too much for you to attend Aunt Miriam's annual get-together on Saturday evening. Yet when a friend calls after the event is well underway you feel fine enough to go out for dinner

Back to Nature

Visualization and guided imagery are techniques that can help you relax and change your perception of pain. In visualization, you focus your mind on seeing the source of your pain dissolve and the problem heal. With guided imagery, you envision a scene of relaxation and peace. Both methods are easy to learn and use. See Chapter 14, "Imagine a Healthy, Pain-Free Back," for more information.

Back Basics

Doctors can assess **subjective** experiences, like pain, only according to what you describe to them. By contrast, objective experiences are those that others can observe, such as bleeding.

and a movie. Are you faking? It might seem you are, and justifiably so, if Aunt Miriam's idea of evening entertainment is setting up the folding chairs and showing slides from her summer vacation to the Grand Canyon. In all likelihood, however, your pain is genuine. It just changes.

Pain varies from one person to another, and from time to time within the same person. It just means your pain is *subjective*—how much it hurts depends on how you feel about what you're doing. When you're doing things you enjoy, you're better able to tolerate—and even ignore—discomfort.

This isn't to say you can just will your back pain away. At best, you can will it to the back of your consciousness for limited periods of time. It's this subjective nature of pain that makes it such a challenge for those who suffer from it, whether they stay home in bed or groan their way to work.

Back Basics

When the pain in one place in your body is caused by a problem somewhere else, this is **referred pain**.

Back Basics

Ultrasound and **CT scanning** (computerized tomography) allow doctors to see what's going on inside your body without opening it up. Ultrasound does so by sending focused sound waves into the body. A **CT scan** uses a sequence of computer-generated x-ray images to generate dimensional images.

It's Pain *in* Your Back, but Not *from* Your Back

Sometimes the pain in your back is *referred pain* that signals a problem somewhere else in your body. It's very common for a toothache to masquerade as ear pain, for example, or for an ailing knee to pose as hip pain. Referred pain occurs when the same sensory nerve serves both the site of your pain and the location of the problem causing it. That it's referred doesn't make it any kinder or gentler—referred pain can be every bit as excruciating as direct pain.

How does your doctor know whether your pain is direct or referred? Every symptom tells a story, and your doctor will want to hear all about yours. This helps pin down the real culprit. Problems that you might feel in your back include kidney infections and stones, inflammation of the pancreas, menstrual cramps, and endometriosis.

Kidney Problems

Your kidneys are a pair of fist-sized organs lying one on each side of your spine at the back of your abdomen. Under the protective cover of your ribs, your kidneys filter toxins, salts, and fluid from your blood. They return substances your body needs to your blood, and eliminate what your body doesn't need in the form of urine.

Sometimes the salts crystallize inside the kidney, forming kidney stones (technically known as calculi). When they get large enough to block the flow of blood or urine, they cause pain. You're most likely to feel this pain, which can be excruciating, in the low-middle part of your back just under your ribs—right where your kidneys call home. Other kidney problems can cause pain, too, such as infection and cysts.

Laboratory tests and occasionally imaging exams such as *ultrasound* or *CT scanning* help narrow the diagnosis fairly quickly. Once treatment begins for the primary problem, the back pain goes away.

Pancreatitis

A serious condition that sometimes includes back pain among its symptoms is pancreatitis, an inflammation of the pancreas. The pancreas is a large gland behind your stomach. It produces digestive enzymes and insulin. Your pancreas can become inflamed from a virus, as a result of gallstones (which block the flow of enzymes from the pancreas), or as a consequence of heavy drinking (alcohol). Movement makes the pain worse. You're also likely to feel nauseated. Prompt medical treatment is crucial and could save your life, but acute pancreatitis usually heals without complications.

Menstrual Discomfort

It's not quite that time of the month, but you can feel it coming in the small of your back—that persistent, annoying ache that no change in position seems to relieve. Back pain is unfortunately a common component of premenstrual and menstrual discomfort. It's a referred pain; your back is not actually injured. Often, over-the-counter pain or anti-inflammatory medications can squelch the pain. Heat also helps some women, though it makes others feel worse. If your back pain seems tied to your menstrual cycle, get a thorough checkup from your regular doctor or women's health care practitioner. Approaches to reduce menstrual symptoms overall usually reduce related back pain as well.

Endometriosis

Women who have endometriosis, a condition where fragments of the tissue lining the uterus lodge throughout the abdomen, often have excruciating back pain during their periods. The pain may start a few days before your period and be more intense than cramps. As with cramps, back pain with endometriosis is referred pain. Heat, over-the-counter pain or anti-inflammatory medications, and sometimes other therapy specifically to treat the endometriosis can help with related back pain.

Turn to Chapter 25, "Women and Back Pain," for more specific information on the special concerns of women and back pain.

When to See a Doctor

Your back hurts. Is that enough to schedule an appointment with your doctor? Most of us think so—visits to the doctor for back pain trail only those for colds and flu as the most common reason to see the doctor.

You should see a doctor right away if:

➤ You could've fractured your back in a fall, accident, or as a result of osteoporosis, or have an injury that puts your spinal cord at risk.

➤ You have a history of cancer (your pain could be from a tumor).

➤ You have numbness or tingling in one or both legs or feet.

➤ You have any symptoms that suggest your problem could be a kidney or bladder infection or kidney stones (especially fever).

You can do just as much for yourself for most minor sprains and strains—take it easy for a few days, take an over-the-counter pain reliever or anti-inflammatory medication, and apply heat or ice to the area. If you're not feeling at least somewhat better after three to five days, then schedule an appointment with your doctor.

Visiting Your Primary Care Physician

So you've done the ice, the medications, the rest—and every movement is still a real pain in the back. Now it's time to call on the experts. If you're like most people, you'll start with a visit to your regular or primary care doctor. In fact, back pain is the second most common reason people go to the doctor, right behind colds and flu. (Some people head for other health care providers, which we discuss in later chapters.) What should you expect?

First, a few words about what NOT to expect. Don't expect immediate x-rays or other tests. (They usually don't tell your doctor any more than your "history" can, unless there's clear evidence of a specific problem.) Don't expect an "instant" fix. (There's no such thing.) And don't expect your doctor to tell you exactly why your back hurts! (Most of the time, there's no clear reason.) So now that we've left you with no hope (just kidding), what should you expect? More often than not, immediate empathy for your situation—doctors, just like everyone else, also get back pain. Your doctor knows how miserable you are, and will do whatever is possible to help you feel more comfortable. And your doctor will have lots of questions for you.

Back Basics

Palpation means "to examine by touch." **Symptoms** are subjective (not observable) evidence of your problem or condition.

Tell Me About Your Back Pain

Be prepared to describe when your pain first started and what you were doing (if you know), how often and when you have pain, how you would rate your pain's severity, and what you've already tried in terms of treatment, either by yourself or with another caregiver. Depending on where your pain is, and what other *symptoms* you have, your doctor might move your legs and perform a few basic tests to check your nerve function. Your doctor may or may not feel the place on your back where it hurts—though it seems a logical thing to do, *palpation* doesn't always provide any useful information (and may aggravate your pain). Again, it depends on your symptoms.

Let's Chat—Your Health in General

When your doctor asks you about your job and your family and what's going on in your life and whether or not you wear seat belts, he or she isn't just being nosey. Your doctor's gathering information that provides insight into your health in a broader context. Many of your responses, though they may seem irrelevant, give your doctor important clues about what might help your back pain. For example, if your job is computer programming, you have three teenagers at home, and you commute by bicycle, your doctor can surmise that you sit most of the day, have some stress in your life, and get regular exercise. These are all factors that can influence back pain.

Do You Need a Specialist?

Doctors first consider what could be the most likely cause of your problem (for low back pain, that's strain or sprain) as well as what chance there is that it could be something serious (the worst case scenario, "red flag" land). If your symptoms suggest an underlying problem that needs specific treatment, of course, your doctor will order the appropriate tests, and may refer you to a specialist (a doctor with additional training and expertise in a certain area, such as orthopedics or neurology).

For most back pain, however, "watchful waiting" is the most effective approach. We know the last thing you want to hear from your doctor, especially if you've been dealing with your hurting back for a while already, is "let's give it a few weeks." But this just might be the best course of treatment, supported by efforts to help you feel better while you're waiting for your back to heal.

Back Talk

Disappointed that your doctor didn't order x-rays to assess your back problem? Maybe you should be relieved. A typical set of lower back x-rays delivers a dose of radiation to your sex organs (man or woman) that is the same as getting a chest x-ray every day for six years! While this level of radiation is well within safe levels, this perspective reminds us that we shouldn't take any test or procedure casually.

We know this sometimes isn't very satisfying. After all, you've come to the doctor because what you tried on your own didn't work, and your doctor wants you to give it a little more time. It's not that your doctor is trying to get rid of you, or save money.

An important aspect of allopathic medicine is the Hippocratic Oath, through which doctors pledge to "first, do no harm." Doctors don't want to put you through tests or treatments that might be harmful if your back is likely to heal itself (nature's way).

Other Health Professionals

Many people find chiropractic or osteopathic manipulation helps their back pain feel better faster. Several studies support this, suggesting that chiropractic manipulation, especially for acute pain due to strain or sprain, provides effective pain relief. Physical therapy and therapeutic massage can also provide relief. Whether your body actually heals any faster isn't clear. After all, your body heals at its own pace, and in some respects there's little you can do to influence that beyond supporting its natural mechanisms. We do know that when you feel less pain, you feel better in general. And feeling better lets you take a more positive role in your healing.

What You Can Do for Yourself

Back pain can be excruciating. Yet 85 percent of the time, it will go away without any intervention from either modern medicine or ancient healing methods. This raises many questions for health care providers about how and when to intervene and has produced a general tone of conservatism in treatment. If you're going to improve in time anyway, perhaps the best approach is to simply keep yourself comfortable while your body heals itself.

The Least You Need to Know

➤ Pain is a complex process that involves your body, brain, mind, and emotions.

➤ Pain is both subjective and relative. Only you can feel your pain, and how much it hurts depends on many factors not necessarily related to the condition causing the pain.

➤ Sometimes other ailments, such as kidney problems and endometriosis, can cause back pain.

➤ Less is more when it comes to back pain. Time is really the best healer.

Part 2

When Your Back Betrays You

If I had the use of my body I would throw it out the window.
—Samuel Beckett, Irish playwright and novelist (1906–1989); Malone Dies *(1951)*

"But I didn't do anything!" you wail. "There's no reason for my back to hurt!" You could be right. Most of the time, it seems, your back hurts for no apparent reason. Sometimes, though, the reason is clear.

Part 2 looks at what can go wrong with your back, and how doctors try to determine the cause of your back pain. Posture, activity (or lack of), and the normal aging process all play roles.

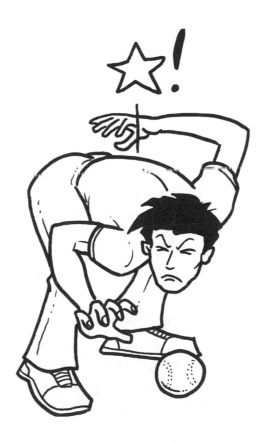

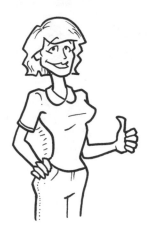

Posture Perfect

The words of grouchy elders shattered your slouching thousands of times when you were younger. "Stand tall! Suck in that stomach! Sit up straight!" Geez, you may have thought as you thrust out your chin and threw back your shoulders in exaggerated compliance, why don't they find something real to worry about? And now that you're an adult, you can slouch all you want—and probably do far more than you realize.

As it turns out, those grumpy commands weren't just about appearances. Poor posture is a real worry. When you slump, your back humps outward and your shoulders roll forward. Your spine takes on curves not in keeping with its natural design. While certainly you won't "freeze" into awkward positions just because your poor posture puts you in them for prolonged periods of time, over time you will find that your muscles complain when you try to change.

Think of poor posture as somewhat like a cast. When a broken arm or leg is first put in a cast, the muscles ache from being held in the same position. After a while, however, they get used to this new position. And by the time the cast comes off, those muscles have gotten quite accustomed to their static existence and they resist movement. Poor posture isn't nearly so confining as a cast, of course. But a day's worth of awkward sitting can make you feel like you've been frozen in place.

Stand Up Straight: A Posture Self-Test

Are you a leaner, a sloucher, a huncher, or a ramrod? Breeze through this self-quiz to see where your posture stands!

1. When I'm walking, my hands are usually...

    a) In my pants or jacket pockets.

    b) Carrying things.

    c) Behind my back.

    d) Swinging at my sides.

2. When I'm standing on the corner waiting for the crosswalk light to turn green, I can look straight down and see...

    a) What I had for lunch on the front of my shirt.

    b) The books and papers in my arms.

    c) My knees.

    d) A quarter on the ground between my feet.

3. The position you'll most likely find me in when I'm watching my favorite television show is...

    a) Curled in a ball in the armchair I rescued from my grandmother's garage.

    b) Lying on my side on the sofa.

    c) Stretched out on my stomach on the floor, looking up at the TV.

    d) Relaxing in my recliner.

4. My office has an ergonomically designed, fully adjustable chair with a five-arm wheeled base and armrests. If you sneak a look at me during the day, you'll find me sitting...

    a) On the floor—I can't figure out how to work the adjustment controls.

    b) With my feet propped on the base and my elbows on my desk.

    c) With my shoes off and my feet curled under me.

    d) With the small of my back against the chair's back and my feet flat on a small stepstool under my desk.

5. It's my day to work the customer service counter, which means seven hours on my feet. To make this easier on my back, I...

    a) Call it quits after two hours, and tell my boss my back just can't take the stress.

    b) Lean on the counter as much as possible to take the weight off my feet.

    c) Sit in a chair whenever there's no one at the counter.

    d) Wear flat, comfortable shoes, change positions frequently, and take a couple minutes every hour to stretch.

6. The checkout lines at the supermarket stretch all the way back to frozen foods. While I'm waiting, I see my reflection in the glass door of the freezer and I'm...

   a) Wearing socks that don't match.

   b) Leaning on my cart, with my elbows on the handle, my chin in my hands, and one foot propped on the lower rack.

   c) Sitting cross-legged on the floor in front of my cart.

   d) Shifting my weight from one leg to the other with my hands resting lightly on the handle.

7. I'm driving all day. To keep my back from aching, I...

   a) Take off my shoes so I can prop my foot on the dashboard.

   b) Put a pillow behind my back.

   c) Stop every couple hours to get out of my car and walk around.

   d) Use the seat adjustments to sit fairly upright, with moderate lumbar support in the seat back.

8. When I walk, my feet...

   a) Hurt.

   b) Scuff and shuffle.

   c) Slap against the floor.

   d) Step briskly, heel to toe.

9. When my back starts to feel tense and tight at work, I...

   a) Call it a day and go home.

   b) Take a couple ibuprofens.

   c) Stretch my arms over my head, move my head to flex my neck, and wiggle my feet.

   d) Take a short break and find a quiet place where I can lie down on a firm surface for a few minutes.

So what's your posture quotient? This is one report card where Ds rule. If you circled five or more D answers, treat yourself to a massage—you could be the next poster child for good posture. If you have five or more C answers, loosen up your ramrod ways—you spend too much time with your joints locked into stiffness. Did you choose mostly A and B answers? If you're sore at the end of the day, little wonder. Straighten up and stop leaning, slouching, and hunching your way through the day!

What Feels Right May Be Wrong

Everybody loves a soft, cushiony chair or sofa. It's a haven of comfort to flop into after a long day at work, both a place and a way to unwind. But is it really? Sure, sinking into those cushions puts your body in a different position than it's been in all day. And it feels good. What happens, though, if you fall asleep in that position? Your muscles are more than a bit cranky when they wake you up. Soft surfaces that let your body collapse—chairs, sofas, beds—may feel good at first, but they fail to provide the support your muscles need.

Driving Comfort

It's not just your comfy easy chair that's a problem. Many sitting surfaces that at first appear supportive turn out to be major letdowns. Automobile seats, for example, are often fine for the short commute to work. But head out on the highway and your back might try to hitch a ride home—not to mention your shoulders, neck, and even thighs. Car seats are often more fashionable than supportive. Those nifty "lumbar supports" that hug your side do little to bolster your back. Many seat surfaces are too short to give good support under your thighs, leaving you squirming to find a position your entire body can agree is comfortable.

It's hard to get beyond cosmetics when you're buying a new car. But if you spend more than 30 minutes at a time in your car, doing so is a worthwhile effort. Take a long enough test drive to get a sense for how the seat feels. Generally if you'll let the salesperson ride along, you can be gone for 30 or 45 minutes. Pay attention to the little signals your back sends. Are you fidgeting like a five-year-old? Can you adjust the seat position to make yourself comfortable? Sure, you could add extra seat cushions and back supports after you buy your car. But you shouldn't have to.

When you're on the road, change your position every so often, however slightly. If your car is equipped with cruise control, use it. Doing so not only gives you better gas mileage, it gives you more ways to move your gas pedal foot. And if your drive is a long one, stop every couple hours to get out and walk around. You'll feel more alert when you're driving, and less stiff when you reach your destination.

Office Chic...or Back Disaster?

Do you like the armrests on your chair at work because they make you feel like Captain Kirk, firmly in command and obviously a leader? Unless they're adjustable, those armrests might only be causing your back to ache. Do your shoulders go up when you put your arms on the rests? If so, the rests are too high for you. You'll soon have your feet on the chair's base to compensate, and before you know it, you'll look like the top contender in a human pretzel competition.

Many businesses are willing to invest in *ergonomic* furnishings to help reduce work-related injuries. (More on ergonomics and the workplace in Chapter 23, "Back to Work.") That doesn't mean your boss will order you that $1,800 massage chair you saw at the Feel Good Back Store. Beyond a certain point, there is little relationship between an item's cost and its effectiveness. Obviously a $29.95 steno chair lacks the

adjustment capability of its more expensive coun-
terpart—this is just common sense. Before requisi-
tioning the $1,800 chair, shop around. Test-sit
several models, and play with the adjustments.
You're likely to find something just as supportive
at a much lower cost—though it probably won't
give you a massage.

Even if your chair does support your back and legs
in all the right places, get up and move around
every hour or so. Walk for a minute or two, even if
it's just in circles around your desk. At the very
least, stretch and give your muscles a chance to
change position. No design, however sophisticated,
can ease the ache of muscles held too long in the
same place.

Back Basics

The science of ergonomics is
sometimes called "human engineering." Objects that are **ergonomic** are
designed to interact with people in
ways that make tasks easier and
more efficient, and often with
reduced risk of injury.

Don't Hunker Down...Lift Up!

How often do you find yourself sitting all scrunched up like you're hiding from a
potential attack? Your shoulders brush against your ears, your chin nearly touches your
chest. If you're at home in your favorite easy chair, you've probably got your knees
tucked up, too!

If you're not already sitting this way, try it now. Then take a deep breath. Deeper!
Can't? If your lungs and diaphragm could groan, they would! But they can barely
expand enough to pull in the air you need just to supply your body with oxygen. Stay
in this position long enough, and your body will force you to stretch to take a deep
breath. Trying to stop it is like trying to stifle a yawn—your body's need for more air is
just too great.

Okay, now sit up straight. Hold your chin high—not so high that you look like a snob,
just out there enough to separate your head from your shoulders a bit. Feel your
shoulders pull back? Straighten your back and tighten your abdominal muscles. Now
take a deep breath. Feel the difference? Take a couple more, just for goodness sake (not
so many that you feel dizzy, though—we don't want any hyperventilating).

Years of inadvertent practice make hunkering second nature. If you're really good, you
can even do it standing up! This throws the natural balance of your skeletal system out
of whack, unevenly distributing your weight. Not only can this put you off balance, it
can also create stress on major joints like your knees and hips. Proper posture keeps
your body in alignment, letting all your organ systems work more efficiently and
effectively. And oddly enough, it seems to expand your attitude, too.

You may think you're sitting or standing up straight when you're really not. It's just that the perspective you've grown used to is the one you perceive as correct. Stand up and imagine someone is pulling a string through your body and tightening it up through the top of your head. Straighten as the string tugs upward. Balance your weight on both feet.

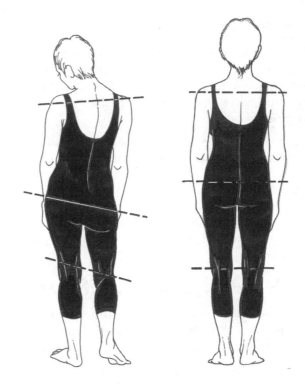

Sitting Postures

How often do you find yourself either perched on the very edge of your chair...and not because you're watching a late-night horror flick? You often become aware of this awkward posture when your backside goes numb, by which time, of course, it's too late to do much except stagger around the room until your muscles forgive you and let you straighten up.

If you slide into a slouch after 15 or 20 minutes in a chair, odds are it's not a good fit for your body and your task. Even if all you're doing is watching television, your seat should provide good support. Many people find that and comfort, too, in a well-built recliner. An office or desk chair should let you sit with your back against the chair's back and your feet flat on the floor (or a stepstool) so your thighs are perpendicular to the floor. If you can swing your feet, your chair's too high. Armrests should be just that—cushions where your arms naturally rest as you sit.

Some people find a "kneeling chair" provides a back-friendly way to work at a desk for prolonged periods of time. This design distributes your weight across your shins just below the knee. Such a position all but prevents poor posture, allowing your body to align itself naturally. If you have a herniated disk, sciatica, or other diagnosed back problem, check with your doctor before using this kind of chair. And before you buy one, check it out. Like the $29.95 steno chair, the cheap versions aren't likely to meet your needs. Shop for a kneeling chair at a reputable back-care store or furniture store. Some will let you borrow one for a day to see how well it works for you.

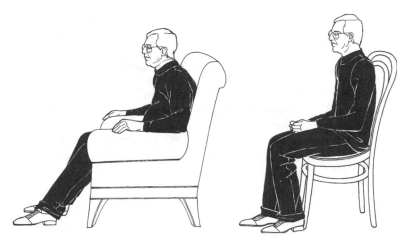

The difference between slouching and sitting up properly can make all the difference in the world to healing your back pain. As you build back strength, you'll find that sitting up straight is actually more comfortable than slouching. It's true! So get off that couch…

Standing Postures

The James Dean look worked well in the movies because it didn't last—the director said "Cut!" and the slouch was over. In real life, far too many of us present that infamous slouch, usually without even realizing it. We stand with shoulders forward, chin down, belly out—and not exactly looking like movie stars.

Today's shopping malls are great places to catch glimpses of your standing posture in action. Mirrored walls and storefronts intended to give the impression of spaciousness have the unintended effect of also allowing us to see ourselves as others see us. All too often, what we see is not what we imagine we look like. The next time you find yourself staring at "the stranger" in the mirror, don't look away in horror hoping that no one else sees you.

Take advantage of this opportunity to straighten up and stand tall. Let your feet bear your weight equally (though if you're standing for a long time, shift your weight from one leg to the other or put one foot on a stepstool to vary your position). Don't lock your knees. Suck in that belly and tighten those buns. No matter what your body shape and size, good posture makes you look (and feel) better.

Back Off!

People whose jobs require them to spend a lot of time bent forward or twisted are more at risk for low back pain. If your job leaves you contorted, be sure to change your position frequently. Something as simple as shifting your weight from one foot to the other, or putting one foot on a stepstool, can make a major difference.

Walking Upright

Walking seems like such a simple activity. It's just one foot in front of the other, with a little arm action for balance. Yet many of us are as out of balance when we walk as we are when we stand and sit. Again, pay attention to your shoulders. If they're hunched forward, you're hunkered down again. This puts a hump in your upper back and pushes your lower back outward, rendering unrecognizable the natural curvature of your spine.

Finishing schools of yesteryear taught young gentlemen and ladies to walk properly by having them balance a dictionary on their heads. Those who could walk across the room without sending the book crashing to the floor had both poise and good posture. You might give this old-fashioned technique a try when no one's watching, just to see how well you do. (Use an abridged dictionary, though, or maybe a paperback novel, to keep it light.)

Lying Down on the Job

Tell your boss you'd like to lie down on the job, and you're likely to get that look you know so well—one eyebrow raised with a half smile to match. Yet doing just that is likely to invigorate and refresh you, improving your alertness and maybe even your productivity (we can only vouch for the alertness part; you're on your own for productivity). We're not talking about a nap here—just a horizontal stretch break.

Of course, be discreet! Don't just sprawl in the hallway. If you have an office with a door, close it. Or find an unoccupied corner of the break room or employee lounge. A firm exercise mat makes a good surface that you can take with you anywhere, though a clean carpeted floor works fine.

Lie down on your back with your arms at your sides or with your hands resting on your abdomen. Lie with your knees up, so the small of your back is flat against the floor. Then lower your legs and feel your pelvis tip forward slightly, and your shoulders pull up. Feel the tension flow from your body as your muscles relax. Take a few deep, slow breaths.

Back Care

No matter how fashionable they are, high heels are never good for your back...or for your knees, hips, and feet, for that matter. Whether stiletto or clunky, big heels distort your body's alignment. Trade them in for flat or low heels. Someday it'll be fashionable to be good to your back.

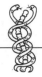

Back Care

Like the idea of stretching out on your back during the day, but not so sure you want to lie where the feet of others trample? Buy an exercise mat that you can roll or fold and take with you wherever you go. Look for one with a high-density filling for firmness and a surface you can easily clean.

Raise your knees again for a moment before getting up. To get up, turn onto your side and pivot into a sitting position—don't do a sit-up! Use your legs to push you to your feet, with a chair (no wheels!) for support if you like. (If you've been lying on the carpet, you might want to dust your back just to be sure you're not wearing paper trimmings or staples.) Just a five-minute "floor break" a couple times a day will make your back—and the rest of you—much happier.

Five Posture-Perfect Exercises

It's easy to improve your posture. Here are five exercises (three traditional, two yoga) that anyone can do anywhere, any time.

Pelvic Tilt: Yes, You Elvis!

This exercise relieves lower back discomfort and helps strengthen the structures of your pelvis, which improves their ability to better support your back.

1. Stand with your back against a wall. Place your feet shoulder-width apart, with your toes pointing straight ahead and your heels six to eight inches away from the wall.

2. Tighten your buttocks and pull in your stomach so the small of your back touches the wall. You may need to bend your knees slightly. Hold for 10 seconds, then slowly release. Repeat six times.

Back Stretches

During the day, your back often gets tense and tight from being held in the same position for too long. Back stretches relieve this pressure and help your back return to its normal position. There are three parts to this exercise; you can do any or all.

1. *The Chicken*: Stand up if possible. If you can't stand, sit up straight. Slowly move your chin out from your neck as far as you can, then move it back as far as you can. Keep your shoulders square and your head level. Repeat six times.

2. *The Runner*: Stand up straight. Put one hand on your hip, with your elbow pointing straight back. Raise the other hand to your head as though you're holding your ear, with your palm in and your elbow pointing straight ahead. Slowly move your arms until your arms trade positions—your "hip" hand goes to your head, and your "head" hand goes to your hip. Repeat six times.

3. *Belly-Out*: Stand up straight. Put your hands on your waist in the back (on the small of your back). Slowly bend backward, keeping your hands in place, pushing your belly out. Repeat six times.

Seated Bend-Over

This exercise is great for stretching your back muscles and relieving the tension poor posture or prolonged sitting causes.

1. Sit in a chair with your feet resting flat on the floor and your knees apart.

2. Raise your arms above your head, elbows straight. Slowly sweep your arms downward between your knees, reaching toward the floor.

3. Hold for 10 seconds, then slowly bring your arms back up. Repeat six times.

61

Tadasana: Mountain Pose

This yoga movement doesn't look like much at first. But looks are deceiving, because tadasana requires both concentration and balance. If you're a sloucher, leaner, or huncher, the mountain pose will help you stand tall.

1. Stand with your feet together, toes pointing forward. Let your arms hang at your sides, with your palms facing in toward your body.

2. Imagine that there's a loop on the top of your head with a string tied to it. Now envision the string tightening, gently pulling and lengthening your spine.

3. Without lifting your legs, pull your thigh muscles up (this takes concentration) and lift the front of your body. Consciously relax your hands, arms, and face. Take a deep breath in, slowly, and let it out.

4. Envision the string slowly going slack, releasing your spine and body as you return to a normal position.

Yoga's mountain pose is a posture enhancer that leaves you feeling strong and confident.

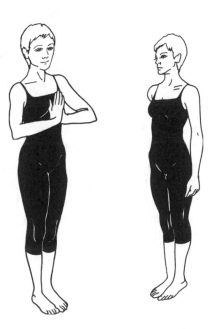

Trikonasana: Triangle Pose

This yoga movement tones and strengthens your spine as well as your waist, legs, and ankles.

1. Stand with your feet about three feet apart. Point your right foot forward, and turn your left foot out.

2. Extend your arms out from your shoulders, elbows straight. Bend slowly to the left, reaching for your left ankle or foot. Keep your shoulders straight, as if they were pressed against a wall. (It's okay if you can't quite touch.) Your right arm should stretch up toward the ceiling or sky.

3. Slowly stretch the muscles in your neck by looking upward or straight ahead. Take a deep breath in, slowly, and let it out.

4. Slowly return to a standing position.

5. Repeat to the other side.

Back to Nature

The trikonasana (pronounced *trih-koh-NAH-sah-nah*) yoga movement is called the triangle. When your hand reaches toward your ankle, your body forms several triangles.

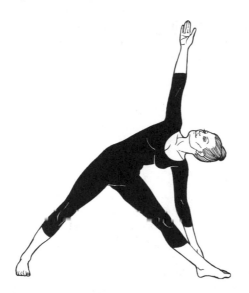

The triangle pose builds strength, increases balance, and gets the internal organs of the torso to participate, too.

Sleep Right, Not Tight

You spend about a third of your life sleeping. So pay attention to how and where you do it! While it might be comforting to sink into that soft mattress you've had since you moved into your first apartment, that body-sized dip in the middle is anything but comfortable for your back. Your bed should support your back in its natural curvature.

What's your favorite sleeping position? If you feel stiff and even sore in the morning, you could be falling asleep flat on your back. Sleeping on your back with your legs straight causes an exaggerated arch in your lower back. Back care experts recommend that you sleep on your side with your knees bent. If it's more comfortable, you can place a pillow between your knees.

Not Too Firm, Not Too Soft

While what constitutes a "good" mattress is to a large degree a matter of personal preference, look for one that is firm without being hard. Coil count is one way to compare different brands; generally, the more coils, the more consistent the support. A good mattress set is a significant investment, so shop around before making your choice.

Quality hotels typically feature high-end mattress sets; if you sleep on one you like, ask which brand and model it is. Often the hotel can steer you to a retailer that carries the same (or a similar) product.

Futons—fabric casings filled with natural or synthetic batting 6 to 10 inches thick—present an alternative to a traditional mattress and box spring. A good futon's filling provides comfortable back support as your weight displaces the batting. Many people place their futons right on the floor for maximum firmness. Others use specially made frames, some of which fold when not in use, turning the futon into seating. Like a regular mattress, a futon will serve you best when you turn and flip it regularly.

What About Waterbeds?

What started as a fad in the 1970s has acquired a small but faithful following among those with chronic back pain. Featuring a thick vinyl casing filled with water to the preferred firmness, a waterbed lets your body "float" through the night. Your body weight displaces water so you lie in natural alignment. While the original waterbed was simply a vinyl envelope filled with water, most waterbed mattresses today incorporate some sort of baffling system that reduces or eliminates waves. Waterbeds are also heated, which can be comforting to tired muscles.

If your sleeping arrangements change, the water volume you've become accustomed to may no longer be right. A bed filled to firmness with two people sleeping on it, for example, will not provide adequate support for just one person. Likewise, a bed perfect for one will be too firm for two—and may even roll one of you out if it crests too high above the bed's frame. And remember that water "goes flat" with time. You'll need to "burp" out the air every now and then, and occasionally add water to restore volume.

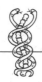

Back Care

Don't try to fix your sagging bed by putting a board between the mattresses. Industry experts warn that doing so interferes with whatever support system remains in your box spring. They recommend buying a new mattress every 10 years or so. To get longer life from your mattress, turn it and flip it once a month. Get someone to help you, so you don't hurt your back!

Back Off!

A waterbed can be great for your back...but very bad for gastric reflux, a condition in which stomach acids flow back into your esophagus when you lie down. Since your body weight displaces water in a waterbed, it's hard to elevate your head as doctors recommend to control gastric reflux.

Back in Balance

When it comes right down to it, a back out of balance often signals a lifestyle out of balance. Are you wound tight by the time your work day ends—not just physically, but mentally? Your state of mind influences your body's wellness more than you might realize. It's important to find ways to unwind both your body and your mind.

Many people find yoga and martial arts are effective for stress relief as well as physical fitness. Others use meditation and visualization to transcend the pressures of hectic living. It's important to find balancing methods that are easy for you to do as well as healthful. In Chapter 14, "Imagine a Healthy, Pain-Free Back," we'll talk more about stress and relaxation, and show you some ways to ease the tension in your life...and your back.

The Least You Need to Know

➤ Proper posture expands your chest, allowing your lungs and diaphragm to bring in more air with each breath. It also permits your skeletal system—bones, muscles, ligaments, tendons—to function with optimum efficiency.

➤ Where the mind goes, the body follows. Yoga and martial arts are among the methods that help keep each fit and relaxed.

➤ Learning a few basic exercises that you can do anywhere, anytime, gives you natural ways to relieve back stress and discomfort.

➤ A good mattress supports your back and your body so you can get a good night's sleep.

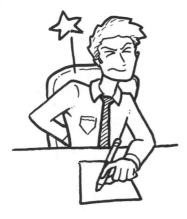

Chapter 6

Not Just for Athletes

In This Chapter

➤ The activities of living

➤ Everyday movements that are hazardous to your back

➤ Back risks for weekend athletes

➤ Activities that strengthen your back

Nothing is more important for your overall well-being than activity. Regular exercise keeps your heart pumping strong and the rest of your body following its lead. Weight-bearing exercise, in fact, is crucial for maintaining bone density and reducing your risk for osteoporosis. In fact, being fit reduces the risk of straining your back in the first place. And some experts believe that muscle activity and flexibility help reduce muscle tension and spasm that contribute to pain.

Regular activity has an advantage beyond fitness, too. Keeping yourself in motion actually reduces aches and pains, if for no other reason than it distracts you from them. But there are other reasons. Activity improves blood flow to your muscles, helping to keep them well nourished. Regular flexing and contracting tones your muscles. And exercise releases natural substances, called endorphins, in your body that tell your brain you feel good. Even if you have chronic back pain, gentle movement can loosen stiff muscles and joints and improve your mood.

Everyday Challenges to Your Back

Housework, desk job, manual labor—whatever you do, your back plays a major role. You sit, stand, lift, bend, and twist all day—most days without any problems. But some days, these challenges get to your back.

The Perils of the Bend-and-Twist

Ah, there it is, under the edge of the counter—the bottle cap that flew out of your fingers. You bend and swoop to grab it—and get stabbed in the back for your effort, a sharp pain that comes out of nowhere to freeze you in your tracks. The suddenness of bending and twisting is more than the average back can bear. Bending from the waist without bending your knees immediately stresses your lower back, stretching your muscles—and a stretched muscle is a vulnerable muscle. Add a twist to the bend, and you could end up in pain.

Though it's all too easy to do, twisting is hard on your back no matter how you do it. You reach behind you to grab a file from the cabinet, lift a box from the floor, and put it on a shelf beside you, all in a single move. Your back really doesn't like this movement, and is likely to send you a pain message in response. To protect your back from injury, keep all your body parts facing the same direction when you move. Instead of letting your torso pivot at the waist like one of those toy action figures, turn your whole body together, from head to feet. This keeps your skeleton and the muscles that support it in alignment and in balance.

When you bend, stoop down so your knees bend, too. Don't bend over at the waist. Not only does this present an unflattering view from behind, but it also makes your back scream. Keep your back straight and your shoulders squared. And as tempting as it is, don't twist when you bend. Take a little more time to turn first, then bend. Straighten, then turn.

Bending properly and turning your body instead of twisting may feel awkward at first. But changing your ways will help correct what are really awkward postures and moves for your back and your body.

Reaching Risks

It never fails. Whatever you want is on the top shelf, a fingertip beyond your reach. You stretch just a little more, maybe raise one foot for added thrust, and—pop! There goes your back, usually a muscle or group of muscles that just can't take the stretch anymore. And what you get is a strain or sprain that may hurt badly enough to limit your activity for a few days and ache for a few months.

Save yourself some anguish—get a stepstool or sturdy chair to extend your reach. Be sure not to stand on anything with wheels or anything not sturdy enough to support your weight. Try to get yourself shoulder-level with the object you're trying to reach, so you can handle it with control. Get someone to help you with items that are large or unwieldy. If you're, shall we say, vertically challenged, you might invest in one of those folding stepstools that have two or three steps.

"But All I Do Is Sit!"

Odds are, you're sitting right now. Stop for a moment and notice how. Where are your feet—flat on the floor, up on an ottoman, or tucked under you? If you drew a straight line from the ceiling to the floor, where would it intersect your body? Would you find your head to the right of the line and your hips to the left? Is your head tipped down to see the book you're holding in your lap, or are you eye-level with the print? Now that you know how you look, how do you feel?

Most of us think of good posture as something related more to standing and walking. But it's equally important when sitting. When you're on your feet, you have a natural tendency to shift around a little bit. This gives your back somewhat of a break. But how often do you sit in the same position for so long that a body part goes numb? This is not a good thing! It is amazingly easy to do, however. Often what you're doing when you're sitting occupies you beyond distraction until muscles everywhere howl for relief.

Your chair should evenly distribute your weight, with good support for your lower back. Its surface should be soft enough to cushion you, but not so cushy that you sink into it. Different bodies do better in different styles of chairs, so you may need to try several before finding what works for you. Even after you find the ideal chair, don't rely on it alone to keep your back free from pain. No matter how ergonomic your chair is, it cannot overcome the reality that your back was not designed to sit for long periods of time under any circumstances. At least shift your position every 20 minutes or so, and stand up once an hour. Add a short walk around your desk for even greater relief.

Back Care

Your favorite recliner might not be so bad for your back, especially if you sit in a reclined position. Firm cushions for contoured support, especially with an adjustable lower back support (or a rolled towel), could be just what a tired back needs. Old and sloppy doesn't cut it, though—such a chair, recliner or not, will make your aches only worse.

Lifting

"Bend your knees to lift with ease." The saying is familiar to anyone who's gone through workplace injury-prevention training. It's a slogan business owners and risk managers wish employees would both memorize and implement—60 to 80 percent of sprained backs happen during lifting, usually when you try to straighten up with your load. There's a little more to proper lifting than just bending your knees, though.

The ideal bending posture is one in which your knees are somewhat bent (not in a deep knee bend position), your back is straight, and you're holding the load you're trying to lift close to your body with both hands. Lifting an item weighing 10 pounds by holding it an arm's length away from your body gives that item an equivalent weight, in terms of the work your muscles have to do to lift it, of more than 150 pounds. Keep your shoulders and your toes facing the same direction so you don't twist—move your feet if you have to turn your body.

*Correct bending posture
for lifting.*

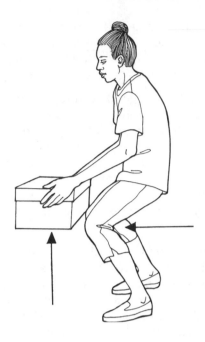

Back Talk

Each year nearly 500,000 Americans have back pain attributed to work, about 10 percent of whom are disabled. At a cost of over $60 billion a year in direct health care costs as well as lost productivity, back injuries are the most expensive occupational injuries for employers.

"But I can't pick up very much like that!" goes the common protest. Yes indeed, that's true—and that's the point. If what you're trying to lift is larger or heavier than is comfortable with this posture, you shouldn't be lifting it alone. Get someone to help you—or better yet, get a hand truck, dolly, or cart. Don't try shortcutting by pushing or pulling an object you can't lift, either.

Weekend Warriors, Beware!

So much to do, so little time—weekends are just not long enough for all you want to do. If you could, of course, you'd engage in your favorite activities all week long. But few of us get paid to play, so the weekends become playtime. If you get regular exercise during the week—walking, jogging, aerobics—you're probably in pretty good shape for your weekend games. If pushing papers is the closest you get to exercise, however, cramming your weekend full of your favorite pastimes could hurt more than it helps. A body that cruises through the week on passive autopilot is ill prepared for the transition to a rigorous workout come Saturday.

To avoid those aches and pains come Monday, try some gentle stretching before you exercise or participate in an activity. This will increase blood circulation to your muscles, bringing them oxygen and other nutrients. Gentle stretching again after you've given your muscles a workout has the same effect, and also carries away the by-products of muscle activity.

When Bodies Collide: Contact Sports

When you think "football," do you think pass plays and touchdowns, or grunting blocks and crashing tackles? Many of our favorite sports involve some level of physical contact—some coincidental, some intentional. In the heat of the game, however, few players are thinking about protection. Many contact sports use protective gear to thwart the force of blows to various body parts. Football and hockey players dress as if they're going into outer space. Soccer players wear shin guards. Coaches teach body position techniques to lessen impact—such as in football or wrestling. Combined with physical conditioning, these factors reduce risk in organized activities.

Back Off!

Some people attempt to head off minor aches and pains with a pre-exercise dose of an over-the-counter pain or anti-inflammatory medication (such as acetaminophen or ibuprofen). This is a dangerous practice. Intense exercise draws fluid from your body as you sweat, putting you at risk for dehydration. Yet you need extra fluids to help flush such medications through your kidneys.

Few "pickup" players have the advantage of such safety features, however. You don't often see pads and helmets at weekend scrimmages. Your body is simply out there, exposed to whatever hits it. And being hit isn't the only risk. Delivering a hit to an opponent could stop you both in your tracks. Back injuries that can occur as a result of being hit or hitting include sprains, strains, bruises, and occasionally fractures.

Holes and Pins: Golf and Bowling

Ah, tee time (on the green, not the queen's variety). Americans who groan and roll over for another five minutes of groggy sleep when the weekday alarm signals the start of another workday bound from bed on the weekends, eager to hit the course. Unfortunately, a good game can turn into a bad back with a single, errant swing before you even know what's happened.

In full swing, the golf club hits the ball at an astonishing 60 to 160 miles an hour or more. To reach this velocity, the golfer bends and twists with great speed—two of the actions your back likes least. Body position is critically important, not just to get off a good shot but also to protect your back from injury.

Back problems among golfers are legendary, striking players as prominent as Tiger Woods as well as countless anonymous fairway amateurs. So how do you play your favorite game and still keep a healthy back? General fitness makes a strong foundation. Regular exercise to strengthen and tone your back, abdominal, arm, and leg muscles puts them in optimal condition to work with one another (instead of conspiring to work against you). Next, take lessons. Learn how to hold your club and plant your feet and swing with your whole body, not just your torso (upper body). Most golfers who hurt their backs can remember the precise moment their pain struck—which more often than not was the precise moment the club struck the ball.

Hurling a 12- to 15-pound bowling ball down a narrow channel of highly polished wood is little better, from your back's point of view. While an excellent form of exercise, this other favorite American pastime also demands good technique for a good score—and for a healthy back when you leave the lanes. That ball at the end of your arm (held by just your thumb and two fingers) gains tremendous momentum by the time it swings from behind your back to in front of you just before release.

Strains and sprains are the most common back injuries among both golfers and bowlers. While fitness and conditioning certainly help, these sports stress the structures of every back. Reduce your risk of hurting your back by investing in lessons to help you position and protect your body.

Back to Nature

Love the snow, but not sure flying down the side of a mountain is the way to enjoy it? Cross-country, or Nordic, skiing is a kinder, gentler way to play outdoors in the winter. It actively involves your entire body since you're responsible for most of your movement (though of course there are nice downhills to reward your efforts). This reduces the strain on your back and also gives you a good aerobic workout.

Hitting the Slopes: Downhill Skiing

What's more exciting than flying down a mountainside, your skis or snowboard barely skimming the snow and the wind frosting your face? Those unexpected sudden stops, for one! They can certainly jolt your heart—not to mention your back and other body parts. Even your run-of-the-mill swooshing can leave your back stiff and sore the next day if your technique and position are off.

Downhill, or alpine, skiing demands exceptional performance from your body. Olympic ski champion Picabo Street you may not be, but it's not uncommon to hit 25 or 35 miles an hour on a good slope. If your position is solid—back straight, shoulders squared with hips, knees slightly bent and together—you'll do just fine. Just as most of us slouch when we sit, however, we tend to get sloppy on skis. Tenseness adds to the problem, tightening your muscles when you most need them to be loose and relaxed.

In the United States, we ski for fun and for exercise. We could learn a lesson or two from our European counterparts, who get in shape to go skiing. It's important to maintain strength and flexibility through regular exercise to keep activities like skiing enjoyable. If you don't use it, you'll lose it when it comes to fitness. Skiing is the leading winter recreational activity in the United States, which any emergency room near a ski resort can confirm. Common back injuries from skiing include sprains and strains. A hard fall can certainly crack vertebrae, too.

It doesn't take long for your back to complain when your downhill position is off. First there's that sharp ache between your shoulder blades, which quickly spreads to involve your lower back. You try to straighten your knees to relieve your discomfort, which is the wrong move and threatens to give you a close-up view of the moguls (those bumps of snow that look so small and harmless when you're standing at the top of the run). You'd like to stop and stretch, but your freshly waxed skis are beelining for the lodge—your only stop would be sudden and your stretch horizontal, which isn't quite what you had in mind.

If this is how your skiing adventures go, you already know you're probably going to hurt for a few days after. You don't have to continue this pattern, though, even if you can escape to the slopes only a few days a month. Starting today (even if winter is months away), prepare for your next ski getaway with a regular routine of back-strengthening exercises. Some legwork would be good, too, to keep your back from compensating for wobbly knees. Turn your exercise into recreation by adding in-line skating and bicycling to your routine. These activities work the same muscle groups that skiing calls on, and give you a good aerobic workout as well.

Back Off!

Alarmed by the dramatic rise in serious head injuries related to skiing accidents, doctors and many ski professionals recommend wearing a helmet when you ski. Ski helmets generally cover the head including the ears, and some have face guards as well. Some ski areas require children to wear helmets

Back Off!

Because both feet go on the same device, one behind the other, snowboarders are more likely to fall on their tailbones when they go down. Resist the temptation to brace yourself with your wrists. Casts will end your season in a snap, not to mention make even getting dressed a challenge.

Wheels and Blades: Skating

In some cities, inattentive pedestrians are the least of your worries when you step onto the sidewalk. In-line skating has become a popular transportation alternative across the United States, especially in mild climates that permit the activity year-round. High-tech plastics and polymers make these skates (with their four wheels in a line, like an ice skate's blade) fast, sturdy, and relatively inexpensive. From college students to retirees, skaters enjoy the easy access in-line skates offer. All you do is strap 'em on, put on your pads and helmet, and roll away. Small gear bags can contain and hide your wheels during the day.

As long as you stay on your blades or wheels, skating is great exercise. It's easy to get off balance, however. Even if you don't fall, the jerking and twisting you go through to try to regain your balance can pull or sprain your back. Rink skating, either ice or roller, generally offers a more controlled environment and surface.

Back Off!

Be prepared for the unexpected when in-line skating in an uncontrolled environment. A helmet, elbow pads, wrist protectors, and knee pads should be part of your regular attire when you skate. Gravity remains a common (and painful) means of stopping.

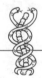

Back Care

Wrap up your strenuous workouts with a soak in the Jacuzzi or hot tub, or a nice, hot shower. This increases the blood supply to your tired muscles, bringing much needed oxygen and nutrients and clearing out waste products. Be sure to drink plenty of water, especially if you've had a hard workout (a pint every 15 minutes), to keep your body from dehydrating.

Holding Court: Racquet Sports

Racquet sports are really just high-end bend-and-twist events. You're out there on the court, stooping low, stopping sharp, and swinging with all your might to return the last volley. Whether you make the shot or not, you're likely to feel your back complaining. Unlike the bend-and-twist activities that challenge your back during routine activities, racquet sports add force to the formula. That racquet extending out from your hand does more than stretch your reach. It also intensifies the force of your swing—a force that reverberates back through your arm and down your back.

Be good to your back by stretching and warming up before you take to the court. Relaxed muscles respond better to the extremes of your sport, giving you greater flexibility with less likelihood of injury. If your sports club offers such a service, consider a sports massage after your match to gently stretch and soothe your tired muscles. Sprains and strains are the back injuries most common in racquet sports. And the tremendous forces created with the sudden stops and quick twists of games like squash can even herniate a disk.

Hoops and Spikes: Net Sports

You're on the court, ball in hand. Everything around you ceases to exist as you realize you're poised to make the perfect shot. The ball arches up and drops straight through the net; the only sound it makes is the gentle rustling of the nylon cords of the net as the ball passes through. As long as you're the only one shooting hoops, your risk of back injury is slight. Add enough players to have teams, and the risk shoots higher than your jump shot. Stories of player back injuries fill the sports pages, particularly among pros. Their oversized bodies collide like meteors in a game that has become fast and physical, subjecting them to injuries of all kinds. A few, like Isaiah Thomas, can make near-miraculous recoveries in just a few days from injuries that end the careers of others.

Net sports like basketball and volleyball add reach-and-stretch risks to bend-and-twist perils. You're leaping and swatting and swooping and throwing—fast and furious. And yours is a rare game indeed if there's no body crashing on the way to the net. Strains and sprains are the most common injuries. Pregame warm-ups, even just a few stretches and a jog around the court, will help loosen your muscles before the game puts the pressure on them.

What *Can* You Do Without Hurting Your Back?

We don't mean to make it sound like all your favorite activities are just waiting to ambush your back. Regular exercise—activities that get you sweating at least 30 minutes four or more times a week—is good for your body, your spirit, and of course, your back. As we've tried to stress in this chapter, a fit body is far less likely to be injured no matter what you're doing. And with proper warm-ups, positions, or technique, and warm-downs, you greatly reduce risk during strenuous activities. You needn't give up the activities you enjoy just because they're on the "high risk" list. Just get your back in shape!

The first step to reduce your risk of back injury in *any* activity is fitness. This doesn't mean you have to pump iron five hours a day. While that might give you a buff appearance, looks aren't everything. You can get a healthy, fit back through regular, basic exercises. This will get and keep your back ready for most of the action you want it to carry you through.

There are many activities you can engage in without undue risk, too. Walking, swimming, and stationary bicycling rank right at the top of the list—and can give you a good aerobic workout at the same time.

In the previous chapter we gave you five easy exercises you can do anywhere to improve your posture (the foundation of back fitness) and tone your back. In Chapter 12, "Exercise Does a Back Good," we'll tell you all you need to know about improving your back's strength, stability, and flexibility.

Back Care

When you walk, wear shoes with good support and adequate padding to cushion your steps. The heel supports sold in sporting good stores can do a good job of stabilizing your feet and are less expensive than custom orthotics. If your feet hurt even after trying insoles, get an evaluation from your doctor or podiatrist.

Just Walk!

It's so simple, yet so effective—walking may well be the ideal activity. It's so simple, in fact, that many people overlook (and even scoff at) its effectiveness. But just 30 minutes of brisk walking a day (a pace of three to five miles per hour) tones and strengthens nearly every muscle group in your body—and gives your heart and lungs a good aerobic workout, too.

When you walk, pay attention to your posture. Hold your head high and your shoulders back. Swing your arms in rhythm with your legs. Take steps that are long enough to have your front foot's heel just coming down as your back foot's toe is releasing, to give you smooth and powerful strides. Feel the muscles in your back move as you walk. Vary your routes to keep them interesting. Companionship keeps walks interesting, too, even if the only partner you can coax into accompanying you is your dog.

Back to Nature

You don't need fancy electronics to tell whether your walking is a workout. Can you sing while you walk? If so, you need to pick up the pace—you've got more of a leisurely stroll going. Once you get going, can you talk? If all you can manage is words between huffs, back off a bit—you're pushing too hard.

Back to Nature

Want more of the real adventure in your indoor cycling? Try rollers. This device uses fixed rollers that you balance your bicycle on, riding as though you were on the street. Though at first you might feel like a hamster in a wheel, once you get the hang of it rollers offer realistic riding performance.

Don't overlook the abundance of natural opportunities to hoof it. You can park a few blocks from your office or at the back of the parking lot at the store and walk the rest of the way. Take the stairs instead of the elevator. Walk to lunch, or around the block after lunch. It may not seem like much, but the cumulative effect can be a tremendous boost to your fitness.

C'mon in, the Water's Great: Swimming

The best thing about swimming is that your body feels and acts half its weight in the water. This lets you get a good workout without nearly the stress of land activities. It's also much harder (though certainly not impossible) to fall into poor postures in the water. Since your body moves so effortlessly, it falls into its natural alignment. The odds of hurting your back swimming are pretty small. Unless, of course, you take up diving—that changes everything.

Riding Nowhere: Stationary Bicycling

Sure, the scenery leaves a lot to be desired—but you'll never get wet or run off the road. Stationary bicycling gives you all the benefits of a good ride without the hazards. You can ride an exercise bicycle designed just for indoor use, some of which have synchronized moving arms so you get a full body workout as you pedal. You can also use a special training stand that lifts a regular bicycle's rear wheel off the ground and provides a spinning cylinder to give it resistance as you pedal. This also stabilizes your bike so you don't have to worry about balance.

Some stationary bicycles come with a small fan setup to simulate the breeze you'd generate if you were really riding, or you can set one up yourself. You will work up a sweat, so the fan's a big help in keeping you cool. Remember to vary your position, particularly if you're using your regular bicycle on a track stand. This will keep your muscles from tensing and your hindquarters from getting saddle sore.

Outdoor cycling is good exercise for your back and for the rest of you, too. If you live where the weather's generally moderate, you can get out regularly. Outdoor riding has the disadvantage of traffic and road hazards.

An Eastern Influence: Yoga and Martial Arts

Yoga and gentler forms of martial arts can improve both the condition of your body and state of your mind. These methods bring an Eastern perspective to our Western views of fitness and conditioning. With an emphasis on control and slow, conscious movement, these approaches are ideal for toning, limbering, and strengthening your back.

If the word "yoga" conjures an image of an old man with a flowing beard contorting his limbs into configurations that would make a pretzel run for cover, it's time to update your perspective. The word "yoga" comes from an ancient Sanskrit word that means yoked or joined. It embodies the philosophy of the practice of yoga, which is to unite and integrate body and mind. Yoga emphasizes awareness of what's happening with your physical body—how your muscles feel as they stretch and relax. It also focuses your mental awareness, helping to reduce stress.

And if "martial arts" brings to mind a solitary ninja defeating dozens of bad guys with a few well-placed kicks, you're watching too many late-night movies. Certain forms of martial arts, such as t'ai chi and QiGong, look more like graceful dancing than fighting techniques. Like yoga, these methods emphasize awareness and the body/mind connection. The movements tone and condition the physical body, while meditation elements do the same for the mental and spiritual being.

There's more on these topics in Chapter 14, "Imagine a Healthy, Pain-Free Back."

The Least You Need to Know

➤ Even though bending, twisting, reaching, and lifting are common, everyday activities that threaten your back's well-being, you can protect your back by keeping it fit and conditioned.

➤ Contact sports, racquet and net sports, golf, bowling, skiing, and in-line skating are popular pastimes that are great exercise, yet can be hazardous for your back. Stay active and exercise the proper precautions to keep your sport back friendly!

➤ Walking, swimming, and stationary bicycling are good activities to strengthen your back.

➤ Yoga and gentle forms of martial arts integrate body and mind to condition both.

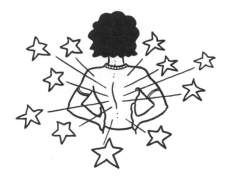

How Does It Hurt? Let Us Count the Ways!

That body of yours is an amazing, living machine. It keeps you moving through the activities of your life, mostly without you even noticing. Your bones, muscles, tendons, and ligaments hold you upright and give you structure, strength, and movement. By the time you think about getting up out of your chair to get another cup of coffee, your brain has already sent millions of instructions to these body systems via an intricate "intranet" of nerves.

When you maintain and treat it with care, your body machine is more reliable than any mechanical machine. Days, weeks, months, and even years can go by with everything working just as it should. Then something goes wrong—it could be minor, or it could be more serious. You discover that the body machine that propels you so effortlessly through your day can break down—and it hurts. Fortunately, most injuries heal with time and TLC (tender loving care).

Strains, Sprains, and Spasms

You hurt your back—playing racquetball, lifting a box of books, reaching for a stray sock in the bottom of the washing machine. You're fairly certain nothing's broken, but you're not sure what other damage you might've done. How does your doctor figure it out? While you might be expecting x-rays and other tests, one of the most effective diagnostic tools your doctor can use is listening.

The majority of back injuries involve damage to muscles, tendons, and ligaments—your back's *soft tissues*. Most people will be back to their regular activities within a few weeks, though it may take several months to feel entirely normal after a back *strain* or *sprain*. Other problems involving your back, such as degenerative disk disease or osteoarthritis, can be a more of a bother over time. Since most back problems are soft-tissue injuries that will heal whether you do anything about them or not (treatment aims to make you comfortable while healing takes place), it's not always important to know what kind of back problem is giving you pain.

Doctors diagnose soft-tissue problems, sometimes called *mechanical strains and sprains*, as much by what you tell them happened as by the symptoms you have. Strains, sprains, and pulls don't show up on x-rays or more sophisticated and expensive imaging techniques such as MRI, either (though MRI is very useful for diagnosing some soft-tissue problems such as torn ligaments in the knee). Rarely, a soft-tissue injury can involve a serious muscle tear or ligament separation. Such an injury, if severe, might require surgery to repair it, though this almost never happens in the back.

There isn't much your doctor can do for most soft-tissue problems beyond what you can do for yourself at home—ice or heat, over-the-counter pain or anti-inflammatory medication, and limited activity (do as much as you feel able to without pushing it) for a few days. After three or four weeks, you should feel better and have a sense that you're still getting better, even if you still have some lingering pain. If you don't, consider seeing your doctor to be sure there aren't any underlying problems. Physical therapy, therapeutic massage, chiropractic manipulation, or acupuncture might provide relief if your back is taking longer to heal.

Not all soft-tissue problems are the same, of course. Even if you and your best friend, who have everything in common, hurt your backs in exactly the same place while doing exactly the same thing, your course of recovery is likely to be one of the areas where you differ. How much an injury hurts is very much an aspect of your expectations and past experiences. And even if you and your best friend have been playing tennis on Wednesdays for the past 15 years, you each bring a different body to your games. You could be ready to volley in two weeks, while your friend can barely pick up a racquet. This variability is one of the most frustrating aspects of back pain for both people with it and the health care providers trying to treat them.

Back Basics

Soft tissues are your muscles, tendons, and ligaments—body parts that are "soft" compared to bone. Soft-tissue injuries account for about 80 percent of all back pain. **Strains** are muscle injuries; **sprains** are ligament injuries.

Back Basics

Mechanical strains and sprains affect the way in which your back functions, though they don't alter its structure. Such problems in the soft tissues in your back often occur during movement, particularly lifting, twisting, and bending.

Back Talk

Ever wonder what a trillion might look like? Stand in front of a mirror and you can see 40 times that—about 40 percent of your body's 100 trillion cells are muscle cells. Though they make a hair appear thick by comparison, muscle fibers are incredibly strong, capable of supporting up to 1,000 times their weight.

Strains

A common cause of back pain, strains affect muscle tissue. You can strain a muscle when you suddenly stretch or reach, causing the muscle fibers to stretch abnormally. On rare occasions, the injured muscle fibers can tear and bleed (usually too little to see), which can create an irritation—and gives you pain. Unlike with injuries to your arms and legs, you'll almost never see a bruise emerge unless you've had something hit you or have been in a car accident with a sudden impact. A mild strain is sometimes called a pulled muscle.

You can reduce your risk for back strains by stretching and warming up before exercise. If you're chuckling to yourself right now, thinking there might be an advantage after all to living a sedentary life, the joke could be on you. You might consider preparing for everyday activities as though you're warming up for a basketball game. (Seriously.) A few gentle stretches throughout the day will at least help you feel more relaxed and alert and could save you a backache.

Strains are most likely to affect your lower, or lumbar, back. By now you should know what we're about to say—you can reduce your risk of injury by staying fit. Fit muscles are better able to help each other out, as well as more resistant to injury. Weak abdominal and leg muscles put the full burden of lifting on the structures of your back, which really weren't designed to handle such stress.

Back to Nature

Make your own "ice rub" blocks by filling paper cups about two-thirds full and putting them in the freezer. When you need to ice an injury, just pull one out, peel away enough of the paper cup to expose the ice, and rub the ice directly over where it hurts.

Back Care

If you think you strained your back, ice the spot that hurts as soon as you can. This reduces swelling, which helps limit the injury and the pain it causes. Apply ice for 20 minutes every couple hours for the first 24 to 48 hours, and as needed after that if it makes your back feel better (or switch to heat).

Most strains feel better in a few days, although it can take weeks or even a month or more for you to return to good-as-new status (with depreciation for the wear and tear that comes with growing older, of course). Follow your body's cues—if an action or movement stops you in your tracks, back off.

The reality is, you're unlikely to remember any precipitating event. However, you'll be more likely to remember if you're trying to lift something, since that's what we've all been taught is the biggest risk (we'd like to put this in the "most likely myth" category).

Sprains

Sprains affect ligaments, the tough tissue that connects muscle to bone. You can sprain your ankle, for example, when you step down and your foot rolls to one side. Your ankle suddenly finds itself bearing your full weight, and—ouch! You can sprain your back, too, when a sudden, forceful movement gives a ligament more than it can handle. Prime culprits when it comes to pointing the finger at a cause include lifting and activities that involve forceful twisting (such as golf, basketball, and racquet sports).

You could resume most of your regular activities in a few days to weeks after a back sprain, though it could be several months before you feel completely normal again. While wrapping a sprained ankle helps support the structures as they heal, this is seldom practical for a sprained back. Although many health care providers recommend neck or lumbar supports, recent studies have been unable to show that these tools make a difference in healing or affect pain in any significant way for the majority of people. A cervical collar (a soft, thick pad that wraps around your neck) *may* help when a sprain involves your cervical or upper thoracic spine. Wearing a cervical collar can increase stiffness, decrease neck mobility, and weaken your muscles if you wear it too long, however. Sometimes a lumbar support can help if your sprain is in your lower back.

Back to Nature

If "raw" ice is just too cold for you, try a bag of frozen peas or corn. This usually isn't quite so cold, and the bag flexes to mold to the area of your injury. You can refreeze the bag as needed. Label the bag so you don't eat from it, though!

Back Off!

Motor vehicle accidents cause many upper-back sprains. Your cervical and thoracic spine areas are at greatest risk. *ALWAYS* wear a seatbelt (lap and shoulder combination when possible) when riding in a vehicle. Adjust your headrest so it's directly behind your head, not your neck. Even a minor fender-bender can exert tremendous force on your neck and back.

During the initial, or acute, phase of a back sprain, ice and anti-inflammatory or pain medications can give you some relief. Rest also helps, though don't take to your bed. Change your position every hour or so while you're awake. If you wake up at night, get out of bed and walk a little. This will help loosen your back muscles and keep painful spasms at bay.

Back Talk

"Whiplash" is a catch-all name for a variety of injuries involving the upper spine. Often, such injuries occur in motor vehicle accidents when your neck is "whipped" (snapped from front to back) and "lashed" (jerked from side to side) from the forces of the accident. Like other soft-tissue injuries, whiplash can be mild or severe and can involve muscles or ligaments, or both.

Spasms

There you are, just minding your own business, when all of a sudden you feel like an iron fist has grabbed a handful of your back and is squeezing and twisting. You can't seem to escape, and before long more muscles are hurting. This describes a muscle *spasm*.

Skeletal muscles, like those in your back, are always in a state of partial contraction. It's this tension that allows them to support other structures and keeps them ready for movement. A spasm happens when a muscle or muscle group stays too contracted, often in response to pain. It becomes tight and rigid, which you can sometimes feel as sort of a lump. Though the word "spasm" might conjure an image of twitching, it really has more to do with nonmovement.

Spasms go away when the muscles relax, which often isn't as simple as it sounds. Once a muscle spasm starts, it's easy to get into a cycle of exacerbation—it hurts, which causes you to stiffen and try to hold the area still, which causes the muscle to tense even more…and so on. Your doctor may prescribe a muscle relaxant medication to help break this cycle. Heat and therapeutic massage often provide relief, too. Once the spasm starts to go away, gentle movement helps return regular blood flow to the muscle, which restores

Back Care

Give your sprained back the same treatment Olympic and professional athletes give theirs: relative rest. Instead of resting your entire body because your back hurts, just give your back a break but keep the rest of your body active. As your pain improves, add gentle stretching to restore your back's full range of motion.

Back Basics

A **spasm** occurs when a muscle stays in a state of contraction. The word "spasm" comes from the Latin word *spasmus*, which means "to pull or draw."

the chemical balance the muscle needs to maintain a normal state of tension. Regular movement and activity are particularly important during healing. Guarding the sore area tends to encourage the spasm's return.

Back Talk

The term "charley horse" comes from seventeenth-century England, a time when constables were called "Charleys" since they were in the service of King Charles I and King Charles II. Aching legs were an occupational hazard among these local police officers, who spent their days walking. Today "charley horse" refers to painful muscle cramps that can occur during or after intense exercise.

Muscle Fatigue

Muscles get tired, too. After a lot of contracting and expanding, they need a little rest to recover. If you're working them too hard, as often occurs during intense exercise, they'll begin to feel heavy and even numb. Though you might not know it, your muscle fibers are becoming less and less efficient—even as you need them to exert more power with each contraction, they exert less. Your muscles warn you that they're going into overload by sending pain signals. If you ignore these signals, which is easy to do in the heat of competition or when you've got just one-half mile to go in the marathon for which you've been training for months, you could end up with a muscle strain. Acute muscle fatigue from overuse generally makes itself known as an aching soreness that can last a few days.

Back Off!

Most muscle relaxant medications relax your brain a bit, too, affecting your reaction time and level of alertness. For your well-being and the safety of others, don't drive, operate machinery, or drink alcohol while taking muscle relaxants. If you feel sleepy, take a nap.

It doesn't take an intense physical workout to generate muscle fatigue, however. Static stress—stress that affects your muscles when they're not moving much—and repetitive motion can also cause muscle fatigue. Office workers who often sit or stand in the same position may find their muscles feeling tired and sore by the end of the workday. Those who do repetitive tasks, such as typing or key entry, may start aching after just a few hours. To reduce your risk of muscle fatigue on the job, think of your work as an athletic event (even if you're just a desk jockey). Start your workday with a stretching routine. Try to stand and stretch for a few minutes every hour. At the end of the day, go through your stretching routine again.

Fatigued muscles often have too much lactic acid (a by-product of the work your muscle cells do). Getting more oxygen into your blood gives your cells the energy they need to remove lactic acid. When you feel tiredness set in, breathe—take a deep, slow breath in, then slowly let it out. Do this five or six times. It might be difficult to breathe slowly if you're engaged in strenuous exercise, but be careful not to breathe in deeply and rapidly. You'll hyperventilate, which can make you feel lightheaded and woozy. Slow, deep breathing expands your lungs, bringing in more oxygen for your blood to carry around your body's systems. It also helps relieve stress, which can contribute to muscle tension.

Rarely, muscle fatigue can be a symptom of a more serious condition. If your muscles feel heavy and tired for longer than a few weeks, or without apparent cause, schedule a checkup with your doctor.

It Hurts, but No One Knows Why

Sometimes the pain lingers, and no one can find a good reason for you to hurt like you do. Maybe your pain started with an injury that has since healed, or maybe it just grew on you. In either situation, your pain rules your life. There are several *syndromes* involving back pain that encompass collective, chronic symptoms. Diagnosis is difficult, and doctors often arrive at it by ruling out other possible causes.

Some syndromes are as mysterious to health care providers as they are to the people who have them—there is no clear identification of the cause of the symptoms, no tried-and-true treatment that eliminates the symptoms, and no understanding of why or how the symptoms occasionally just disappear. While doctors, chiropractors, and other health care providers are familiar with muscle-related pain syndromes, yours might refer you to a physiatrist for diagnosis and treatment. A physiatrist is a physician (M.D. or D.O.) with specialized training in physical medicine and rehabilitation. Most people eventually get better with persistent treatment and return to their usual activities. Sleep disturbances are common in these syndromes, so it's wise to avoid caffeine and alcohol (these substances interfere with sleep).

The three syndromes we briefly discuss here—myofascial pain syndrome, fibromyalgia, and tension myositis syndrome—are complex conditions with many variables in diagnosis, treatment, and prognosis (outlook). We mention them because back pain is a primary symptom of each.

Back Basics

A **syndrome** is a collection of symptoms that collectively describe a disorder. Most people who have a syndrome have multiple symptoms.

When Muscles Keep Hurting: Myofascial Pain Syndrome

Myofascial pain involves the fascia and muscle. Fascia is a thin, membrane-like tissue that covers and connects muscles, tendons, ligaments, and other tissues. Fascia also separates specific muscles, allowing them to slide past each other easily. Though an odd word, fascia is probably familiar to you—if you've ever prepared chicken for dinner, fascia is that filmy, stretchy stuff that clings to the meat. In your body, when you tear or cut fascia as a result of an injury, it tenses and tightens and loses its elasticity, or allows muscles to rub together. This causes pain.

Unfortunately, no one knows for sure what causes myofascial pain to continue after the initial injury heals, or to exist when there has been no apparent injury. Myofascial pain can be local (affecting a single site), regional (affecting an entire area of your body), or generalized (affecting your entire body). Other symptoms that often accompany muscle pain include difficulty sleeping, stress, and what doctors call *trigger-point* sensitivity (especially sensitive nerve endings that can trigger severe pain with very little stimulation).

Most treatment approaches attempt to offer a holistic approach, often incorporating physical therapy, trigger-point massage, heat or ice, ultrasound, biofeedback, medication (including antidepressants to promote sleep, muscle relaxants, and analgesics or anti-inflammatory agents for pain relief), and regular exercise to improve body mechanics and posture. Acupuncture sometimes provides pain relief, as does injecting trigger points with a local anesthetic (drug to numb the area) or a procedure called "dry needling" (a sterile needle inserted at the trigger point without injecting anything) to desensitize it. Treatment teams often include a psychologist who can address the stress and mental-health issues that typically arise when pain becomes chronic. And some people get relief from chiropractic or osteopathic manipulations. What works in the way of treatment seems as variable as the symptoms.

Back Basics

A **trigger point** is an overly sensitive area within a muscle that reacts to pressure by sending signals of referred pain.

Back Basics

Greek and Latin root words can help you *identify* the meanings of many medical terms. *Myo* means "muscle." *Algia* means "pain." *Itis* means "inflammation" (irritation and swelling). *Fascia* means "band" (like a belt, not the marching variety). *Fibro* refers to "fiber." Something that is **myofascial** involves both the muscle and fascia. **Fibromyalgia** is pain of the muscles and fibrous tissues. **Myositis** is inflammation of the muscles.

Fibromyalgia: Aching All Over

Fibromyalgia, formerly called fibrositis, is a more widespread pain condition than other pain syndromes. It involves muscles throughout the body as well as other symptoms. Some researchers believe fibromyalgia is related to, or even part of, a generalized syndrome called chronic fatigue syndrome. An estimated five to seven million Americans have fibromyalgia (2 to 5 percent of the general population), and 70 to 90 percent are women. About 80 percent eventually recover, though it can take several years to be back to normal.

Though its symptoms have puzzled physicians since Victorian times, no one really knows what causes this painful and distressing condition. Many theories abound, but no one theory has a preponderance of supporters. Those who have fibromyalgia generally experience numerous and varied symptoms, including debilitating pain in the back, arms, and legs (with multiple painful "trigger points"), sleeping problems, depression or anxiety, and stress. Fibromyalgia is sometimes difficult to distinguish from myofascial pain syndrome; some practitioners consider the two syndromes aspects of the same condition. As with myofascial pain syndrome, treatment approaches are holistic and often involve various specialists and providers.

Polymyalgia Rheumatica (PMR)

Polymyalgia rheumatica (*PMR*), a rare disorder, can be confused with fibromyalgia or other causes of muscle pain. It causes stiffness and soreness primarily in the neck, shoulders, thighs, and hips. It's more common as you get older (the average age of sufferers is 70), and can be associated with fatigue, severe headaches, jaw pain during chewing, and even vision loss. Doctors don't know the precise cause, but believe it's probably an immune reaction to an unidentified virus. PMR is treated with steroids (prescription medications to reduce swelling and inflammation).

Back Off!

There are many alternative treatments advertised to treat chronic pain syndromes. A few might actually help, but at best most will do no harm (or good). And a few can cause even more problems. Thoroughly research alternative treatments before trying them, and discuss those that interest you with your regular health care provider.

PMR can be very serious (even fatal) if left untreated. For this reason, it's important to distinguish it from fibromyalgia and other chronic pain syndromes.

Wry Neck: Torticollis

Torticollis (from the Latin words meaning "twisted" and "neck") in adults often results from a muscle spasm or an injury. Your head tilts to the side where the muscles are contracted. This soft-tissue condition improves with heat, and sometimes physical therapy or therapeutic massage, to relax and stretch the muscles. Occasionally your doctor may recommend a cervical collar to give your neck additional support while the injury heals.

There is a form of torticollis that appears in infants, usually caused by an awkward position in the uterus or an injury to the neck muscles at birth. Gentle stretching usually restores the affected muscles to normal, though sometimes the baby may need additional physical therapy.

The Least You Need to Know

➤ The majority of back injuries involve soft tissues (muscles, ligaments, and tendons).

➤ The majority of soft-tissue injuries heal in time, with or without treatment. Most treatment approaches aim to improve comfort and mobility while healing takes place.

➤ A quick return to activity, even if your back still hurts, seems to shorten the healing time.

➤ Though chronic pain syndromes are frustrating, most people eventually recover or adapt and can lead relatively normal lives.

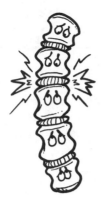

Chapter 8

Structural Distress: Bones and Disks

In This Chapter

➤ When joints become inflamed

➤ Disk problems

➤ When bones break

➤ The special risks of osteoporosis

Though soft-tissue injuries account for most back pain, most serious back problems involve vertebrae and intervertebral disks. Your spine is a complicated structure that will serve you well through much of your life. The older you are, however, the more likely you are to have problems.

A certain amount of degeneration occurs as part of the natural aging process. Regular exercise, especially weight-bearing activities like walking and running, can delay or minimize many of these changes by keeping your bones strong and dense.

Flare-Ups: Joints and Inflammation

Your joints are marvels of engineering. While artificial joints are increasingly common (particularly hips, knees, and knuckles), researchers have yet to develop a mechanical substitute that works as well as the ones that came with you as original equipment. However marvelous they are, your joints do eventually wear out. And when they do, they can cause you pain (though certainly not always).

Facet Joint Inflammation

They spend your entire life keeping your spine both erect and flexible, hinging your vertebrae together. Every time you move, your facet joints come into play. These fluid-filled cartilage caps cover the bone ends, providing a lubricated surface for smooth movement. Over time, the pressures of lifting and stretching irritate the cartilage and can cause it to rupture. Without its film of fluid protection, the joint surfaces become irritated and inflamed.

A few days of limited activity, ice, and over-the-counter anti-inflammatory medication can help you through the acute phase of pain. Proper lifting methods protect against, though can't entirely prevent, future inflammations. Many people also find relief from chiropractic manipulations, which may restore facet joint and vertebrae alignment.

A vertebral pair.

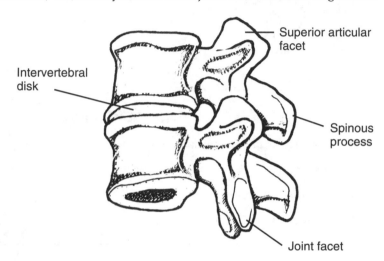

Intervertebral disk

Superior articular facet

Spinous process

Joint facet

Osteoarthritis

As cartilage deteriorates, it makes the joint less stable. One way your body compensates for joint deterioration is to generate bony growths, called osteophytes, to brace the joint. As ideal a plan as this compensation appears to be on the drawing board, it overlooks your desire to remain flexible and mobile. Activities once easy and pain free become difficult and painful as the tissues surrounding the joint swell and stiffen. Most people first notice osteoarthritis in their hands or knees. But since we're talking about backs here, osteoarthritis most often affects vertebrae in the lower back.

Though typically a consequence of aging, osteoarthritis can attack younger joints (and not just in your back). This is most common when you've had an injury that leaves a vertebra vulnerable. Treatment focuses on relieving pain and stiffness, and may include anti-inflammatory medications, ice or heat, physical therapy, and therapeutic massage.

Exercises that gently stretch your back and keep your muscles conditioned, such as yoga and t'ai chi, can ease discomfort and improve flexibility. Some people get relief from acupuncture and chiropractic manipulation.

Rheumatoid Arthritis

Rheumatoid arthritis is another beast altogether, in which your body's immune system attacks your joints as though they were invaders. No one knows why this happens. While in osteoarthritis, your body tries to protect a deteriorating joint by laying down more bone tissue (which causes swelling and pain), in rheumatoid arthritis your joints become inflamed (which causes swelling, pain, and often deformity). Rheumatoid arthritis most commonly strikes joints in your fingers, wrists, knees, hips, shoulders, and cervical spine. Untreated, it destroys and deforms joints as the tissues around them weaken. Other symptoms usually accompany rheumatoid arthritis, including fatigue, generalized aching, and fever.

Most people with rheumatoid arthritis have specific antibodies in their blood. These antibodies, collectively called the rheumatoid factor, are somewhat like shell casings left after an attack. They are evidence that your body's immune system has declared war on your joints. Treatment may include various medications, heat, and physical therapy. Yoga helps keep your back as flexible as possible, and acupuncture and chiropractic manipulation sometimes provide pain relief.

Back Off!

Beware of products that promise to "cure" arthritis. As yet there is no cure, though many treatment approaches can relieve symptoms. Some purported "cures" are harmless enough, but others can endanger your health or life. If a new or alternative treatment interests you, check it out through independent resources (such as not-for-profit organizations) that have nothing to gain or lose because of the product.

Ankylosing Spondylitis

Ankylosing spondylitis is a rare (one third of 1 percent) form of arthritis that affects the spine and sacroiliac joints (where your spine joins your pelvis). You're more likely to have this condition if you're a man between ages 20 and 40, and if others in your family have it. The joints between your vertebrae become inflamed, causing pain and stiffness.

You're likely to first feel ankylosing spondylitis in your lower back, with symptoms that are worse in the morning. Unlike most other back pain, the pain caused by ankylosing spondylitis improves with exercise.

When the stiffness becomes permanent (called ankylosis), the involved vertebrae become fused together. The affected part of your spine loses flexibility. Ankylosing spondylitis can also affect other joints, such as hips and knees. Therapeutic massage, physical therapy, heat, and regular exercise (like swimming) to strengthen and condition your back muscles can help keep symptoms in check.

Disk Problems (and We Don't Mean Your Computer)

Ah, it's that "as we grow older" tune again. Sorry. But with increasing age come certain changes in our bodies.

Back to Nature

Are you a heavy walker? Each step you take "weighs" as much as you do in terms of the pressure your body feels. You can lighten your body's perception of this pressure by stepping more lightly. Walk across the room and listen. Can you hear your footfalls? Practice walking in such a way that you no longer hear your feet thudding as they hit the floor.

Back Off!

Do you smoke? If so, your back will likely take longer to heal, and hurt more, than if you don't. Smoking reduces the level of oxygen and other nutrients your blood can carry to body tissues, and your disks get less blood than many other body parts to start with. Smoking also seems to interfere with your body's ability to release natural pain-relieving chemicals.

Natural Deterioration

We get many years of good use from these bodies of ours, but eventually they wear down. (This becomes crystal clear even to those who want to deny it, when your arms are no longer long enough to hold reading material so you can see it.) In your back, the cartilaginous cushions that hold your vertebrae apart get stiffer and less resilient. The outside of these intervertebral disks harden like old leather, and inside the gel-like core thickens. As this happens, the disks flatten somewhat, allowing your vertebrae to move closer together.

Unfortunately, you can do as little about this as you can about your changing vision. Many people notice their changing backs when they realize they have more aches and pains than they used to. You may feel more of the jolts and shocks of activities like walking, as your intervertebral disks are less able to shelter you from them. You may also find your back becoming more sensitive to other activities it once tolerated, like sitting or standing for long periods of time. For most people, however, the changes of an aging back don't result in any significant changes in lifestyle.

As hard as it might be for you to acknowledge your back's reminders that yours is an aging body, respect the message. Be kinder and gentler to your back. Learn ways to ease its burdens. If you golf, take lessons from someone who can show you how to get the most effort and least resistance from your swing. If you sit behind a desk most of the day, set a timer on your watch or your computer to remind you to stand, stretch, and walk around for a few minutes every hour. If you watch a lot of television, get up and walk around during the commercials (which are getting longer and more frequent to give you more activity breaks).

Sleep on a comfortable bed that offers good support. Try yoga to keep your back flexible and to gently stretch your muscles. Walk as much as you can, and try other activities that keep you on your feet, like dancing or low-impact aerobics. Weight-bearing exercise is one of the best ways to maintain bone density, which helps you resist another age-related problem, osteoporosis (which we discuss a little later in this chapter).

Protruded Disk

The disks that separate and protect the bones in your back, your back's natural shock absorbers, take quite a beating. Just the shock that reverberates up your spine with every step you take causes them to flex and compress, absorbing the energy of your footsteps. Imagine what they go through when your activity level goes up!

All this pounding makes your intervertebral disks vulnerable to damage. A disk's thick, fibrous wall can weaken, stretch, and crack, allowing its jelly-like center to bulge through. When this bulging, called a protruded disk, puts pressure on the nerves leaving your spinal cord at the involved vertebra, it can cause pain. It's also entirely possible and, in fact, common, to have a protruding disk that causes no symptoms.

Though they can be extremely painful when they first occur, the majority of protruded disks heal themselves in time. Physical therapy, chiropractic manipulation, heat, ice, limited activity, yoga, and medication are all treatment approaches that can provide pain relief while healing takes place. With numerous studies showing that no one approach is necessarily better or more effective than others in speeding recovery, many doctors now advocate a "watchful waiting" approach coupled with a gradual return to regular activity as the acute pain subsides.

Herniated Disk

A herniated disk (sometimes called a ruptured disk) occurs when there's a tear in the disk's outer covering that allows the inside gel to ooze out. This irritates nearby nerves, causing pain in the area of the rupture and often radiating down the back of your leg (sciatica). A herniated disk is somewhat like an overnight best-seller (though decidedly less pleasant)—it happens seemingly instantly, though it's often been years in the works. A disk can also herniate from trauma, such as a fall or auto accident.

Like protruded disks, most herniated disks heal on their own with time and rest. The tear gradually scars over to seal the leak, and your body replaces the lost gel. Healing in your intervertebral disks can take longer than healing, say, a deep cut on your arm. This is largely because your disks have a more limited blood supply.

While you might find a day or two of bed rest helpful immediately after the herniation happens, you'll feel better faster if you get up and get moving (gently, of course). Follow your doctor's advice for activity and medication.

Though surgery to remove a herniated disk was once the treatment of choice, doctors now operate only when conservative approaches fail to relieve your pain over time, or when the disk presses on nerves that affect movement and sensation in your legs.

*A normal disk and a
herniated disk.*

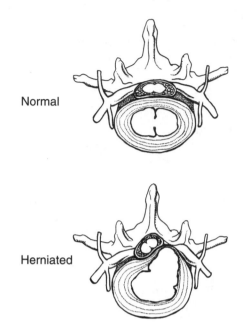

Normal

Herniated

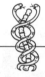

Back Care

Wonder what you're doctor is up to when he or she raises your leg to see if it causes pain? This maneuver is called the "straight leg raise," and it helps your doctor identify whether a prolapsed disk is affecting the nerves in your leg, and to what extent. The height to which you can raise your leg (measured in "degrees of elevation") helps differentiate pain from a pulled muscle in your thigh (or other causes of numbness and tingling in your leg) from nerve root pain caused by pressure from a disk.

Sciatica

Sciatica is a real pain in the rear—literally. This pain follows the sciatic nerve down your buttock and the back of your leg to below your knee. Sciatica usually (but not always) signals a disk herniation or rupture in the lower back, with the disk pressing against the spinal nerves that form the sciatic nerve. You can end up with sciatica from other reasons, too, from sitting too long in a position that compresses your sciatic nerve to conditions such as diabetes.

Diagnosing sciatica is fairly straightforward, based on its unique symptoms. Finding its cause, however, can be challenging. Treatment for a first episode generally focuses on relieving the pain. If sciatica becomes a regular visitor, your doctor will probably do more testing to look for the cause. The treatment for sciatica—a few days of rest and anti-inflammatory or pain medications—will also help a problem disk, so often treating the symptoms treats the underlying cause as well.

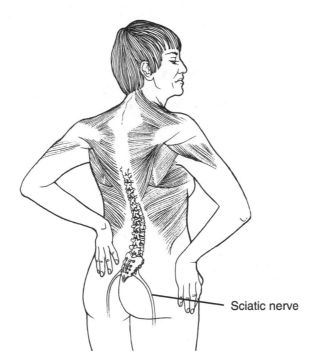

Sciatica causes pain that follows the sciatic nerve.

Sciatic nerve

Going Around the Curves

Your back has five natural curves—three that curve in, and two that curve out. These curves help your spine function properly. Sometimes your curves head off on a different path, which causes problems not just for your spine but also for other body systems in sort of a domino effect. Whenever possible, treatment attempts to bring the curves back within normal range.

Scoliosis

When you look at your spine square on from the back (a tricky thing to do, so you can look at someone else's if you want), you should see pretty much a straight line. A tilt to one side or the other anywhere along the line signals scoliosis. Most commonly, there are two sideways curves, one offsetting the other. Mild scoliosis generally doesn't create any problems, and you may not even know you have it unless your doctor mentions it to you during a physical exam.

Hip pain and problems bending are often clues that scoliosis is present. For mild and moderate scoliosis, treatment targets pain relief and muscle strengthening through exercises. Severe scoliosis may require wearing a brace to straighten the spine, and rarely, surgery. Chiropractic manipulation may also help.

Lordosis and Kyphosis

Everyone has both lordosis and kyphosis to some degree—these are the curves you see in your spine looking at it from the side. Lordosis is the inward curve in your lumbar spine and kyphosis is the outward curve of your thoracic spine. They become a problem only when they become exaggerated, which can happen as a result of chronically poor posture, osteoporosis, or congenital defect.

Lordosis and kyphosis often appear together, since what happens to the curvature in one segment of the spine often affects others because they must compensate for the off-line segment to keep your spine working. In most situations, lordosis and kyphosis cause soft-tissue aches and pains, particularly as you grow older and the abnormal curvatures become more pronounced.

When poor posture is the problem, treatment includes corrective and strengthening exercises to restore your spine to normal curvatures. When kyphosis or lordosis are present from birth, doctors may try bracing or even surgery in adolescents who seem to be getting worse. Severe kyphosis can put pressure on the spinal cord, which creates neurological problems. Lordosis is less likely to do this.

Adults with kyphosis or lordosis are seldom candidates for surgery, unless the condition causes nerve problems. Chiropractic manipulation or physical therapy may improve both discomfort and the degree of curvature.

Kyphosis in the elderly, especially women, can be a sign of painful spine fractures, usually involving thoracic vertebrae. This is most often a result of osteoporosis.

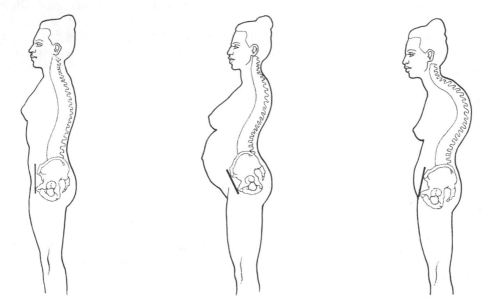

Left to right: Correct spinal curvature; lordosis, a condition common in pregnant women or in overweight individuals; kyphosis, a condition common in the elderly.

Spinal Stenosis

The medical term for narrowing is "stenosis." Spinal stenosis results from narrowing or impingement of the spinal canal itself—compressing the spinal cord or nerve roots (in the lumbar spine). As your aging disks become thinner and less resilient, they allow the vertebrae to move closer to one another. This, or bone spurs, can narrow the channel through which the nerves exit, putting the squeeze on those nerves. A key symptom of spinal stenosis is pain (of course!) that improves when you sit down and worsens when you walk.

Severe spinal stenosis causes numbness or tingling in the leg on the affected side, and can even interfere with movement. If the stenosis is in your neck, you may feel similar symptoms in your arms on one or both sides. Surgery is the usual treatment for spinal stenosis that reaches this level. Until function becomes a problem, treatment aims to relieve pain.

Spondylolisthesis

Ten bonus points if you can get this one to roll smoothly off your tongue! Spondylolisthesis (pronounced *SPON-da-low-lis-the-sis*) is the tongue-twisting name for a painful condition in which one vertebra slips over the top of another. This can put pressure on the spinal nerves and sometimes the spinal cord, causing pain. Spondylolisthesis most commonly involves lumbar (lower back) or cervical (neck) vertebrae. Sciatica and pain that hurts more when standing are clues that spondylolisthesis might be the problem (or neck pain and arm numbness or weakness when cervical vertebrae are involved).

Injury, improper formation of the vertebra (called spondylolysis), osteoarthritis, and rheumatoid arthritis (especially in the neck) can cause spondylolisthesis. X-rays are helpful in diagnosis. Treatment may include medications to reduce pain and inflammation, and traction coupled with physical therapy. Chiropractic manipulations are often especially effective in getting vertebrae back where they belong.

Occasionally spondylolisthesis is severe enough to warrant surgery to fuse together the affected vertebrae. According to allopathic experts, the only way to correct severely slipped vertebrae in spondylolisthesis is with surgery. In the chiropractic view, the pain from spondylolisthesis goes away in most people once the upper slipped vertebra returns to its rightful position with chiropractic adjustments. Hopefully, future scientific studies will help doctors and chiropractors decide when to try these approaches for different degrees of spondylolisthesis.

Back Care

If you can glue that ceramic mug back together, why not your broken back? That might be among the treatment options your doctor offers you. A special medical cement shows great promise for stabilizing back fractures, especially those that occur in people with osteoporosis. The surgeon can inject the cement into the bone without major surgery or a lengthy hospital stay. This treatment is still experimental, however.

Exercises to strengthen the muscles supporting your spine in the affected area can help keep the condition from coming back.

When the Bone Breaks: Fractures

Spinal fractures are no laughing matter. The unstable bone segments can bruise or cut your spinal cord. It's not that easy to break your back—it typically takes a considerable blow or force. The one exception is if you have osteoporosis. With this condition, your bones are quite brittle and can break spontaneously (without any outside trauma).

Back Talk

Your bones may appear solid and hard, but inside they're spongy and resilient. This helps them resist breaking under the tremendous forces that they encounter every day. Overall, your bone tissue is about 75 percent water.

Back Off!

DO NOT ATTEMPT TO MOVE anyone who might have a back fracture. Back fractures can happen whenever there is an intense blow or force to the back. Motor vehicle and bicycling accidents, diving accidents, and workplace accidents can cause back fractures. So can tumbling down the steps. Summon emergency aid, then help the injured person remain still and calm until help arrives.

Traumatic Fractures

Fractured vertebrae usually show up on x-rays. Treatment may require a brace or cast, traction, or surgery to add supporting rods or plates to the damaged area. A broken back will likely put you out of commission for several weeks to several months. If there is no damage to your spinal cord, however, you can expect a full recovery once the fracture heals. Sometimes soft-tissue injuries accompany a spinal fracture. A comprehensive rehabilitation program can help restore function and strength, though recovery can take time.

Compression Fractures in Osteoporosis

Compression fractures act more like crushed cans—the weakened bone collapses. Fractures that develop as a result of osteoporosis receive different care than do traumatic fractures of the spine, usually a few days of bed rest and pain medication. Although they can be very painful, these fractures very seldom put your spinal cord at risk, so there's no reason to immobilize your back (though occasionally a brace can provide comfort, especially if several vertebrae are involved). About 700,000 people with osteoporosis have compression fractures of the vertebrae each year.

Weak Bones: Osteoporosis

For much of your life, bone replacement is an automatic process. Old bone cells, like other cells in your body, die off and new bone cells grow to replace them. Unfortunately, this process slows by the time you reach age 35. The older you get, the less new bone your body produces. So as bone cells die off, fewer new bone cells replace them. By the time you reach age 70, your skeleton has only about two thirds of the bone mass it had when you were 35.

Osteoporosis is the condition that results when this process reaches a critical level. Because it happens so gradually, you may not realize you have a problem until you break a bone. Over 25 million Americans have osteoporosis, including half of women over age 45 and 90 percent of women over age 75. In addition to aging, numerous factors influence the severity of osteoporosis, including a diet poor in calcium, lack of exercise, excessive alcohol use, hormones, and smoking. X-rays, CT scanning, or bone densitometry (x-ray assessment of bone density) can detect the extent of osteoporosis.

The Calcium Factor

In addition to slowing its efforts to replace old bone cells with new, your body also becomes less efficient at moving calcium into your bones. Calcium and other minerals are what make the outer surface of bone tissue so hard.

Back Off!

If you've ever had compression fractures or you have osteoporosis, avoid any strong manipulations of your spine such as chiropractic or deep-tissue massage. These usually beneficial techniques can turn harmful when your bones are fragile. It takes very little pressure—sometimes just rolling over in bed—to generate a compression fracture if you have osteoporosis.

Back Basics

Osteoporosis comes from the Greek words *osteon*, which means "bone," and *poros*, which means "passage." Medically, osteoporosis is the condition that results when bones lose their density and mass, becoming weak and susceptible to breaking.

While you can't replace lost bone tissue, you can strengthen the bone tissue that remains by increasing your intake of calcium. From age 25, men and women need at least 1,000 milligrams of calcium a day. Pregnant women, women past menopause, and men past age 65 need 1,500 milligrams a day. You can get the calcium you need

Back to Nature

Weight-bearing exercise provides a particular benefit for bone strength and density. Good weight-bearing exercises include walking, hiking, jogging, dancing, and climbing stairs. It takes at least 30 minutes of moderately intense weight-bearing exercise three or four days a week to strengthen your bones.

through a nutritious diet. Dietary supplements containing vitamins and minerals can help you maintain adequate calcium intake.

The Estrogen Factor

The hormone estrogen, which women's bodies produce freely before menopause, helps bones retain calcium. When estrogen production falls off after menopause, calcium drains quickly from the bones. Estrogen replacement therapy (ERT) restores the body's ability to hold onto calcium longer. Women *not* on ERT are twice as likely to have osteoporosis-related fractures as women who are. ERT is not risk free, however, so if you're a postmenopausal woman considering it, discuss the benefits and risks with your doctor. Even with ERT, performing weight-bearing exercise and adding calcium to the diet remain important aspects in strengthening bone tissue.

The Least You Need to Know

➤ Most disk problems heal in time. Treatment aims to help you feel better while this healing takes place.

➤ Exercise and proper posture can help maintain a healthier back.

➤ Spine fractures from trauma can damage your spinal cord if not treated promptly and properly. NEVER move someone who might have a broken back.

➤ Compression fractures of the spine can occur suddenly and without warning if you have osteoporosis. Weight-bearing exercise and adequate calcium in your diet are your best defenses against osteoporosis.

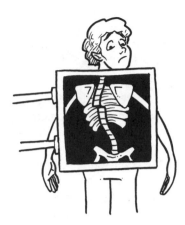

Chapter 9

What the Tests Tell

> **In This Chapter**
>
> ➤ Examining your back
>
> ➤ What x-rays show—and don't show
>
> ➤ Getting an inside look with imaging procedures
>
> ➤ The challenges of interpreting findings
>
> ➤ What comes after the tests?

When your back pain is severe, or doesn't go away after four to six weeks, it's time to find out why. There are a number of diagnostic tools at your doctor's disposal, from physical exam to sophisticated imaging.

Checking You Over: Physical Examination

A physical exam is the starting point in the search for the source of your pain. Though it seems pretty basic, your back exam may begin like any other physical examination, with a check of your temperature, blood pressure, and pulse. These measurements, sometimes called your vital signs, give a quick glance at your overall well-being. In particular, having an elevated temperature (fever) alerts your doctor to the possibility of an infection (though this is not a common cause of back pain, it's worth ruling out). Your doctor will then examine your back by looking and feeling for anything unusual, focusing on the area where you're having pain.

Simple tests can activate certain *reflexes*. Two tests your doctor is likely to do are the knee-jerk reflex, in which your lower leg kicks out when the doctor taps just under your kneecap with a small rubber hammer, and the ankle-jerk (Achilles tendon) reflex when the doctor taps at the back of your ankle. These tests can show whether your back problem is interfering with the nerves controlling your legs and feet. A third reflex, the Babinski reflex, in which your toes curl when the doctor strokes the bottom of your foot, if abnormal, may reveal a problem in your spinal cord.

Your doctor might also check certain *dermatomes* (places on your body that are supplied with nerves coming from the spine) to look for sensory changes in your skin. These changes might be tingling or numbness, and often indicate a prolapsed (ruptured) disk at the level in your spine that correlates to the affected dermatome. A common dermatome runs down the outside of your lower leg (on each leg and then over to your big toe, correlating to your fifth lumbar vertebra [L-5]). Another runs down the very outside and bottom of your foot, correlating to your first sacral vertebra (S-1). Your doctor will likely test your ability to feel a finger or cotton swab (light touch) and a pinprick in these areas, if there is any concern about numbness and tingling (possible nerve damage) in those areas.

Back Basics

A **reflex** is a body reaction over which you have no conscious control. **Dermatomes** are areas of your body supplied by certain root nerves from your spine.

Also, your doctor may have you try certain movements, such as raising your leg up straight while you're lying on the exam table. The point at which this hurts can point to—or rule out—a herniated disk as the culprit causing your pain. The doctor may also have you flex and stretch your foot to test your ankle strength. Difficulty pushing against the doctor's hand, or pointing your big toe back toward your body, can also signal disk problems.

Details, Details

Your doctor will want to know what you were doing when you hurt your back. Not to be nosy or to embarrass you, but because this can shed light on what's wrong. Stay brief and to the point, but don't leave out information just because it doesn't seem very important to you. Give your doctor the details, and let him decide what's relevant. Were you golfing, lifting a box of books, reaching into the washing machine for a stray sock, lying in bed, raking leaves, walking the dog, playing catch with the kids? What happened when the pain hit? Did you freeze in your tracks, crash on the couch, or keep going without noticing that you hurt until later that night when getting ready for bed?

What kind of pain you're having provides clues about its causes. Is your pain sharp or dull? Constant or intermittent (comes and goes)? Worse with certain activities or positions, at certain times of the day, or when the weather turns stormy? Do you feel pain, tingling, or numbness in either leg? Are you having trouble with bladder or bowel control? Is your pain preventing you from doing things you did before? Have you missed work? What, if anything, gives you relief now? Have you had this particular pain before? What helped it go away? Do you have arthritis or pain in other joints such as your knees or hips?

Your doctor will also ask you about your general health, and about any stress you might be having in your life at the time. This information is important because other health circumstances can have an effect on your back, or provide insight into why your back is bothering you. Tension and stress eventually take a toll on your body and can aggravate chronic conditions. Your doctor will also ask about your work and activities, since what you do all day (and how you do it) can make your back ache.

In Quest of Evidence

In most situations, back pain stems from some sort of problem involving your muscles and connective tissues or an intervertebral disk. If this appears to be the case for you, and you're not showing any signs that your nerves are affected, your doctor will probably just recommend treatment to improve your comfort while your back heals. Don't feel slighted; most of the time, the best treatment is to let nature take its course. Don't push for x-rays, an MRI, or other tests if your doctor doesn't think they're necessary. Just because Joe at the gym had a full-scale encounter with medical technology for his back pain doesn't mean you need one.

In some situations, your doctor may decide to order further tests. Don't be afraid to ask what and why. What does your doctor expect to learn from these tests? What risks are there for you in undergoing the tests? How will knowing this information make a difference in your treatment? "Just so we'll know" may not be reason enough, unless the findings will influence your doctor's treatment recommendations. Remember, your health—and health care—should be a collaboration involving you and your health care providers. You won't offend your doctor by asking questions. (And if your doctor does take offense, you might consider changing doctors.)

If you've previously had any of the tests your doctor wants to order, or other tests because of back pain, let your doctor know. Earlier findings might offer clues about what's going on this time, or could keep you from unnecessarily repeating a test.

Back Talk

German scientist William Conrad Roentgen (1845–1923) discovered x-rays in 1895 while conducting experiments with electric current. He noticed that when he sent a current down the inside of a tube containing a vacuum, a chunk of barium (a natural metallic element) sitting on the counter nearby would glow. He didn't know at first what caused the effect, so he named it "x-radiation," using the algebra symbol for an unknown. Roentgen received the first Nobel Prize in Physics in 1901 for his discovery.

Snapshots of Your Bones: X-Rays

In the 1940s and 1950s, shoe stores all across America proudly featured the newest equipment for fitting shoes—a fluoroscope. This device used *x-rays* to show a picture of how feet looked inside shoes. Toes too close to the edge got a new size—and a new picture. Of course, we didn't know then what we know now, that overexposure to radiation of any sort, including x-rays and the sun, is harmful. (But we Americans really love our technology. Despite this knowledge, states had to pass laws making fluoroscopy for fitting shoes illegal.)

William Roentgen, the scientist who discovered x-rays, took an x-ray of his wife's hand using a 30-minute exposure to get a somewhat grainy image of the bones inside as well as of the large ring she wore on her finger. Today, we measure x-ray exposures in fractions of a second and get crystal-clear images. An x-ray image on film is sometimes called a roentgenogram, in honor of its discoverer.

X-rays work by passing a beam of low-dose, *ionizing radiation* through your body. As they do, various tissues absorb them at different levels. Soft tissue, such as muscles and ligaments, absorb very little. Bones, which are far more dense and contain a high level of calcium, absorb nearly all of the x-rays that pass through them. Tissues that absorb a lot of radiation display a light or white image on x-ray film; tissues absorbing less radiation display as a darker image.

Healthy body tissues absorb x-ray radiation at predictable rates, which makes it easy to identify abnormalities. An x-ray shows a fracture, for example, because the location of the fracture doesn't absorb nearly as much radiation as regular bone. What you see as an x-ray is really a shadow of the body part recorded on film.

What X-Rays Show

X-rays show your bones. They can show if your vertebrae are out of alignment, as happens with spondylolisthesis, fractures, and sometimes with a herniated or ruptured disk. X-rays show most fractures, some bone tumors (which are very rare, causing less than 1 percent of all back pain, though they become a consideration if you've ever had any form of cancer), bone changes due

Back Basics

X-rays are a form of electromagnetic energy that have very short wavelengths and very high frequencies. The energy that makes up x-rays is called **ionizing radiation**. As this energy passes through an object, it temporarily creates an electrically charged particle called an **ion**. An x-ray image shows these ions.

Back Off!

If there *is* any chance, however remote, that you could be pregnant, tell your doctor *before* she orders x-rays. Though the radiation you receive from x-rays is usually not significant, it could be enough to harm a developing baby because its cells divide very rapidly. Normal tissue cells in an adult divide much more slowly, and so are not affected by brief radiation. A series of back x-rays is the equivalent of several hundred chest x-rays to your ovaries, which is a pretty high dose of radiation.

to arthritis, and can indicate osteoporosis. They also show abnormal curvature of the spine, such as scoliosis, lordosis, and kyphosis (see Chapter 8, "Structural Distress: Bones and Disks").

Some doctors order x-rays "just to see" the first time you come in with back pain, particularly if you're older than 50 and could have osteoporosis or arthritis. Such x-rays, especially if the findings are normal, can provide a baseline for future problems. Most doctors are becoming more hesitant to order tests like x-rays, however. They prefer to wait, unless you have "red flags" (such as severe nerve problems the first time you're seen or a history of cancer) because the x-rays aren't likely to help. Every time you have an x-ray, you're exposed to radiation. Though the amounts can be small, there's no reason to have the exposure at all if it's not going to tell your doctor something about how to treat your back pain. When soft-tissue injury is the likely culprit, your doctor will probably try a course of conservative treatment first before ordering x-rays or any additional tests.

Back Care

Keep your own records of when you have x-rays, why your doctor orders them, and where they're taken. If you see a different doctor, you can share this information. You'll have access to previous x-rays for com-parison purposes and can avoid unnecessary duplicate x-rays.

What X-Rays Don't Show

There's really more that x-rays *don't* show. For starters, unless it's a bone problem, you won't see it in white on black. Strains and sprains involve soft tissues, which don't show up well on x-ray. And your nerves and disks don't show up on x-rays. One study, conducted in Sweden over a period of 10 years, found that x-rays produced useful findings in only about one in 2,300 patients. Standard medical practice is moving away from routine back x-rays unless certain circumstances exist (such as an injury that could cause a fracture).

Often, even when an x-ray shows an abnormality, it doesn't bring you any closer to a diagnosis. Hyperkyphosis (an exaggerated thoracic curve), for example, by itself doesn't tell you what's causing your pain, though it does point the finger at muscle or liga-ment strain. X-rays don't show all fractures, either. Compression and hairline fractures can be especially difficult to detect, and may require additional tests to be sure. And sometimes even the experts don't agree on what an x-ray shows, particularly when findings are inconclusive.

A Closer Look: Imaging Procedures

Modern technology gives us many ways to "see" inside your body without cutting it open, using *imaging procedures*. Most combine computer enhancement with an energy source to produce dimensional images. Some imaging techniques involve injecting dye into a suspect intervertebral disk or an area around your spinal cord. Others are noninvasive (nothing enters your body). And sometimes doctors use diagnostic

Back Basics

Imaging procedures provide a look inside your body without cutting you open.

procedures in combination with one another to show problems either procedure alone might not detect; for example, myelography (dye injected around your spinal cord) in combination with CT scanning (a CT myelogram).

Imaging procedures are generally safe, though those that involve an injection carry the risk of an allergic reaction to the injected substance. They are quite expensive, however, and don't always show the reason for back pain. Imaging procedures are most appropriate when you're already a candidate for surgery to confirm the location and extent of abnormalities surgery will attempt to repair.

CT Scan

Computed tomographic scanning, commonly called a *CT scan*, puts the power of computers to work to get more mileage from x-rays. A computer combines dozens of flat, two-dimensional x-ray pictures taken from multiple angles to produce progressive "slices" of, say, your spine. This presents your spine, soft tissues, and body organs all in the same picture.

Like imaging procedures, CT scanning is noninvasive (the x-rays are just passing through). There's no special preparation beforehand. After changing into one of those

Back Basics

A **CT scan** uses a computer to compile multiple x-ray images into "slices" of images to give a dimensional perspective of your spine. **MRI** uses a strong magnetic field to accomplish a similar feat.

stylish, tie-in-the-back hospital gowns, you lie on a table that slowly moves you through the opening of a large, doughnut-like machine. You don't feel anything. Doing a CT scan of your spine takes about 15 to 30 minutes. The risks of CT scanning are the same as those for standard x-rays—brief exposure to low levels of radiation.

CT scanning with injection of contrast dye (CT myelogram), can also show problems such as herniated disks. No matter how you slice them, however, the x-rays that form the basis for CT scanning have the same limitations of standard x-rays—soft tissues don't absorb them. CT scanning is more useful for showing problems that affect your bones, like fractures and cancers involving the bone.

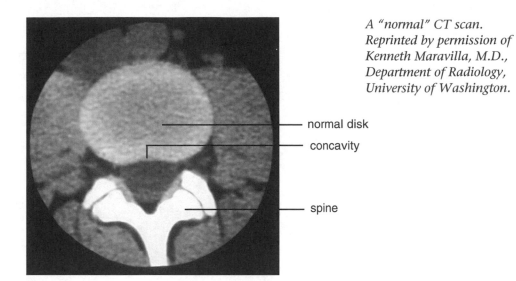

A "normal" CT scan. Reprinted by permission of Kenneth Maravilla, M.D., Department of Radiology, University of Washington.

— normal disk

— concavity

— spine

MRI

Magnetic resonance imaging, or *MRI*, is a newer technology that might eventually replace CT scanning, especially to help diagnose muscle and nerve problems. Instead of x-rays, MRI sends out radio frequency signals that create an electromagnetic field. As your body passes through this field, its tissues respond by sending back signals of their own. (For those of you whose inquiring minds want to know a little more, the MRI's magnetic field temporarily realigns the hydrogen molecules of your body, which has a lot of them since it's mostly water.) A computer collects and assembles these signals into images that show internal body systems.

Like CT scanning, MRI is noninvasive. However, it's important that you have no metal on your person when having an MRI. You'll need to remove all jewelry (including wedding rings and earrings). Don't try to stash your wallet under your hospital gown—the MRI will erase the magnetic strips on your credit and bank cards. (Most imaging facilities have a place to secure valuables; ask about this when you change your clothes.)

While MRI is especially useful for diagnosing injuries such as serious muscle or ligament tears in other locations, such as your knee, it's not very helpful for diagnosing similar problems in your back. MRI does show back problems such as herniated and prolapsed disks, spinal stenosis, and tumors, as well as problems involving bone such as fractures.

Back Off!

If you have a pacemaker, coronary or arterial stent, sternal wires (after open-chest surgery), aneurysm (surgical) clips, or "hardware" from a fracture repair, tell your doctor before you go for an MRI. Because they contain metal, these objects will interfere with the procedure. Your doctor may want to order a different imaging test that doesn't involve an electromagnetic field.

107

An MRI of an asymptomatic patient with degenerative disk disease. Several desiccated (dried out, degenerated) disks are shown, with an area of prolapse. Although this patient has a very abnormal MRI, the patient has no symptoms! Reprinted by permission of Richard A. Deyo, M.D., M.P.H., University of Washington Medical Center

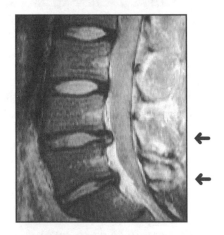

normal disk

desiccated disk

"herniated" prolapsed disk

An abnormal MRI of the spine showing disk herniation of two disks. The prolapsed disks are pressing on the spinal cord, causing typical symptoms. Reprinted by permission of Kenneth Maravilla, M.D., Department of Radiology, University of Washington.

A "normal" MRI of the spine showing mild disk degeneration. Reprinted by permission of Kenneth Maravilla, M.D., Department of Radiology, University of Washington.

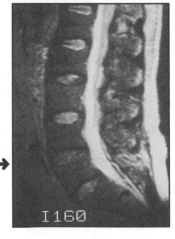

degenerative disk (less bright) ➡

I160

Bone Scan

Sometimes bone problems are difficult to detect with x-rays and even CT scans. Another type of imaging is a *bone scan*, which uses a nuclear medicine camera to take pictures of your body after injecting a *radionuclide* into your vein. The way your bone tissues absorb the dye paints a picture of what's going on within your vertebrae and other bone structures.

Because a bone scan involves an injection, it's considered an invasive procedure. There is a very slight chance you could have a reaction to the dye. You might also get a bruise where the needle goes into your arm.

Your doctor might order a bone scan to look for a compression or hairline fracture, a tumor, or an infection. A bone scan is usually a second or third level of testing, done after other imaging procedures fail to show the problem your symptoms point to and your pain continues.

Back Basics

A **radionuclide** is a radioactive substance that, when injected into your body, releases energy that your tissues absorb at different levels. A nuclear medicine camera records the patterns of absorption. In a **bone scan**, the injected radioactive substance concentrates in your bones to show bone density (only when used for bone density tests for osteoporosis—and this is a different test called bone densitometry) and any fractures or tumors.

Myelography

Myelography uses a dye injected into your spinal column to outline the structures of your spine. X-rays then show those structures. During myelography, you lie facedown on the x-ray table. The radiologist numbs an area in your lower back with a local anesthetic, then uses a fine needle to enter the fluid-filled space around your spinal cord. After injecting an opaque dye (which looks white on the x-ray), the radiologist slowly tilts the x-ray table to gradually move the dye up your spine toward your head. The procedure takes about 20 minutes, after which you lie with your head slightly elevated for a few hours until the fluid level in your spinal column returns to normal.

Because myelography involves injecting a substance into your body, it's considered an invasive procedure. There is a slight risk of reaction to the local anesthetic or to the dye, and the injection site may be sore for a few days. About 20 percent of those who have myelograms get a moderate to severe headache afterward, which is a consequence of increasing the pressure in your spinal column by injecting the dye. The radiologist usually removes a small sample of spinal fluid at the time before injecting the dye, to minimize pressure changes.

Back Basics

Myelography uses a dye injected into the fluid around your spinal cord to highlight the structures of your spine. In **diskography**, doctors inject dye into a suspected prolapsed disk (and several normal disks for comparison) to determine whether the suspect disk is causing your pain.

CT myelogram of disk prolapse showing displacement of the spinal cord. Reprinted by permission of Kenneth Maravilla, M.D., Department of Radiology, University of Washington.

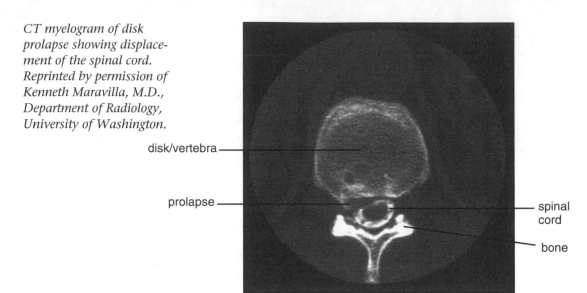

disk/vertebra

prolapse

spinal cord

bone

Your doctor might order myelography to see where and how much pressure a herniated or prolapsed disk is putting on your spinal cord. Because its invasive nature carries the potential of side effects, myelography is usually reserved for situations where you're not a good candidate for CT scanning (your problem likely won't show up) or MRI (you have metal in your body).

Diskography

Diskography is similar to myelography, except the radiologist injects dye into a suspected painful degenerative disk. She also injects dye into several "control" (normal) disks for comparison. She will ask you if the injections reproduce your pain *exactly*. If the procedure stimulates an attack of sciatica and gives you the exact same pain you've had, then spine fusion may relieve your pain from that disk. Diskography's preparation and risks are the same as for myelography, though you're not as likely to experience a headache afterward.

Back Basics

An **electromyography** measures and records the electrical activity of your muscles, helping to determine whether there's any damage to the nerves or muscle tissue that affects the muscle's ability to contract and relax.

Electromyography and Nerve Conduction Studies

Just as the electrical patterns of your heartbeat can paint a picture of your heart's health, so can the electrical impulses of your muscles tell the story of what's bothering them. An *electromyography* (EMG) measures the way your muscles respond to the signals they receive from your brain and nerves to contract and relax. Nerve conduction studies assess the responsiveness of your nerves to external electrical signals.

EMG and nerve conduction studies are often done together. Though there's no risk, the procedure can be uncomfortable at times. A technologist attaches electrodes to your muscles, sometimes on the surface of your skin and sometimes via very thin needles inserted into the muscle. The electrodes connect to wires that connect to the EMG machine, which records the electrical impulses the wires feed to it. The technologist takes readings while you're lying still, then while asking you to move certain muscles in certain ways. The tests usually include stimulating your muscles and nerves with mild electrical shocks to measure their responses. The procedures take between 30 and 60 minutes. They can detect damage but not irritation.

Evaluating Test Results

After you have your imaging procedure, a specialist reviews the findings and reports to your referring physician. This generally takes a few days to a week. Your doctor will either telephone you to discuss the results, or ask you to come in (this is a more a matter of the time needed to go over the results and options than an indication of how serious the findings are).

One challenge in evaluating the results of x-rays and other imaging procedures is that they can show physical changes in your back that have nothing to do with the pain you're experiencing. In numerous research studies, MRIs and CT scans done on people with no back pain show herniated disks, osteoarthritis, and even spinal stenosis—all conditions that often do cause pain and other problems, yet for some reason have no effect on many people. For example, among healthy people in their 20s and 30s, 25 to 50 percent will have a protruding disk. It's sometimes difficult to determine what's relevant to your situation and what's just coincidental. Sciatica, for example, is a far more significant sign of a herniated disk than is an MRI finding alone, because the sciatica is evidence that the herniation is causing problems.

Abnormal Findings

Not all abnormal findings will cause your doctor to shout "Eureka!" and dance on the exam table. As we've said before, it's entirely possible—and common—to have a herniated or degenerated disk that's *not* the cause of your pain. But some findings will pinpoint your problem, and from there you can move to treatment options. (You didn't think this was going to be simple, did you?)

There are various treatment approaches for most back problems. Different specialists often have different opinions about what works best. If you were able to walk into your doctor's office, it's very unlikely that your back problem requires you to make a decision right away. Take enough time to understand and research your doctor's recommendations before choosing a course of treatment, and seek another opinion if you're uncertain. Only a few rare conditions, such as some tumors or a huge herniation that's pressing against your spinal cord, require immediate action.

Normal Findings

Don't be surprised if the tests show nothing at all. After all, muscle and ligament injuries cause most back problems, and they don't usually show up on any tests. Normal, or negative, findings don't mean there's nothing wrong with you. They just mean that you have a problem that doesn't show up on the tests.

In all likelihood, your doctor will recommend an approach of watchful waiting coupled with measures to help you feel better while your back heals. Inappropriate intervention could end up causing more harm, which violates the first rule of medicine—"first and foremost, do no harm." Don't hesitate to contact your doctor if your pain gets worse, but give your back some time to get better.

What Next?

Often, what your test results show depends on who's evaluating them. An orthopedic surgeon, for example, looks at findings from a different perspective than does an internist or even a neurosurgeon. A physiatrist (specialist in physical medicine) has a different perspective still. How do you know who's right?

All of them could be right. There are different ways to interpret the same findings, and they don't necessarily exclude each other. Yet you're the one who's in pain—what do you do?

You've heard the saying, "knowledge is power." Learn as much as you can about your back problem, particularly if it's been with you for a while. Your doctor may have patient education materials for many common conditions, and you can learn more about yours in an afternoon at the library. The more you know, the better equipped you are to make informed decisions about your care.

And do what you can to take care of yourself. Once the pain subsides, get moving. Ask your doctor about exercises to strengthen and condition your back and other muscles. Lift with caution, and watch your posture. Trite as these recommendations sound (especially when you're still in the stage where you can barely move), they really are effective.

The Least You Need to Know

➤ Your history and physical examination are the most useful diagnostic tools for your doctor.

➤ Sophisticated imaging procedures are amazing but not necessary for the majority of back problems. If the findings won't make a difference in your treatment, you probably don't need the procedure.

➤ Imaging procedures can show structural abnormalities that have nothing to do with your pain (and can show abnormalities in people who are having no pain at all).

➤ Often, there is no single course of treatment that's best for your condition. Learn as much as you can before making a decision.

Part 3
Pain, Pain, Go Away

There was a faith healer of Deal
Who said, 'Although pain isn't real,
If I sit on a pin
And it punctures my skin,
I dislike what I fancy I feel.'
—*Anonymous,* The Week-End Book *(1925)*

While at least pain lets you know you're alive, it's a reminder most of us prefer to do without, thanks just the same. Back pain has been around for as long as humans have walked upright, with references to it in writings that are thousands of years old. Some approaches to relieving pain are just as old, and some spring from recent advances in (and reevaluations of) medical technology.

The chapters in Part 3 present different approaches to relieving back pain. You might be surprised at what works—and what doesn't.

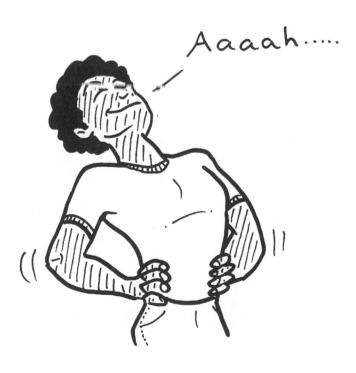

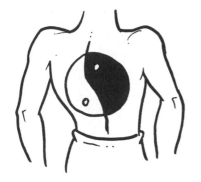

Chapter 10

Eastern Philosophy, Western Technology

In This Chapter

➤ The ways of Western medicine

➤ The ways of Eastern medicine

➤ How to blend the best of both worlds for your health and wellness

➤ When and how to use nutritional and herbal remedies

Do you go to a chiropractor, acupuncturist, herbalist, or use "home remedies" for minor ailments? If so, you're far from alone. Americans, increasingly, are interested in complementing traditional health care with alternative therapies and treatments. Ongoing research at major medical schools and institutions such as the National Institutes of Health are studying the effectiveness of alternative medicine techniques. Researchers are working to determine how, and whether, to integrate alternative therapies into conventional treatment plans for patients.

Allopathic and Alternative: Two Approaches

According to a study done by Dr. David Eisenberg and his colleagues at Beth Israel Deaconess Medical Center in Boston, Americans made 639 million visits to *alternative health care* providers in 1997—about 50 million more than the visits they made to *allopathic* primary care physicians. In the same year, we spent $27 billion on alternative health care therapies not covered by health plans and insurance companies—roughly the same amount of money we spent on all kinds of allopathic care combined.

Two in five Americans use some form of alternative health care, most often for back pain, headaches, and anxiety. Yet fewer than 10 percent of them tell their regular doctors that they also see chiropractors, acupuncturists, herbalists, massage therapists, or even yoga instructors. Why? "I'm afraid my doctor will either laugh at me or get mad," is the most common response.

Do we have to do things one way or the other? An increasing number of practitioners on both sides of the philosophy line say no. East and West can marry. Like all marriages, there'll be ups and downs. But in the end, life could be better for all.

Back Talk

Early Western physicians found it difficult, if not impossible, to follow in the footsteps of their mythological predecessors. Asclepius, son of the sun god Apollo, was a healer who often visited his patients in their dreams to deliver them from their ailments. His sons, Machaon and Poldalirius, initiated the fields of surgery and medicine, respectively. Machaon gained fame healing battle wounds, while his brother Poldalirius acquired a loyal following for his understanding of how diseases affected the human body.

Back Basics

Allopathic is the term for conventional Western medicine, practiced by those who graduate from medical school with an M.D. degree. The word comes from the Greek terms meaning "other" and "diseases." It was coined to separate conventional medical practices from **alternative** (or **complementary**) **health care**, which, in Western cultures, encompasses all other approaches to health care.

The Body as Machine

To the Western eye, the human body looks like a machine—intricate, sometimes even mysterious, but still a mechanism with predictable processes and responses. From the time of Hippocrates (460–377 B.C.)—known as the "Father of Modern Medicine"—physicians searched for insight into the workings of the human body, hoping to understand them in health so they could heal the body in sickness.

It was a daunting process, as Hippocrates himself wrote in the introduction to his medical textbook *Aphorismi*: "Life is short and the art long, opportunity fleeting, experiment dangerous, and judgment difficult." Unlike the gods before him, Hippocrates recorded his failures as well as his successes, providing the first written documentation of symptoms and treatments.

The teachings of Hippocrates formed the core of the practice of medicine for another four centuries. As the world gained more experience in the battles of war, surgeons learned more about the workings of the human body. The Roman physician Galen (A.D. 130–200) was the first to openly challenge the Hippocratic practices. Wounded soldiers helped him demonstrate that the body's vessels carried blood, not air as Hippocrates had taught.

Despite a few fundamental flaws (Galen believed the liver, not the heart, directed the body's circulation), Galen's teachings guided the practice of medicine until a young anatomy professor named Andreas Vesalius (1514–1564) published the landmark work "On the Fabric of the Human Body." Vesalius established the understandings of *anatomy* and *physiology* that are the foundation of Western medicine as we know it today.

Back Basics

Anatomy is the study and knowledge of the body's structure. **Physiology** is the study and knowledge of how the body works.

It's the Matter That Matters

All this interest in body parts—what they look like, how they function, how they work together in systems—established a philosophy in Western medicine that centered on matter. Physicians relied on observable evidence and symptoms to both understand the healthy body and treat an ailing one. Everything had a plausible, tangible explanation (even if some sound quite far-fetched to us today).

Discarding the Hippocratic notion of maintaining balance among the four humors (blood, phlegm, black bile, and yellow bile, which we'll discuss in more detail in Chapter 22, "Unproven Remedies"), evolving Western medicine shifted to a model of achieving physical balance in the body. Everything had a role and a place. If a physician could not heal the body, it was because the body had a malfunction the physician couldn't identify or lacked the resources to repair.

"We Can Fix It"

Something happened to Western cultures with the tremendous medical advances that came during the twentieth century. We shifted from viewing injury, illness, and death as normal (if unpleasant) aspects of life to elements over which we could and should have considerable control. Scientists had the diseases that wiped out entire families early in the century—pneumonia, tuberculosis, polio—pretty much under control by the time Alan Shepherd blasted off for a unique view of our home planet. We could put a man in space and defeat infection...life was good.

Now we've come to expect that doctors can mend just about anything. Because, actually, they can, mostly. From broken bones to damaged hearts and beyond, medical technology offers a fix—and often, a replacement part. Thousands of Americans can walk again (except through airport metal detectors) thanks to screws, rods, and plates that have replaced their damaged vertebrae. Death rates over the span of the twentieth century have plummeted; life expectancy more than doubled from age 40 to over age 80.

In reality, of course, doctors and surgeons can't fix everything, regardless of how gifted they are. Certain deteriorations and consequences are an inevitable aspect of living, no matter how hard we work to deny them. The hard part is knowing when you've reached the limits of modern medicine, when it's time to accept what you (and modern medicine) cannot change.

Empirical Evidence

It's no accident that some of the most popular games and books in our culture involve trivia. How tall is the Empire State Building? What's the fastest speed a land vehicle has ever traveled? How many bones are in a giraffe's neck? (If you've been paying attention as you're reading, you know this one! And if you haven't, tsk, tsk!—take a stretch break, then turn back to Chapter 2, "Back School.")

Back Basics

Empirical evidence is that which can be observed, objectively measured, and repeated. It differs from anecdotal evidence, which people report but is not verified. The word "anecdotal" comes from the Greek word for "unpublished."

It's the Western way to measure everything. And we love consistency. These traits show in our approach to medicine. If you buy a bottle of aspirin, you expect (rightfully) for every single tablet in that bottle to look, feel, and weigh the same, and have exactly the same action when you swallow it. This is how it is, and this is how it should be.

In Western medicine, it's not enough to see that there's a positive outcome from a particular treatment—we need to know just how the treatment created the cure. What actions did it have on the body, and how did the body respond? Can you touch it, see it, repeat it? Can others use your methods and obtain similar findings? This is the nature of the *empirical* study that characterizes Western practices—observable, verifiable, repeatable results.

Manipulating the Body

With an emphasis on evidence comes a focus on the mechanical. Its basis in the body-as-machine school of thought means allopathic medicine often relies on approaches that alter the physical body in an observable way. Medications, for example, induce biochemical changes. Physical therapy moves joints and limbs. Surgery can move—or remove—just about anything, making it perhaps the ultimate bodily manipulation.

> ### Back Talk
>
> The three Celestial Emperors, China's earliest known rulers, gave their culture the practice of medicine. The first, Fu Hsi, founded China's first dynasty in 2953 B.C. and created, among other important developments, the concept of cosmic opposites known today as yin-yang. The second, Shen Nung, investigated and catalogued medicinal and poisonous plants and herbs. The third Celestial Emperor, Huang Ti, developed the first system of medical philosophy and authored the *Nei Ching*, the first ancient Chinese medical textbook.

The Body in Balance

Like its Western counterparts, Eastern medicine comes from a history steeped in a blend of fact and mysticism. According to legend, a man came to the great Chinese surgeon Hua T'o (A.D. 145–208) with a severe headache. While he usually treated headaches with acupuncture, Hua T'o found a tumor on the man's forehead. When he sliced it open, a canary flew out and the headache disappeared. Most procedures were less dramatic, however, and focused on restoring the body's energy balance—the foundation of Eastern medicine.

Everything Is Energy

Eastern healing systems view the human body not as an arrangement of parts and organs, but as a collection of energy. Energy is a dynamic force, existing at different vibrational levels. Some energy, such as electricity, vibrates so rapidly that you can't see it. The body acquires a physical presence because its energy vibrates at very slow frequencies the eye can perceive.

Eastern medicine believes that energy must flow freely within the human body (and indeed the entire environment) to maintain its correct balance. Blocked energy unbalances and distorts the system, even though you can't see or feel it. This disruption creates discord in your body, just as electrical surges through the power lines can wreak havoc on the appliances in your home, even though you can't see the changes in energy directly.

"Remove the Obstacles, and the Body Will Heal Itself"

Healing is not a process of fixing the outward symptoms, or what's wrong with the matter, as is the focus of Western medicine. Rather, healing is a process of locating and removing the blockages to restore the flow of energy and let the body heal itself.

In Eastern medicine, your body doesn't need an outside force or substance to come in and right what's wrong. In fact, this can worsen the problem by creating other blockages. Most Eastern healing methods are noninvasive, minimizing intrusion upon normal body functions.

Back Talk

In diagnosis and treatment, the Hindu physician of 800 B.C. to A.D. 1000 used his sense of the natural and the supernatural. He noted what he could see, hear, touch, smell, and taste—the objective details. And he noted what animals or other people he encountered on the way to see the patient—the mystical elements he believed would influence the patient's situation. The physician's role was to restore balance among the body's three divine universal forces—spirit, phlegm, and bile. Treatment used herbs and medicinal plants to restore their balance. These antediluvian healers were also master surgeons who used instruments that even today's surgeons would envy.

Sometimes Mysterious Ways

Though theories attempting to explain energy-system healing abound, no one really knows how Eastern therapies such as acupuncture work. The need to know this is a Western perspective; from the Eastern perspective, the "how" doesn't matter. What does matter is that they do work.

Many Eastern therapies appear quite mysterious or mystical to the Western world. We're not accustomed to manipulating what we can't see or touch. Yet we have little trouble plugging a power cord into the wall to allow invisible energy—electricity—to surge into a box with a window on it, beaming television into our homes! The difference is that, thanks to electron microscopes and other technologies, scientists can actually see the energy particles that make electricity possible. So far, we haven't been able to do the same with the energy that makes the human body possible.

Manipulating the Energy

Eastern methods of diagnosis and treatment center on the energy system of *chi* (also spelled "qi" and pronounced "chee" for either spelling). Chi flows through unseen channels in the body called meridians. There are 12 primary and eight secondary meridians, also called extraordinary or homeostatic (balancing). Traditional Chinese Medicine (TCM) identifies 365 points along the meridians where the practitioner can gain access, though modern acupuncture uses 2,000 points. Each meridian point corresponds to a specific body region, organ, or problem.

When the meridians are clear and unobstructed, chi flows freely and you enjoy harmony and health. When a meridian becomes blocked, the disrupted flow of chi causes disharmony and alters the energy balance (sometimes called yin-yang). This can show itself as disease or pain. To remedy the problem, the practitioner must identify and release the blockage. This restores the flow of chi.

If this seems confusing, go back to our analogy of electricity. When you turn on your television and nothing happens, what do you do? Go jiggle the plug in the outlet! Sometimes the connection isn't quite right, and the electricity can't get through to the appliances it's supposed to operate. You manipulate the carrier or container—the power cord—to restore the flow, and voilà! You have energy, power, and picture (function). The energy in your body operates in a similar, though more subtle, way. By manipulating the carrier or container—through acupuncture, massage, or other therapies—you free the blockage and release the energy flow.

Back Basics

Chi, also spelled "qi," means energy. It's pronounced *chee* either way it's spelled. Chi is both physical and metaphysical, an animated and nourishing force that sustains all life and existence. Chi is sometimes referred to as "cosmic breath."

Does It Have to Be One or the Other?

Even Hippocrates, with his intense scientific focus, encouraged his students to do only what was necessary to assist the body in healing itself. "Our natures are the physicians of our diseases," he wrote in one of his many medical textbooks.

Sometimes, differences are more philosophical than functional. For example, physical therapy, chiropractic, and therapeutic massage all focus on restoring your body to full function and movement using physical manipulations. Yoga, t'ai chi, and traditional exercise all emphasize maintaining health and fitness. Where these methods differ is in the "whys" of what practitioners do, not the "hows."

Back Talk

In 1992, the United States Congress created the National Institutes of Health Office of Alternative Medicine, which funds 10 Centers of Alternative Medicine Research. The Office and its Centers are working to establish a centralized information center for material about commonly used alternative therapies, their applications, and their risks.

Complementary Medicine: Blending East and West

The famous sixteenth-century surgeon Ambroise Pare served four French kings, yet remained humble about his power to heal. "I dressed him, God healed him," Pare was fond of saying. As confident as he was in his abilities to use the science of his day to treat battle wounds, Pare had no qualms about playing a shared role in his patient's care.

A 1998 article in *Archives of Internal Medicine*, a widely respected medical journal, reported the findings of a 13-year survey of nearly 4,000 physicians in countries where Western medicine dominates health care practices (including the United States). Among them, 53 percent said they had referred patients to acupuncturists, 43 percent to chiropractors, and 40 percent for therapeutic massage.

The study's authors, researchers at the Stanford Center for Research in Disease Prevention (California), point out that individual practice patterns vary widely—some physicians seldom make such referrals, while others do so frequently. Nonetheless, they say, the study highlights a key shift in professional opinion about what is becoming known as *complementary*, rather than alternative, medicine.

Some approaches go a step further than sharing responsibility for patient care. For example, allopathic doctors who aren't too sure about acupuncture are often more willing to consider a Westernized version of this ancient healing method—percutaneous electrical nerve stimulation, or PENS. Using fine needles inserted at traditional acupuncture points, PENS delivers a mild electrical stimulation to the needle. The Western theory behind this therapy is that the gentle shock disrupts the ability of the nerves to transmit pain impulses. What your brain doesn't know about doesn't exist—no signal, no pain.

Back Basics

Complementary medicine refers to treatment methods that, while philosophically different from conventional Western medicine, are often useful in a collaborative, integrated, and holistic approach to healing and health.

What to Choose and When

How do you know what therapies will complement each other in helping you heal? One way, perhaps the most important, is to select practitioners who are willing to work cooperatively with you and each other to heal your back pain and improve your health in general.

If you prefer to work with a conventional primary care physician (Western medicine), be sure he is open to complementary therapies such as acupuncture and chiropractic. If there seems to be hesitation, ask more questions. Does your doctor object to complementary medicine in any shape or way, or is there something about your particular condition that raises a red flag? In turn, be open with your doctor about alternative therapies you're either using or considering.

If you prefer to have a complementary practitioner as your primary care giver, select one who is well educated in her practice area as well as knowledgeable about Western medicine. Does the practitioner understand and accept that there are often multiple approaches that could be effective, and is she willing to accommodate your desires to blend East and West? Does the provider seem opposed to particular treatment approaches without regard for the conditions they might treat? If the practitioner appears uncomfortable at the thought of working with an allopathic physician, ask more questions.

No matter what practitioner or philosophy you choose, your health care provider should:

➤ Be willing to consider both Eastern and Western therapies

➤ Have appropriate professional credentials (board certification, license, evidence of education)

➤ Not claim to cure all ailments, or any condition for which there is no evidence-based cure

➤ Understand potential drug and herbal interactions

➤ Share your views about your involvement in your own care, explain your diagnosis and treatment options in ways you understand, and respect your right to decline a recommended procedure or therapy

Back Care

If you're new to complementary medicine, read up on the therapies that interest you before going to a practitioner. You'll have a better idea of what to expect and what questions to ask. And if you know of someone who uses the approach that interests you, ask whom she sees for care. A direct recommendation says more about a practitioner than any advertisement can.

Herbal Remedies

While you might be more familiar with sage and chives as food seasonings, these two herbs do more than add zip to marina sauce and zing to baked potatoes. They are among the oldest of herbal remedies, with their medicinal uses dating back thousands of years in both Eastern and Western cultures. Today's *herbalists* use thousands of plant-based remedies for healing and prevention. Herbal remedies are a key component of Traditional Chinese Medicine (TCM, sometimes also called Traditional Oriental Medicine or TOM). Herbalists generally develop individualized herbal preparations for each patient's specific and unique needs.

Even though herbal remedies have been around for centuries, there's more we don't know about most of them than we do know. We do know, for example, that herbs can interact with medications

Back Basics

An **herbalist** is someone who uses herbs for healing purposes.

in unexpected, and sometimes hazardous, ways. What we often *don't* know is how, under what circumstances, or with what results.

Americans spend nearly $3 billion for herbal remedies each year, buying preparations to treat everything from acne to warts. The U.S. federal government doesn't regulate herbal remedies in the same way it oversees medications, which causes concern among some health care professionals. While many brands of prepared products adhere to strict purity and consistency standards, others don't. To help safeguard yourself, buy herbal remedies from reputable manufacturers and dealers.

If herbal therapies interest you, talk with your doctor about ways to integrate them safely into your regular routine. In particular, use caution if you regularly take any medication—sometimes when you're taking the same drug every day, you lose sight of the fact that it is, in fact, a regular medication. This includes drugs for thyroid conditions, high blood pressure, and heart conditions as well as any you might be taking for your back pain, particularly prescription antidepressants. And don't stop taking your regular medication to switch to an herbal preparation. Suddenly stopping certain drugs can be very dangerous.

Dietary and Nutritional Therapies

A nutritious diet is essential for good health, of course. Some treatment approaches advocate certain kinds of diets, either in general (such as vegetarian) or for specific conditions (such as meat and dairy restrictions for arthritis). For the most part, diet is a matter of personal choice. Vegetarian diets are especially low in cholesterol and fat, which benefits many health conditions. If your arthritis feels better when you stop eating red meat, you're not doing yourself any harm (and your heart will thank you).

The Least You Need to Know

➤ Western medicine focuses on matter and measurable outcomes, while Eastern medicine focuses on energy and processes.

➤ Learn as much as you can about therapies that interest you. The more you already know, the better equipped you are to ask questions and make sense of the answers.

➤ Integrating East and West for healthy living requires open communication with all your health care providers.

➤ Herbal remedies and conventional medications can interact with each other to create unexpected problems. Be sure to discuss your use of either with all your health care providers.

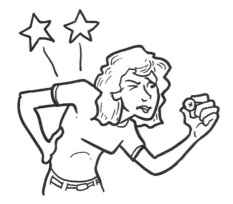

Chapter 11

Rx: Medical Approaches to Back Relief

In This Chapter

➤ Distinguishing fact from fable: a self-quiz

➤ Common medications for back pain

➤ Sending signals to muscles that hurt

➤ Supporting your healing back

When it comes to back pain, modern medicine has an arsenal of treatment options. The challenge lies in choosing the one (or ones) that work for you.

Sadly, even with years of training and the miracles of technology, doctors can't identify the exact cause of back pain in many cases. We don't want to be so trite as to suggest your aching back affirms your status as a conscious, breathing lifeform, but in fact, back pain seems a normal consequence of living. Hang on, though. In the centuries of human existence, we've made some progress. We'll share what's clear and known about back pain with you, so read on. And take heart—doctors and scientists are learning more about back pain and the problems that can cause it every day.

Fact or Fable? A Self-Quiz

How good are you at separating fact from fable? Try your hand at these seven common perceptions about treating back pain.

1. Bed rest is best when you hurt your back.

    Fact _____   Fable _____

2. The more severe the pain, the worse the problem.

    Fact _____   Fable _____

3. Today's technology can tell you what's wrong.

   Fact _____   Fable _____

4. Once a hurt back, always a hurting back.

   Fact _____   Fable _____

5. Surgery is the only cure for a slipped disk.

   Fact _____   Fable _____

6. An exam for back pain isn't complete without an x-ray.

   Fact _____   Fable _____

7. For every back problem, there's a fix.

   Fact _____   Fable _____

If you identified all of these statements as fables, congratulations! Now let's look at the facts.

1. Ten years ago, bed rest was the recommendation of choice for back pain (and much of what else could ail you). It made sense to both doctors and patients—if it hurt too much to move, then don't. Since then, we (doctors and patients) have learned that too much of a good thing is a bad thing. A day or two in bed gives your back a rest break; lying in bed for weeks makes your back stiff and sore, and can actually prolong healing. It may hurt to move around at first, but the sooner you get going, the faster you'll be back to normal.

2. There really is little correlation between how much your back hurts and how badly it's hurt. A minor strain can bring tears to your eyes every time you take a breath, yet a compression fracture may not hurt at all (though many cause intense pain). Muscle injuries tend to hurt because muscle tissue contains a rich supply of nerves.

3. What today's medical technology can tell us about body functions and injuries is truly astounding. Yet for all the capabilities technology offers, your body still has its secrets. As often as 80 percent of the time, you may not know *exactly* why your back hurts. But the likelihood that your back will get better anyway is even higher.

4. Every year, about 15 million Americans experience some sort of back problem— about 50,000 of them are permanently disabled. So if you're among the 14,950,000 folks whose back pain heals, for you this perception is a fable. If you're among the unfortunate few whose back pain lingers, this statement is a sad fact. Even so, you needn't let your pain rule your life—we hope the information in this book gives you renewed encouragement.

5. In the 1970s and 1980s, surgery was a common course of action for numerous back problems, including herniated (you remember, of course, that a disk can't

really slip). Though surgery usually fixed the disk problem, it often created other, sometimes more serious, problems. In seeking to avoid these other problems, doctors bumped surgery to the bottom of their treatment options list—with surprising results. Many patients got better, faster, with conservative treatment. Today, surgery is seldom a first option for most back problems.

6. Unless you or your doctor think you have a fracture or other bone problem, an x-ray is nothing more than unnecessary exposure to radiation. Soft-tissue injuries are the most common cause of back pain, and they're a bit camera-shy, so to speak. X-rays show bones, but don't tell us anything about the muscle problems that are the cause of most back pain.

7. Time is the "fix" for the majority of back problems. Most of what you do to help your back feel better does just that and has little to do with the healing process. Sure, modern medicine is wonderful and can even work miracles at times. Other approaches, like chiropractic care and acupuncture, can ease your discomfort while you're healing. Incorporate basic stretching and simple exercises into your daily routine, too. You'll feel better all over!

If It Feels Good, Does It Help?

Most of the time, if your back feels better because of what you're doing, you're not hurting it any. The one exception is lying in bed or on the couch. No matter how comfortable you feel, lying down for longer than a couple of hours at a time actually prolongs your pain. You may feel stiff and sore, and even hurt, when you first get up and start moving around. Be gentle with yourself, but keep moving. You will feel better once your muscles get used to their upright position.

Rubs and Soaks

How well do those creams and ointments work that you rub into your skin over the body part that hurts? It depends. Most contain a substance that irritates your skin, often a form of salicylate (a chemical variation of aspirin) or oil of wintergreen (that familiar locker-room fragrance), causing it to flush and thereby bringing an increased blood supply to the surface. This makes the area feel warm and relaxed. Very little of the rub's pain-relieving ingredients actually penetrate your skin to get circulated through your body in your blood.

Soaking in a tub of warm water feels good all over, which is especially welcome after a long day at work even if your back feels fine. Keep the temperature moderate—you shouldn't look like a cooked lobster after you've been in for a few minutes. Hot tubs and Jacuzzi-style tubs often have adjustable spray nozzles that you can use to direct a pressurized stream of water directly against areas that hurt. A little bit goes a long way, so be careful. With your muscles relaxed and off-guard in the warm water, it's easy to overdo a water massage and end up hurting more. Injured muscle fibers are quite sensitive (which you, of course, already know all too well). Move around or redirect the jets often to avoid making an area feel worse. Do some gentle stretching exercises when you get out of the water, while your muscles are still warm and too drowsy to complain. (Dry off first, though—your muscles won't like it if you start to shiver.)

Heat and Ice

Ice your aching back for the first 24 to 48 hours after you hurt it to reduce swelling and to numb the area somewhat. Beyond this time frame, doctors generally recommend heat.

Moist heat works better than dry heat because it more deeply penetrates your muscles to help them relax. You can buy a heating pad that produces moist heat. If you're on the economy plan, an old-fashioned hot water bottle works just as well. Use heat for 20 to 30 minutes at a time, then stand and gently stretch your back muscles while they're still relaxed from the heat. This extends the beneficial effects of the heating pad.

Back Off!

Don't fall asleep with a heating pad on your back, or cover the pad with anything other than your normal clothing. Though they're designed with your safety in mind, heating pads can still burn your skin if left in the same place too long.

Back Basics

An **analgesic** is a drug that relieves pain. An **anti-inflammatory drug** relieves swelling as well as pain. **NSAID** stands for "nonsteroidal anti-inflammatory drug." An **over-the-counter (OTC)** medicine is one you can buy without a prescription.

You might find ice continues to provide you more relief than heat—if that works for you, great. Apply the ice by rubbing it over the area that hurts until the area becomes numb. Then stand and do a few basic stretching exercises, gently and slowly, to get those sore muscles moving a bit. You can ice again for a few minutes if your back complains about the activity. Sitting with an ice bag is not a good idea—it's too easy to get your skin too cold, which can trigger a pain reaction of its own.

Medications for Pain Relief

Take a stroll down the "pain lane" at your local pharmacy, and the selections will make your head spin. What's right for *your* back pain?

One reason there are so many different medications available is that not everyone responds in the same way. What helped your neighbor get back in action when he hurt his back two months ago may do nothing for you. As well, different pain relievers act in different ways or at different steps in the pain communication process. If you've taken something for back pain before and it's helped, start with that. If not, or the tried-and-true can't cut it this time, ask your doctor or pharmacist for suggestions.

Medically, pain relievers are called *analgesics*. Over-the-counter *anti-inflammatory drugs* (also called *NSAIDs*) that reduce inflammation (swelling in muscles, for example) also have analgesic properties, though analgesics don't necessarily have anti-inflammatory properties.

Blocking Reception: How Pain Relievers Work

Pain relievers work by interrupting your body's pain signal system. Injured tissues release substances called prostaglandins. Prostaglandins act as chemical messengers that activate cells in your spinal cord and brain called opiate receptors. Opiate receptors then send a signal to your brain that your brain interprets as pain. In some ways, it's like an elaborate version of the childhood game "telephone." An analgesic acts like a curtain or shield, preventing the message from getting through. Most over-the-counter analgesics shut down the prostaglandins or the opiate receptors. Acetaminophen actually blocks pain signals in your brain, preventing you from perceiving that your back hurts.

Getting into Your System

Analgesics that you can buy without a prescription come in three forms: oral (taken by mouth), topical (applied to the surface), and suppository (inserted into the rectum). Oral drugs come in tablet, capsule, caplet (a tablet coated in a gel that turns slimy when it gets wet so it's easier to swallow), and liquid forms. Most liquid preparations are designed for children, so the strength per dose is lower than an adult would take. If there's some reason you need a pain reliever in liquid form, your pharmacist can help you calculate the dose that's right for you.

Some over-the-counter medications come in extended release preparations, so you have to take them only once or twice a day. You need to take others every four to six hours. Again, what works best for you is what's best. Long-acting pills are usually more convenient, but it's more difficult to take less, which means it's more difficult to avoid unpleasant side effects. For example, if high-dose (prescription) ibuprofen bothers your stomach, you can buy over-the-counter ibuprofen and take a lower dose that might still relieve your pain. You have to take short-acting drugs more often, but you can adjust how much you take according to how much pain you're feeling. It's usually a good policy to take as little medication as possible (the exception being post-operative or serious pain where waiting until the pain is horrible makes it harder to get an effective dose).

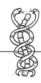

Back Care

Keep your medications in their original (and childproof) containers. That way, you always have the name of the drug, dosage, ingredients, warnings, and expiration date right there. Keep medications in a cool location—the bathroom medicine chest is usually not the best place. And keep them away from curious little fingers and the children attached to them.

Back Off!

Don't drink alcohol if you're taking medication for pain or inflammation. Many drugs irritate your stomach's sensitive lining, and so does alcohol. Alcohol also affects the way medications (over-the-counter and prescription) work. A combination also can make you far more drowsy than either substance will alone.

Follow the Directions

When you're hurting, you want relief RIGHT NOW. Before you pop a couple of pills, take a minute or two to read the label. (Another few minutes won't make a difference to your pain and could save you from further discomfort.) Are you allergic to aspirin, acetaminophen or ibuprofen, or other NSAIDs? If so, talk with your doctor or pharmacist before taking any medication that contains any of these substances. You could also have a sensitivity to substances that are chemically similar.

Most medications reach their maximum effectiveness when there are enough of them in your system to reach what health care professionals call therapeutic levels. It may take several doses to reach this point. With something like back pain, where the usual course of recovery means a few days of pain before you start feeling better, you get the most relief when you take the medication regularly for that time (the acute pain phase). Don't wait until you can't stand the pain before you take a pill—doing so reduces the relief you'll get from the medicine. As you start feeling better, taper off. If you've been taking two tablets for each dose, cut back to one tablet per dose. And once you get to the healing stage where your back hurts on some days but not others, or only with certain movements, you'll do fine by taking something for pain only when you hurt.

NEVER combine different kinds of pain relievers and NSAIDs unless your doctor specifically instructs you to do so. Most of these medications stress your liver and kidneys and can quickly overwhelm your body's normal filtering and excreting mechanisms if you take more than you should or combine drugs. If you're taking medication for your back, be especially careful if you take anything for cold symptoms. Many multisymptom cold preparations contain acetaminophen or ibuprofen. If the label says "relieves aches and fever," check the list of active ingredients. Your pharmacist can help you find a cold medicine that's safe to take with your back medications.

The directions for most pain relievers suggest taking the medication with food or milk. Though you may find it hard to believe, the same stomach that can down three chili dogs and a plate of nachos without so much as a belch of complaint can feel turned inside out by two

Back Care

While allergic response is one form of side effect from pain relievers, not all side effects are allergies. Many medications upset your stomach, for example, and may cause you to throw up. This is not an allergic response; it's a side effect. A true allergic response usually produces hives (a welt-like rash) and may include swelling. Swelling of your mouth and throat tissues is especially dangerous. Get immediate medical attention if this happens to you.

Back Off!

Do you take an aspirin a day for heart disease? Check with your doctor before taking pain relievers or NSAIDs. You could end up with results (and potential complications) you didn't expect. Also check the ingredients of other medications you take, especially over-the-counter cold preparations, since many contain acetaminophen or ibuprofen.

little pills. Believe it! Analgesics, especially NSAIDs, can make your cast-iron stomach feel more like a forest on fire. Take them with a glass of milk, a piece of bread, or before a meal. If you still have indigestion or nausea, talk with your doctor or pharmacist about trying something different. Continued stomach irritation can cause an ulcer.

Common NSAIDs

Chemical Name	Common Brand Names	Comments
Over-the-Counter (OTC)		
Fenoprofen	Nalfon	
Ibuprofen	Motrin IB, Advil, Nuprin, Medipren, Midol 200, Pamprin IB, and generic products	Many combination products contain ibuprofen
Ketoprofen	Orudis	Long-acting
Naproxen, naproxen sodium	Naprosyn, Anaprox, Alleve	Long-acting
Prescription		
Diflunisal	Dolobid	
Diclofenac	Voltaren	Higher reported incidence of liver problems (further studies underway; liver toxicity may be a potential problem with other NSAIDs as well)
Indomethacin	Indocin	
Meclofenamate	Meclomen	
Phenylbutazone	Butazolidin	
Nabumetone	Relafen	Long-acting (once a day)
Sulindac	Clinoril	
Tolmetin	Tolectin	

N-What? NSAIDs

This tongue-twisting moniker is shorthand for the class of medications called non-steroidal anti-inflammatory drugs. You can buy many NSAID (pronounced *EN-sed*) products over-the-counter. Stronger NSAIDs are available by prescription.

NSAIDs came into use in the 1970s, with many formulations becoming available without a prescription in the late 1980s. They represent a major breakthrough in pain relief for millions of Americans, who take them for ailments ranging from arthritis to whiplash—including, of course, back pain. NSAIDs relieve both pain and swelling.

Over-the-Counter Pain Relievers

Chemical Name	Common Brand Names	Comments
Acetaminophen	Tylenol, Datril, many aspirin-free products	Gentle on the stomach; does not reduce swelling; reduces fever
Aspirin (acetyl-salicylic acid)	Bayer, Bufferin, many generic and store brands	Can irritate the stomach; has anti-inflammatory action; reduces fever; comes in different strengths
Other salicylates	Doan's Pills, Empirin, Alka Seltzer, Equagesic, Aspergum, Vanquish	Chemically modified variations of aspirin that are longer acting; there are often added ingredients in these products

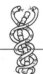

Back Care

Drink plenty of water when you're taking NSAIDs and other over-the-counter pain relievers. Dehydration coupled with these medications can be a dangerous combination for your kidneys.

Back Off!

Don't combine different kinds of NSAIDs and pain relievers. Doing so can seriously damage your liver and kidneys. Even medicines that seem "safe" like acetaminophen and ibuprofen can be deadly when taken in combination or overdose.

Other Over-the-Counter Pain Relievers

The two most common over-the-counter pain relievers are acetaminophen and aspirin (more formally known as acetylsalicylic acid). Both relieve pain and fever; aspirin also reduces swelling.

Aspirin has been around for more than a century, coming about as an accidental discovery in 1899. Acetaminophen hit the market half a century later, providing an over-the-counter pain relief alternative. Even though acetaminophen doesn't have anti-inflammatory properties, it's an effective pain reliever for muscle injuries because of the way it blocks pain signals in the brain (rather than interfering with prostaglandins or opiate sensors as do other analgesics).

Both aspirin and acetaminophen come in different strengths. Each regular-strength tablet has 325 mg; each extra-strength (sometimes called arthritis-strength) tablet or capsule has 500 mg. Aspirin tablets may be buffered to make them easier on your stomach or coated to make them easier to swallow. Some have a special enteric coating that keeps them from dissolving until they get into your small intestine, to protect your stomach. Because aspirin and acetaminophen are so common—we take them for nearly everything that causes us to hurt—it's easy to forget that they are powerful drugs with potentially hazardous side effects. Overdosing on either (by taking too many all at once or too many over a period of time) can cause permanent liver and kidney damage.

Back Talk

Ancient healers might have told their patients, "Take two branches and see me in the morning." Various cultures relieved pain and fever by chewing on willow bark, which contains salicin, a chemical relative of aspirin. Clearly they were onto something! Today you can buy aspirin products just about everywhere, from a gas station mini-mart to a pharmacy.

There are numerous drug formulations available that combine various ingredients. Some target specific kinds of pain relief, such as headache, and include substances such as caffeine. Unless your doctor or pharmacist specifically recommends such a combination product for a particular reason, stick with the straight stuff—it's cheaper, and often the only ingredient that helps is the pain reliever.

Drugs to Relax Your Back

Injured muscles often get tight and tense and can easily cramp or spasm. Muscle relaxants are drugs that interfere with the nerve signals that tell your muscles to contract. Some, like diazepam (Valium) and methocarbamol (Robaxin, Robaxacet, Robaxisal) often cause drowsiness. Because muscle relaxants weaken muscle contractions, taking them for more than a few days can begin to cause problems. Other common muscle relaxants include baclofen (Lioresal), cyclobenzaprine (Flexeril), and carisoprodol (Soma). Muscle relaxants require a prescription from your doctor.

Back Off!

Aspirin and acetaminophen are very dangerous in the hands (and mouths) of children. It doesn't take much of either to be toxic to a child, and unfortunately, aspirin and acetaminophen overdoses are often fatal. Keep these and all medications in childproof containers and in cabinets (locked if young children live in your home) that children can't reach.

Narcotics: Danger Zone

Rarely, your doctor may prescribe a narcotic pain reliever for your back problem. This is more likely following surgery or if your injury is severe. Narcotics are the "heavy artillery" of pain relievers.

133

Narcotics, which require a prescription, have numerous side effects that require caution in using them. Most narcotics cause drowsiness and a sense of altered consciousness, so you can't drive, operate machinery, or do much of anything that requires you to be alert and awake. They often cause nausea and almost always cause constipation. They are addictive if you take them too long.

Back Off!

DO NOT take more medication than the label instructs (over-the-counter or prescription). Too much of any good thing can be bad for you, and you won't necessarily get more relief by taking more pills. If you're not getting the relief you need, ask your doctor to recommend or prescribe something else.

Back to Nature

Constipation can be a problem if you're taking pain medications that contain codeine or other narcotics. Exercise gets your intestines moving along with the rest of you. Get up and walk around for 10 to 15 minutes every hour or so during the day—a short walk outside will refresh your mind as well as your body. And drink plenty of water to ward off dehydration (which will make constipation even worse).

Narcotics commonly prescribed for serious back problems include codeine (usually in combination with acetaminophen, as in the brand name Tylenol #3), propoxyphene (the ingredient in Darvon and Darvocet brand-name medications), meperidine (name brand Demerol), and oxycodone (a morphine derivative in Percodan and Percocet brand-name medications).

Research in pharmaceuticals (drugs and medicines) continues to search for pain relievers that have the pain-killing power of narcotics without the side effects. Several studies have shown that NSAIDs are just as effective as some narcotics in some situations.

Tasty Pain Relief

What if you could get a nutritional boost and knock down pain at the same time? No, we're not talking about vitamin-laced pain pills. Many foods contain the chemicals that laboratories turn into pain medications. Doctors also know that certain foods trigger pain in conditions such as migraine headaches. Red wines, chocolate, aged cheeses, and processed meats contain tyramines and nitrites, chemicals that cause your blood vessels to constrict. This results in a reduced blood supply, which activates a complaint in the form of pain from the affected tissues.

Eat Your Salicylates

Got pain? Try a handful of blueberries, raspberries, cherries, or prunes. Doctors have known for years that these and other foods are high in salicylates, a family of chemicals that relieve pain, reduce swelling and fever, and inhibit clotting. Aspirin is the most common drug compound that uses salicylates. In fact, allergists warn people with aspirin allergies to avoid these foods. Foods that contain moderate amounts of salicylates include dried currants and dates, licorice, most fruits, and paprika.

Caffeine Can Do More Than Keep You Awake

Caffeine, a chemical present in coffee, tea, chocolate, and many carbonated sodas, also works to relieve pain. Caffeine seems to work by interrupting pain signals on their way to your brain. Chemically, caffeine is nearly the same as a pain-signaling chemical already in your body, adenosine. Though the two substances have very different actions, your body seems unable to tell which one is present. If you consume a high enough level of caffeine, your cells accept caffeine instead of adenosine. No adenosine, no pain as far as your brain is concerned. Too much caffeine has a number of unpleasant side effects, however, from jitters to nausea.

Check Out Those Chili Peppers!

Ever wonder how someone can down one spicy-hot chili pepper after another and seemingly feel no pain? Turns out chili peppers contain a chemical called capsaicin, which is a powerful analgesic. Capsaicin first came to the attention of researchers when they checked out a folk remedy for toothache—applying pepper extract to the affected tooth, where it numbed the area. Some pain medications used to treat chronic nerve pain and a form of migraine called cluster headaches now contain capsaicin. Capsaicin works by "shooting" the messenger. It chemically depletes nerves of substance P, which is what they use to send pain messages to your brain. No messenger, no pain.

Straight to the Source: Injecting Pain Relief

Sometimes pain, especially that caused by arthritis or a herniated disk, doesn't respond to conservative treatment. Your doctor may recommend an injection directly into the area. Such an injection usually contains a combination of a local anesthetic (drug that numbs) and a steroid (synthetic cortisone that reduces inflammation). Relief from a direct injection can last several days to several months.

Risks are slight. You might react to the medication, or feel soreness at the injection site for a day or two. And the injection might not work at all for you. Some people are pain free after a direct injection, however.

TENS

No, we're not talking change for a 20. TENS stands for transcutaneous electrical nerve stimulation. A TENS unit about the size of a deck of cards sends a weak electrical signal through electrodes attached to your skin. One theory about how TENS works is that the electrical signals it sends out disrupt the signals your nerves are trying to send to your brain. Once the signals get scrambled, your brain can't interpret them as pain.

Though TENS has been a treatment alternative since the 1980s, health care professionals and patients disagree about its effectiveness. Some people get good relief from TENS; others get none. Research studies are inconclusive, meaning they can't make a determination, either. TENS is most often used for chronic pain.

The first time you use TENS, a physical therapist usually places the electrodes on either side of the area that hurts, and may try different locations to find what works the best. After you're comfortable using the TENS unit, you use it on your own. You control the level and frequency of the TENS stimulation—you should feel a mild tingling but your muscle should not contract. Your doctor or physical therapist will tell you how often to activate a TENS session, which usually lasts about 20 to 30 minutes. Check under the electrodes during each treatment period to be sure there's no skin irritation.

Sometimes your muscles adapt to the TENS stimulation, and TENS loses its effectiveness.

Traction

Ancient Greek physicians tried to help their back patients by lashing them to a flat board and hanging weights from their feet. Today, the equipment is more sophisticated but the concept remains the same. You lie on a special table or bed, and a series of belts attach weights that gently pull your back into alignment. For much of the twentieth century, doctors ordered traction to treat a wide variety of back problems ranging from fractures and herniated disks to serious strains. (And ordered patients to bed until the pain went away, too.)

Now, doctors treat back problems with traction only for certain conditions, most often cervical spine fractures. Traction is often used to try to relieve pressure on nerves (especially in the neck) from prolapsed disks. True to the modern rigorous scientific method, doctors recently compared patients with back pain (and some with sciatica) who got real traction with patients who got "sham" traction (the device squeezed them the same way a real traction device does so they couldn't tell the difference). These studies found that patients who got traction didn't get better any faster or have less pain. Doctors want further tests to make sure they get the right answer. Until then, your doctor or therapist may recommend traction. If done by a skilled person, traction is probably safe.

Corsets, Braces, and Supports

As long ago as 2000 B.C., people wore corsets. Most wore them as a fashion statement, though by A.D. 1700 corsets were available in styles that supported, not squeezed, the back.

The corset remains in the back pain treatment arsenal. Soft corsets combine fabric with plastic or metal stiffeners. Straps and buckles allow easy tightening and removal. By putting more pressure on your abdomen, a corset takes pressure off your lower back. They also keep you from making the wrong moves, so corsets can be useful in protecting against re-injury. A rigid corset (also called a brace) is made of plastic specially molded to the contours of your body and provides more substantial support. Your doctor may prescribe a soft corset for a bad strain or sprain, and a hard corset for a traumatic fracture, compression fracture, or to stabilize and support your back following surgery. Rigid corsets or braces also help correct deformities, such as those that occur with scoliosis.

Lumbar supports have made their way into many workplaces where tasks involve lifting. Similar in concept and design to the back belts weight lifters wear, lumbar supports provide additional protection for your lower back. When worn and used properly, lumbar supports may reduce back injuries (though studies haven't shown that they work—and some studies suggest they may not help). The biggest problem is that people don't like them so they don't wear them. The belts restrict movement (which, of course, is what they're intended to do) and can be uncomfortable. And for the fashion-conscious, they're not especially attractive. Whether or not you wear a lumbar support, the best protection for your back is strong, conditioned muscles (including abdominals as well), and proper lifting techniques.

The Least You Need to Know

➤ Many myths persist about what works best for back pain.

➤ Combining different kinds of medications, or taking more than the label instructs, is hazardous.

➤ Everyone responds differently to medications. There are many pain relievers to choose from, so if one doesn't work, ask your doctor to recommend another.

➤ Most pain treatments help you feel better while nature takes its course. Moving about, or having stronger muscles in the first place, is best for your back.

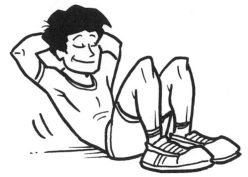

Chapter 12

Exercise Does a Back Good

> ## In This Chapter
>
> ➤ What's your fitness level? A self-quiz
>
> ➤ Stretching and conditioning exercises to keep your back flexible
>
> ➤ Exercises for strength and endurance
>
> ➤ Exercise and weight control

Nothing gets your back in a better mood than a little exercise. Even if you don't really feel like it, your back loves nothing more than some good stretching and moving.

Don't Just Sit There

You're probably sitting right now, which is okay since you're reading. But what were you doing before you sat down with this book? What will you do when you're finished reading it?

Most of us spend more time sitting than in any other position. We sit in a car or bus to get to and from work, we sit at work, and we come home and sit in front of the TV. It's not surprising that more than 40 percent of American adults are overweight—we're not doing much to burn up the calories we take in every day. And we're not doing much to keep our backs and bodies in shape, either. Pushing buttons on the TV's remote control doesn't quite qualify as exercise!

Back Talk

You already know walking is great for your back, but did you know it could lengthen your life? According to one study, people who walk 30 miles or more a week (five miles a day) cut their risk of dying by half when compared to people of similar age who walk five miles or less each week. In addition to the excellent aerobic workout walking gives your heart and muscles, it also controls calories. Each mile you walk burns 100 calories or so, depending on your pace.

How Fit Are You?: A Self-Quiz

So how fit are you? Take this short self-quiz to see!

1. When you get home from work, the first thing you do is...

    a) Collapse on the couch.

    b) Clean up the house or the yard.

    c) Change into sweats and go for a walk or jog.

2. Your office is on the second floor and you have five minutes until your meeting in the seventh-floor conference room. The elevators are shut down for routine repairs. By the time you climb five flights of stairs, you...

    a) Look like you just swam the English Channel.

    b) Sit on the steps of the last landing for a few minutes to catch your breath before going to the conference room.

    c) Stop at the restroom to comb your hair, since the meeting hasn't started yet.

3. You stop at the grocery store on the way home from work to pick up a few things for dinner. You park...

    a) In the handicap spot—it's been a long day, and there's no point in letting such a close spot go to waste.

    b) In the first regular space you find, about in the middle of the parking lot.

    c) At the back of the parking lot, so you can stretch your legs on the walk to the door.

4. You find yourself with 20 minutes of unexpected free time in the middle of the afternoon. You…

    a) Curl up under your desk for a short nap.

    b) Walk to the break room, sit down, and read the newspaper.

    c) Put on your walking shoes and do a couple laps around the block.

5. You look down and notice an untied shoelace flopping around. You…

    a) Know it's someone else's foot—you wear only slip-ons.

    b) Look for a place to sit down, prop your foot up, and retie it.

    c) Kneel down and retie it.

6. How long does it take you to walk a mile?

    a) Walk a mile? Is the car in the shop?

    b) Early in the day, about 15 minutes. After a day at the office, about a half-hour.

    c) Ten minutes.

7. The kids are shooting baskets in the driveway when you come home from work. You…

    a) Honk the horn until they clear the way and one of them opens the garage door for you.

    b) Park on the street—you can move the car into the garage later.

    c) Park on the street, toss your briefcase on the front step, and take a few shots.

Give yourself 5 points for every C, 3 points for every B, and 1 point for every A. If your total is 28 or more, take a victory lap—you're in good shape. If your total is between 18 and 27, you need to put a little more zip in your life. And if you scored less than 17, go get your sweats on. You have some work to do!

Move over, Charles Atlas

So you're feeling a little on the wimpy side these days as you look at the image that stares back from the mirror? While appearances aren't everything, they do offer clues that should catch your attention. Muscles that look flabby and weak are, in all likelihood, pretty much what they appear to be. They don't have to stay that way, though—and you don't need bulging biceps to have better strength and muscle tone. You don't need the movements of a ballet dancer to have improved flexibility, either. What you do need is a regular program of exercise that gives your muscles a good all-around workout for endurance (aerobic capacity), flexibility, and strength.

Stretching and Flexibility

Stretching and flexibility are essential for your back. No series of bones in your body has the range of motion that your spine has. Its facet joints—the connections between your vertebrae—allow controlled movement front to back and side to side. But all this motion happens only in concert with your muscles, tendons, and ligaments—the connective tissues that hold the entire structure of your spine together.

Muscles have a sort of memory. Not memory like your brain, which files away a vast array of experiences and thoughts that you can recall at will (and sometimes against it!). Muscle memory is rather mechanical. You know how a rubber band comes out of the box small and stretches to go around a bundle of mail? If you remove it after a short time, it snaps back to its original size and shape. If you leave it in place for a long time, however, it stays somewhat enlarged and elongated when you remove it. Muscle memory works something like that. Your muscles get used to certain positions that they spend a lot of time in.

Back Basics

An **isometric** exercise uses static resistance (pushing against a non-moving force) to increase muscle strength.

It's important to give your muscles enough variety in terms of activity that they regularly stretch and contract. This helps them to function to the full extent of their capabilities. They don't have an opportunity to "lock" into a particular memory, which keeps them flexible enough to respond to the demands you place on them. And flexibility—controlled range of motion—lets your back do what it's supposed to do for you.

Strengthening

Activities that build muscle strength force your muscles to work against resistance. Over time, this causes the muscle fibers to thicken, which increases both their strength and size (mass). Resistance can be as simple as pressing your hands together with as much force as you can generate, then releasing. This kind of exercise is called *isometric*, and one of its greatest advantages is that you can do it anywhere, any time. Weight lifting also builds muscle mass and strength (more on this in the next section).

Activities that combine endurance with resistance—such as rowing, bicycling, and cross-country skiing—are especially effective for building strength, though not necessarily for improving flexibility.

Conditioning and Toning

Even at rest, your muscles are not completely relaxed. They stay in a state of partial contraction, ready to move when you send the signal. This state is called muscle tone, and improving it is called conditioning or toning. Muscles with good tone are more ready to respond than those with poor tone. Think of it as waiting at the starting line for a race. One runner is just standing there, while the other is crouched on the line. When the starting gun fires, both runners are ready to take off. But the one in the crouch is more ready, with muscles partly tensed and in the positions they need to be in for running. Muscles with good tone tend to look well defined without bulging.

Working Out with Weights

Working out with weights is a good way to build muscle mass and strength. Weights provide increased resistance, forcing your muscles to work harder to perform standard movements. When part of your regular exercise routine, weight training is a nice way to round out your body work.

When weight training makes up the bulk of your exercise routine, however, you can end up reducing both your flexibility and your endurance. Weight training forces your muscles to do more work with less movement, which causes them to get bigger. This doesn't necessarily improve their ability to

Back to Nature

Exercise doesn't just mean working out or going to the gym. Any physical activity that keeps you going for 30 minutes or so qualifies. A half-hour spent raking leaves, washing or vacuuming floors, gardening, mowing the lawn (pushing, not riding, the mower), and even washing and waxing your car can work several major muscle groups—and leave you with something extra to show for your effort.

Back Care

If you're new to weight training, start slow and light. The whole point is to build, not rush. It takes regular and consistent workouts to produce results.

143

move you around. Weight lifting tends to cause muscle fibers to shorten as they thicken, reducing your flexibility. Add stretching exercises to your routine to lengthen muscle fibers. And use aerobic exercise—activities that get your heart pounding—to increase muscle endurance, giving your muscles (and you) stamina.

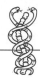

Back Care

Should you use free weights or a weight machine? Most exercise specialists recommend the machine—it's easy to set and adjust, and often records useful information about your workout that you can print out when you're finished. The risk of injury is higher with free weights, in part because you can drop them or lose control of them when lifting.

Back to Nature

Exercise is a great natural stress reliever. The more energy you can put into a quick workout—even just hoofing it around the block—the better you'll feel about whatever's bothering you. Exercise can also quell your anger, giving you a chance to return to rationality before your feelings affect others.

The Importance of Proper Technique

It's absolutely essential to use proper techniques when doing weight training. Making the wrong moves or using the wrong weights can do damage before you even know what happened. Too much weight and too few repetitions, or too little weight and too many repetitions, can make your workout less effective. Unless you've worked out with weights before, we strongly encourage you to join a fitness center or sign on with a qualified exercise trainer. This way, you'll get instruction in how to use weights and develop a personalized program to get you to your goals.

Before joining a gym or signing on with a personal trainer, ask to watch a few classes, especially if you're going to a fitness center that has several instructors. Talk to other people who've used the same gym or trainer. Are there a lot of injuries in the classes? Do the instructors truly work with each individual on a personalized fitness program, or slot you into the standard program?

Bulk Is Not Fitness

You may envy the rippling muscles of the guys (and gals) who seem to live at the gym. Before you decide to sculpt yourself in their image, you should know that bulk is not necessarily fitness. Remember, weight training builds muscle mass and strength, not endurance and stamina. The latter are especially important for overall fitness. If your workouts include regular aerobic exercise, odds are you could run laps around those muscle-bound bodies you so admire.

Extremely bulked-up muscles, such as you see on body builders, can be more fragile in terms of injury than ordinary muscles like yours. Oversized muscles lack flexibility and mobility, making them susceptible to strains and pulls. This tightness also limits joint mobility. When it comes to your back, flexibility and mobility rule—without them, your back can't function as intended.

Remember Those Abs!

You tend to focus on your back muscles when thinking about strengthening and supporting your back—it makes sense. After all, they're the ones that hurt when your back bothers you. But remember that your body's skeletal muscles (the muscles that make movement possible) function in pairs. When one acts, its pair reacts. When you bend forward, your back muscles extend to allow the movement. But it's your abdominal muscles (your "abs") that flex, pulling tight to pull you forward.

Curls (also called crunches) and modified sit-ups provide an excellent workout for your abs. The old touch-your-toes sit-ups are out! Doing sit-ups this way—lying flat on your back with your legs extended and then sitting up while stretching your hands toward your feet—is more likely to hurt your back. It puts tremendous pressure on your lower back. Do modified sit-ups instead: Lie on your back on the floor with your knees raised, and lift your back just enough to raise your shoulders off the floor. You should feel this in your belly as your abs pitch in to do most of the pulling, taking the strain off your lower back.

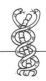

Back Care

When you do sit-ups, lie with your knees up so the small of your back rests flat against the floor. Let your abs do the work of pulling your shoulders off the floor. Try folding your arms across your chest and holding your elbows with your hands as you lift, to keep yourself from pulling yourself up with your arms. Hold your chin forward toward your chest to relieve pressure on your neck as you lift up.

Warm Up, Cool Down

Cold muscles get a little cranky when you place extra demands on them. Asking them to jump into exercise without first warming up is like expecting your brain to balance your checkbook the instant you open your eyes in the morning. You're just not going to get the best results!

Warm up before exercise, even if you're just planning a lap or two around the block. Develop a routine that gently stretches and mobilizes each major muscle group—feet, calves, thighs, hips, back, abs, arms, and shoulders. It doesn't have to be a lengthy routine—five minutes or so should do it. Include activity in your warm-up routine. Walk around a little bit to get your body moving in a synchronized fashion, and if feasible, move through the motions of whatever exercise you're about to begin.

Warm-ups accomplish a couple of things. First, they are a wake-up call for your muscles. Before you

Back to Nature

Yoga postures can be great warm-ups for your exercise routine. Yoga emphasizes slow, gentle movements—perfect for waking those groggy muscles and stretching them out a little bit.

start an activity or exercise, your muscles are pretty comfortable doing nothing. They're semi-contracted—not extended, not flexed. (You know how you feel when you first wake up and the bed feels so warm and comfy that you don't want to stir?) Stretching reminds your muscles of their capabilities and potential. Warm-ups also get blood flowing to your muscles. This brings them vital nutrients to prepare them for their workout, and primes the process that will speed away waste materials (the natural by-products of cell activity).

Repeat your warm-up routine at the end of your exercise or activity, too. This eases your muscles back into normal function just as it eased them into it. It also keeps the blood supply strong, helping remove carbon dioxide, lactic acid, and other substances that accumulate in muscle tissue during intense exercise.

Five Exercises for Back Health

Keeping your back in good shape doesn't require any special equipment or membership in a health club. All you need is a little room and some loose-fitting clothes. If you're under a doctor's care for back problems or any other medical condition, check with your doctor before beginning a new exercise routine.

Before you start exercising, warm up with some stretches or yoga postures. The posture exercises in Chapter 5, "Posture Perfect," and the yoga postures in Chapter 13, "Back Fitness, Eastern Style," are also good to add to your regular routine.

Abdominal Stretch

This exercise stretches your abdominal muscles as well as relaxes the deeper muscles in your lower back. Start with three repetitions if you can, and gradually work up to 10.

1. Lie face down on the floor with your hands next to your shoulders, as though you were preparing to do push-ups.

2. Use your arms and only your arms to raise your upper body off the floor.

3. Keep your elbows close to your body and try to get high enough to straighten your arms completely without letting your pelvis leave the floor.

4. Hold for a count of six, then lower yourself back to the floor.

Back Stretch

This exercise stretches the muscles in your lower and upper back. Start with three repetitions for each leg if you can, and work up to 10.

1. Lie on your back on the floor with your knees bent and your feet flat.

2. Using your hands, pull your right knee slowly up to your chest. (Stop if this creates pain in your lower back.)

3. With your knee still at your chest, tuck your chin to your chest and raise your head.

4. Hold for a count of six, then slowly relax.

5. Repeat with the other leg.

Body Curl

This exercise strengthens your abdominal muscles and stretches your back muscles. Start with three repetitions if you can, and work up to 10.

1. Lie on the floor on your back, with your knees up and your feet flat. Lace your fingers behind your head.

2. Slowly raise your feet, moving your knees toward your chest. At the same time, use your abdominal muscles to raise your shoulders off the floor.

3. Touch your elbows to your knees (or get them as close as you can). Hold for a count of six, then slowly return to your starting position.

Back Leg Lift

This exercise strengthens your lower back muscles as well as the muscles of the back of your thigh and your buttocks. Start with three repetitions for each leg, and work up to 10.

1. Lie face down on the floor with a pillow under your hips. Extend your legs out straight, toes pointed and knees together. Put your hands under your chin.

2. Slowly raise your right leg as high as you can without bending your knee or arching your back.

3. Hold for a count of three, then lower your leg back to the floor.

4. Repeat with the other leg.

Low Back Rotation

This exercise stretches the muscles in your lower back, helping to improve flexibility. Start with three repetitions for each side, and work your way to 10.

1. Lie on your back on the floor with your knees up and your feet flat.

2. Keeping your knees together, rotate your hips to move your knees to your right side. Try to get your knees all the way to the floor (you may not be able to do this at first, so just go as far as you can without pain).

3. Hold for a count of six, then return to your starting position.

4. Repeat, turning your knees to your left side.

Back-Safe Activities

The truth is, most of what you do in the course of a day has the potential to cause problems for your back. It's an unavoidable reality of modern life. What matters more than what you do is how you do it—and that you do it. Any activity is better than no activity when it comes to back health. You're far more likely to end up with a backache from sitting too long without changing positions than you are to get any sort of injury from most physical activities, even those that stress your back.

Keeping your back strong and flexible is the most important move you can make. Such a back is more resilient, better able to withstand the challenges that confront it every day. Your back-health exercise routine should include a mixture of strengthening, flexibility, and endurance activities. Beyond this, keep it fun! Do what you enjoy, and you're likely to do more of it, more often.

On Land or in the Water

Walking is the best general exercise for most people. It's low impact (few jarring movements to damage delicate knees and other joints), requires no special equipment beyond a sturdy pair of shoes, and you can do it just about anywhere.

Back Care

Are you feeling pain when you exercise? Don't give up—just cut back a bit. Reduce the frequency and intensity of your exercise to just below the level that causes pain. Stay at this level for a few weeks, and you'll be amazed at how much further you can go.

Swimming is another excellent activity, especially if you already have back problems. Being in the water offsets the effects of gravity, making movement easier. Water aerobics programs are excellent for your back, as well as any other major joints that bother you. There's no impact, since your feet aren't pounding the pavement. And the water adds resistance while at the same time reducing pressure on your back and joints. Most communities have indoor pools available to the general public through community centers, YMCAs, fitness centers, and often colleges and high schools.

Both walking and swimming exercise your body's main muscle groups, providing an aerobic workout as well as conditioning and strengthening your muscles.

Know Your Pain

How well do you know your back pain? Sure, it's there when you'd rather it wasn't, and sometimes it keeps you from doing what you'd like to do. But you don't want it to stop you from enjoying your life—or to interrupt the regular exercise you need for back health and for your general wellness.

Pay attention to your back pain. Know where it hurts, and how, and if certain movements or activities set it off. When your back bothers you during exercise, compare what you're feeling to your usual pain. If you're feeling the same pain, stop for a few

148

minutes to rest, then continue your workout time with different activities. Just keep moving! If a particular activity continues to trigger your back pain, drop it from your routine for a while and replace it with something else.

If you feel a new pain—for example, your shoulder hurts instead of your lower back—rest for a few minutes. If it lessens or goes away, return to the next activity in your exercise routine. It's usually better to continue even at a reduced pace or intensity. If the new pain becomes a frequent visitor, have a fitness instructor review the activity that brings it on to be sure you're doing it right. You may need to replace the activity with one that doesn't bring on new problems.

Know When to Back Off

You can expect your physical activities to leave you with a little soreness and discomfort at times, especially if you're in less than ideal shape or just starting out. This is normal, and should go away within a day or two.

Regular exercise should make you feel better in general, not worse. Do you:

➤ Have trouble falling asleep at night?

➤ Seldom feel like eating?

➤ Feel exhausted rather than refreshed when you finish your exercise routine?

➤ Exercise like you're training for a marathon, when you're not?

➤ Ache all over, all the time?

If you answer "yes" to two or more of these questions, you might be exercising too much, or at the wrong time of the day. Back off a bit—take a day or two off, and return to half of what you were doing. If sleeplessness is your problem and you exercise in the late afternoon or evening, try shifting your workouts to an earlier time. Exercise too close to bedtime can make it hard for you to fall asleep because your body is too warm and has to cool down before you can fall asleep. If you feel better after a few days, make the changes in your exercise program permanent. If you still feel the same after a week, schedule an appointment with your doctor—there could be an underlying problem that needs medical attention.

The Least You Need to Know

➤ Your back needs a variety of exercise and activity to keep it strong and flexible.

➤ Big muscles aren't necessarily fit or flexible.

➤ Whatever exercise routine you choose, start slow and work your way up.

➤ Choose activities you like, and back fitness will follow.

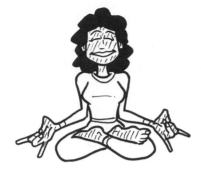

Back Fitness, Eastern Style

When your back pain flares up, whom do you turn to for relief? Your primary care physician? Chiropractor? Acupuncturist? Pharmacist? All of these people can help. But the number one source of relief for the back pain sufferers in a recent survey was none of these. It was…a yoga instructor. Talk about blending East and West!

The "Secret" Language of Yoga

Prana. Asanas. Yamas and niyamas. Yogis. What's with all this "yogaspeak"? Put away your secret decoder ring and your magic translator wristwatch. There are no translations, just interpretations. Yoga words survive from ancient Sanskrit, the 6,000-year-old language of Hindu India. Yoga postures remain as their original words because the languages that followed didn't have words that meant the same thing. So the names simply carried forward into whatever culture adopted yoga.

For our Western convenience, modern yoga instructions include contemporary descriptive titles. We know *parshvakonsana* by its Western name, side angle stretch, for example, not because our description translates the Sanskrit word but because that's what the posture looks like. This is easier for us to both pronounce and visualize, getting us right to the heart of the matter—doing the postures.

Oh, yeah—about the yogaspeak that started this section. *Prana* means life energy or life force. *Asanas* are yoga postures. *Yamas* are not alternative sweet potatoes—they're yoga no-nos. And *niyamas* are yoga-related things you should do. And no, we're not talking about cartoon bears when we mention yogis. A yogi is someone who practices yoga—could even be you!

Back Talk

Sanskrit, the ancient language of yoga, dates back to about 1500 B.C. It's one of the earliest known written languages. A number of Sanskrit documents have survived through the centuries, giving a unique glimpse into everyday life more than 4,000 years ago. In addition to texts describing yoga practices, Buddhist sacred texts, astrological documents, and even literary works have been preserved. Scholars believe Sanskrit evolved from earlier spoken languages. Many of the rituals and beliefs Sanskrit documents discuss existed long before the language that recorded them.

What Exactly Is Yoga?

Yoga is the oldest system of exercise known to humankind. Ancient cultures were far more active physically than their modern counterparts, of course. But yoga has always been something extra, specific postures and activities always done in the same ways—and not while running down game or milling grain. We're not talking jumping jacks and sit-ups here, though. In fact, when you first see someone doing yoga, you might think there's nothing physical going on at all. C'mon, how hard can it be to cross your legs and close your eyes? (Not as hard as staying awake once you did, you're thinking?)

Back Basics

From the Sanskrit *yuj*, **yoga** means "union, to yoke together." As a system, yoga unifies the body, mind, and spirit through a blend of meditation and physical postures.

Don't let appearances fool you. Part activity and part meditation, yoga postures emphasize connecting the body, mind, and spirit. This ancient approach is really more art than sport. There's no competition among participants, no score keeping, no error recording. You just do it (with heartfelt thanks from your body and your attitude).

Yoga is no replacement for *aerobic* exercise. You still need that heart-thumping, chest-pounding activity for

30 to 60 minutes at least three times a week for optimal health. Yoga is considered *anaerobic* exercise. It improves your strength, flexibility, and general fitness. It also relaxes you, reducing stress and promoting a sense of well-being.

The Human-Pretzel Myth

"But you don't understand! With this bad back, I can barely get out of bed in the morning, let alone twist myself into a human pretzel!" We do understand (and we empathize). Certainly many yoga postures are complex, and you might feel you've stumbled into an audition for contortionists when you first see yogis doing them.

Before you bolt for the door, try a new perspective. Think of these advanced yogis as you might think of professional athletes. If Michael Jordan showed up at your Saturday morning pickup game of hoops, would you slink from the court in embarrassment because you couldn't play as good as he does? Or would you smile, dribble a little anxiety slobber along with the ball, and have the time of your life playing with one of basketball's all-time greats?

Some yoga postures are as simple as sitting with your legs crossed and your arms outstretched. Yoga truly offers something for everyone, as well as opportunity for continued and unlimited improvement. What more could a Westerner ask for?

"But I Don't Want My Exercise to Be a Spiritual Experience!"

So you're not really a touchy-feely kind of person, and you don't want a spiritual experience when you exercise? No problem. Yoga postures can certainly condition and strengthen your body without any participation from your mind or your spirit. Yoga can be something you do only in those few spare minutes here and there that sprinkle through your day, if that's what you want. You'll still receive amazing benefits.

Back Basics

The word **aerobic** means "with oxygen." Aerobic exercise gets your heart and lungs working hard, which boosts the amount of oxygen they send to the rest of your body. **Anaerobic** means "without oxygen." You don't stop breathing when you do anaerobic exercises such as yoga and weight lifting, of course—you just don't increase the amount of oxygen getting to your body systems.

Back to Nature

Athletes often use yoga postures to help them "center" before a competition. They know peak performance relies on an absolute integration of body and mind. Yoga, by its very nature, encourages this union.

But if you do allow yoga to stretch and relax your mind and your spirit, too, something even more amazing happens. You begin to understand your body better, to know the subtle signals it sends when it's starting to feel good or starting to feel bad.

153

When chronic back pain is a regular visitor in your life, these subtleties become significant. Because as you already know all too well, nipping a small ache is much easier than trying to turn off a major pain.

In ancient times, physical fitness was a part of everyday life because life demanded it, not because people worked out all the time. Yoga was more a form of meditation that had benefits for the body, not the other way around. It was a way to quietly contemplate the mystery of human existence and one's place in it. (When was the last time you saw a cartoon of a wise yogi sitting on a mountaintop with a caption that read, "Oh, physically fit one, tell me the secret of bulging biceps?")

The need or desire to separate the physical body from the spiritual being is a Western phenomenon. In many Eastern cultures, yoga is a form of religious worship and spiritual expression. But it doesn't have to be if you don't want it to—yet another demonstration of yoga's versatility and timelessness.

Hatha Yoga: Uniting Body and Mind

There are about a dozen core forms of yoga, and dozens more offshoots. Some are very esoteric (internally focused), accentuate mental control, or stress spirituality. The form of yoga familiar to most Americans is hatha yoga, which emphasizes control of the physical body to gain understanding of the body as well as of the mind and spirit.

Hatha yoga is also a system of balancing or joining opposites. Some opposites are obvious and tangible—body and mind/spirit, male and female, contraction and extension, backward and forward, high and low, weak and strong. Others are symbolic representations in the universe as a whole—sun and moon, day and night, hot and cold. Yoga incorporates them all through various postures, always striving for the same goal: balance.

Back Care

Does your back hurt when you do the yoga postures that are supposed to be helping it? First, have a yoga instructor or experienced yogi confirm that you're doing them right. Then analyze the pain you feel while doing the posture. Is it the same pain you have when you're not doing the posture? If so, slow down and take the posture one small step at a time. If it's a different pain, try another posture instead.

Start Slow, Follow Your Own Pace

"Limber" isn't exactly the way you'd describe your stiff, out-of-shape body? Don't worry. While someday it might be, for right now just do what you can with what you have. Start slow, with asanas that gently stretch and tone. If it hurts, stop. You might feel stretched as your muscles move in ways they're not used to, but you shouldn't hurt.

As in distance running, you work up to proficiency in yoga. You don't leap off your couch and into a marathon, and you don't hop out of bed and into maricyasana (spinal twist). You start where you are—a walk around the block, a tadasana (mountain pose). You work up to where you want to be—a 6K walk/run, a vrikshasana (tree pose). You decide how fast you want to go and how to measure your progress.

Set Your Own Goals

How flexible and strong do you want to be? How relaxed and in tune with your whole self? What do you want yoga to do for you? What will your schedule allow you to do?

You set your own goals in yoga, from weight loss to stress reduction. Set small, achievable ones that can serve as stepping stones to your larger objectives. Start with short sessions, just long enough to leave your body wanting more (not begging for a break). Build up to the level you want to maintain. Remember to include time for rest, too.

No matter how long you practice yoga, you'll never run out of challenges. There are more than 1,000 postures, and thousands more variations of them.

Back to Nature

Are you new to yoga? Enroll in a class taught by a qualified yoga instructor. Some classes are just for beginners, to help you get a handle on common terms and basic postures. Others have participants of all experience levels, from novices like you to those for whom yoga is a life philosophy.

Stretching, Strength, and Flexibility, Yoga Style

How do you feel after a rigorous round of calisthenics? If you feel fairly beat up, there's good reason. Though your body needs strenuous activity, Western exercise tends to demand quick, intense reactions from your muscles. Yoga movements are slow and gentle. The idea is to ease into your posture, stretching your muscles along the way so they're always ready for what you're doing. Holding the posture stretches and strengthens your muscles even more. And as yoga strengthens your connective tissues, it builds flexibility in your joints. Your muscles and ligaments stretch farther and hold better, keeping joints stable.

Warming Up

Though yoga isn't very aggressive as far as activities go, it does demand a lot from your muscles. Start with a few basic postures to get your body ready. Do the same postures at the end of your yoga session to help your body "warm down" to return to its normal state.

Using the Breath

Of course you can breathe—it's one of the functions that distinguishes you as a living being. It happens automatically, without your knowledge or effort. Unless you're doing yoga. In yoga, breathing becomes both conscious and active. Yogis call this breath control *pranayama*.

By now it should come as no surprise to you that in yoga, even breathing isn't as simple as it seems. "Prana," you remember, means "life energy." More than just breathing, it's the essence of what gives you life. Breathing moves the air that gives your body life, and it moves the energy that gives your spirit life. Breathing techniques are part of nearly every yoga posture.

Striving for Alignment and Wholeness

As yoga emphasizes balance, it also stresses wholeness. The body—as well as all of existence—consists of pairs of opposites. When these pairs are in balance, you are healthy. When there are imbalances, you have health problems. In yoga, alignment of the body restores balance.

Remember the posture exercises from Chapter 5, "Posture Perfect"? They, too, stress alignment—holding your spine as though a string attached to the top of your head was pulling you up. Even from a Western perspective, balance relieves pressure on your back by distributing the workload evenly among your muscles. Different approaches, same result!

Yoga and Life Energy

Yogis believe there are seven centers in your body, called chakras, that store prana (life energy). Various yoga postures stimulate the chakras, releasing prana. Several chakras are especially important when you have back pain. The Saturn chakra, located at the base of your spine, when activated releases life energy that travels up your spine and into the other chakras. The Jupiter and Mars chakras are also located along your spine. Activating these chakras stimulates other body areas as well.

How Yoga Helps Your Back: A Self-Quiz

All this sounds really great—exercise that's good for the body, mind, and soul. But what does it have to do with your back? Take this fun self-quiz to see how much you know about yoga and your back!

1. When you do yoga, your back...

    a) Responds to a "higher power" and immediately stops hurting.

    b) Goes numb for the duration of the posture, then hurts with a vengeance as soon as it's over.

    c) Can start feeling better after two or three sessions, with steady improvement as you continue your yoga routine.

2. The prana, or energy, that yoga activates affects you and your back by...

    a) Rearranging muscle and nerve molecules.

    b) Surging through your spinal cord to push the happy buttons in your brain.

    c) Refocusing your consciousness to release stress and support healing.

3. Yoga is for people who...

    a) Wear sandals and loose-fitting clothes, and read by the light of a lava lamp.

    b) Work out at the gym four days a week.

    c) Want to gain greater insight into, and feel more in control of, their bodies and their lifestyles.

4. Your muscles respond to yoga because...

   a) The prana makes them.

   b) It hurts if they try to resist.

   c) Yoga movements are gentle and consistent.

5. Yoga can improve an athlete's competitive performance because...

   a) Yoga makes an athlete feel invincible, and as you feel, so you act.

   b) It intimidates other competitors to see the athlete doing yoga postures.

   c) It helps them become centered and one with their bodies.

6. The best way to learn yoga is by...

   a) Reading this book.

   b) Practicing along with a video.

   c) Taking classes from an experienced yoga instructor.

7. The real secret of yoga is that...

   a) One of the postures holds the key to eternal life (you just have to figure out which one).

   b) It gets you to exercise without realizing that's what you're doing.

   c) Anyone can do it, enjoy it, and benefit from it.

How did you do? If you had three or more A answers, go back to the start of this chapter and read it again. If you had three or more B answers, it wouldn't hurt to take a refresher course. And if you had three or more C answers, congratulations—you already know that yoga can be an important part of your back-healthy lifestyle!

Yoga Poses for Back Health

Forward bends are especially good for your back. They stretch and strengthen your lower-back muscles and also your hamstrings. Remember to do these postures slowly and gently. You will improve with time and practice, so don't force yourself into more than your body can handle.

Lightning Bolt Pose and Warrior Pose

These postures are great for relieving upper-back and shoulder tension and pain. For each one, exhale (breathe out) going into the pose and inhale (breathe in) coming out of the pose.

Lightning Bolt Pose

1. Start from the mountain pose (Chapter 5).

2. Raise your arms over your head and bend your knees as though you were getting ready to dive, with your knees and feet slightly apart. Keep your elbows straight, and your palms facing each other.

3. Check your alignment. Your arms and spine should be in line, your hips bent at a 90-degree angle, and your legs parallel to your back. In other words, you should look like a lightning bolt!

4. Hold your posture and feel the tension leave your body, like lightning conducted from the sky (your fingertips) into the ground (your feet).

5. Take in a deep, slow breath, and return to the mountain pose.

The Warrior Pose (Virabhadrasana)

1. From a standing position, move your feet three or so feet apart. Point your right foot out, and let your left foot point slightly toward your right foot.

2. Bend your left leg until your thigh is parallel to the ground and your lower leg is perpendicular. Your knee should have a 90-degree bend.

3. Rotate your body to follow your left leg, aligning so your body is centered over it. Lift your arms straight over your head, palms facing each other. Look to the front of you or up.

4. Be sure your right foot is firmly planted and your right leg straight to hold you in place. Push down on your right heel and take three slow, deep breaths in and out.

5. Reverse your movements to return to a standing position. Switch sides and repeat the posture.

Yoga's warrior pose.

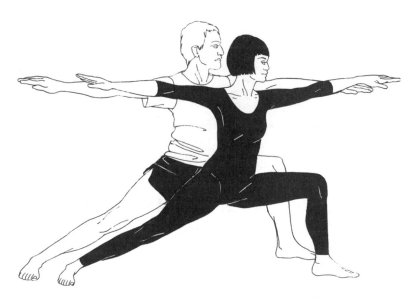

Cobra Pose and Boat Pose

These poses bend your back backward and forward. They target your spine, helping to align your vertebrae and strengthen your lower- and middle-back muscles. Backbends help you feel energized, and forward bends help you feel relaxed and calm.

Cobra Pose

1. Lie on the floor on your stomach, toes and heels together and your nose touching the floor. Put your hands on either side of your chest, as though getting ready to push yourself up.

2. Take in a deep, slow breath. Begin lifting yourself from the floor one section of your body at a time, starting with your forehead. Move slowly and smoothly, and keep your pelvis pressed against the floor.

3. Turn your face upward and breathe out. Slowly return to your starting position.

Back Care

The cobra pose is especially effective for strengthening the muscles along your spine. To measure your improvement, do the pose, and as you turn your face upward, lift up your hands. The more of you that answers gravity's call, the more work your arms are doing. As you practice this pose and your back muscles get stronger, you'll be able to hold more of the position with your hands off the floor.

Yoga's cobra pose.

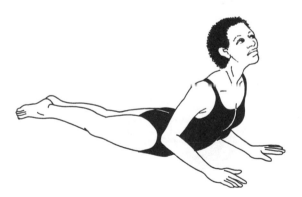

Boat Pose

1. Sit on the floor. Bend your knees, and wrap your arms around them.

2. Slowly lean back until your feet are off the floor and you're balanced on your tailbone.

3. Slowly and smoothly extend your legs so they're straight out with your knees together. Straighten and extend your arms as well, keeping your hands at your knees.

4. Envision yourself bobbing on the water's surface like a little boat. Hold the posture for a few minutes, then slowly reverse your movements to return to your starting position.

Child's Pose and Downward Facing Dog

These poses stretch and relax your lower back to relieve tension and pain.

Child's Pose

Back Off!

If you feel pain behind your knees or in your lower back when doing the downward facing dog, slowly return to your starting position to give your back a break. Then try the posture again, and this time concentrate on lengthening your back rather than stretching your legs. It's okay for your knees to stay bent and your heels to be off the floor until you have the strength and flexibility to hold the full posture.

1. Sit on the floor with your legs tucked under you and your buttocks resting on your heels. Slowly and smoothly bend forward until your forehead touches the floor. (Use a pillow or folded towel under your forehead if it's hard to bend so far forward. If your knees hurt, put a pillow or folded towel under your thighs.)

2. Let your arms rest beside your body, palms up. You should feel completely relaxed and safe.

3. Hold the posture for a few minutes. Breathe in and out deeply and slowly, and feel the breaths enter and leave your body.

4. Slowly reverse your movements to return to your starting position.

Yoga's child's pose.

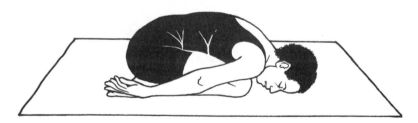

Downward Facing Dog Pose

1. Start on your hands and knees. Lift up as though a string was tied around your waist and pulling you. You'll find yourself balanced on your toes and your hands with your backside pointed to the sky.

2. Drop your shoulders and your head. Slowly drop your heels until your feet are flat against the floor. Straighten your legs as much as you can (if it hurts, you've gone too far).

3. Keep your back stretched and in its natural curves. If your balance is off and your wrists hurt, your back is arched or rounded. Raise your heels off the floor until your back is comfortable.

4. Hold the posture for a minute or so, then slowly reverse your movements to return to your starting position.

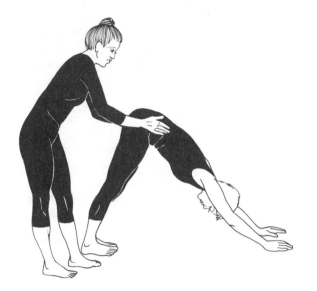

Yoga's downward facing dog pose.

A Kinder, Gentler Martial Art: T'ai Chi

You won't hear any screams or grunts in a t'ai chi class. In fact, you probably won't hear anything at all except the soft rustle of clothing as participants progress through their movements. T'ai chi is sometimes called the "soft" martial art because of its emphasis on gentleness.

T'ai chi almost turns yoga into performance. Movements are slow but continual, and postures flow from one into another in careful choreography. To the uninformed, people practicing t'ai chi appear to move in slow motion—which is the intent. The underlying philosophy of t'ai chi is that while change is constant, it is also slow and steady. Even change that seems to happen instantly is really the culmination of tiny changes taking place over time.

Some people use t'ai chi to slow down their world and at the same time build up their personal flexibility and strength. T'ai chi is gaining popularity especially among seniors, who often practice this graceful form of exercise because it dramatically improves balance, strength, and flexibility. Also known for its stress-relieving capabilities, t'ai chi has found its way into the American workplace as an element of wellness programs and accident-reduction programs.

Back Talk

A recent study sponsored by the National Institute on Aging demonstrated a 25 percent decrease in injuries from falls among elderly t'ai chi practitioners. The study compared several exercise programs to determine whether any could measurably improve balance among fall-prone seniors—injuries from falls are a leading cause of death in people over age 65.

The Least You Need to Know

➤ Though yoga's been around for centuries, it's as relevant in today's fast-paced world as it was in ancient times.

➤ Though slow and steady is the way to healing through yoga, many people with back pain experience prompt and significant relief when they start doing yoga postures.

➤ Yoga offers something for nearly everyone—really!

➤ The Eastern approach to fitness blends mental concentration with physical conditioning.

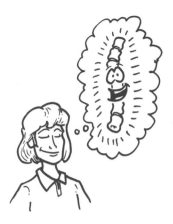

Chapter 14

Imagine a Healthy, Pain-Free Back

In This Chapter

➤ How does your attitude affect your back pain?

➤ Turning the "cycle of sickness" into a "cycle of wellness"

➤ How stressful is your life? A self-quiz

➤ Techniques for relaxation and stress relief

If you've had back problems for a long time, you've probably asked yourself, in your darker moments, if your pain is all just in your mind. Is the agony that keeps you from enjoying your life simply the product of your imagination? Wouldn't *someone* be able to fix the problem if it was truly physical?

First, we want to assure you that there's nothing imaginary about your back pain. We know there are days when you'd trade your right arm—or at least your left big toe—for a healthy, pain-free back. You're no slouch; you want to work and play with everybody else, and this bad-back stuff really gets you down.

Second, we want to remind you that doctors never really know the cause of 85 percent of all back pain. It comes, it wreaks havoc in your life, and it goes. Sometimes you have a spot that's sore to the touch, or an obvious physical problem that shows up on an MRI. But most often, no one knows why your back hurts. It's normal, even expected, to become angry and frustrated when you can't do what you want to do.

Which leads us to our third point. Your attitude—and yes, even your imagination— can enable you to reclaim some, if not most, of the activities and joys that make your life worth living. Your mind is the most powerful instrument of healing in existence. Unfortunately, not many know how to use it to its fullest advantage. We hope to change that situation to put you among those who do!

Pain, Stress, and Attitude

How do you define a good day? (No, you can't cheat by saying it's any day that's not a bad day, or that you don't know because you haven't had one for as long as you remember.) It's a day when everything goes your way, isn't it? You wake up before your alarm, well rested and refreshed. There's plenty of hot water for your morning shower, the toast pops up nice and brown, your orange is sweet and juicy, and traffic moves right along. You arrive at work energized and alert, eager to make the most of your time. Even your back seems happy for a change. You're in a good mood, and it shows.

Okay, now think about a bad day. You sleep past your alarm, can't find socks that match, race out of the house with a mug of coffee that you leave on the roof of your car when you squeal out of your driveway, and end up behind a police car all the way to work. You rush into your morning meeting with toilet tissue trailing from your shoe, only to discover everyone impatiently waiting for the marketing presentation you left lying on the kitchen counter when you poured your coffee. Your head's throbbing, your shoes are too tight, and your back's already knotting up. You're headed for a rough day, and everybody knows it.

It doesn't seem fair, does it, that a good day vanishes before you know it, and a bad day drags on for at least a week? Certainly events make a difference. What good can you find in a speeding ticket or a flat tire? But what really separates a good day from a bad day is attitude. Yours. A negative attitude can sour the brightest day, while a positive attitude can make a dark day at least tolerable, if not actually enjoyable.

Back Talk

Not all stress is bad. Eustress, or good stress, happens when the pressure you feel is positive—the publisher just accepted your book proposal, and now you have to write the book. Distress, or bad stress, results from situations you view as negative—your job's a drag, your boss makes the Wicked Witch of the East look kind, and the school principal wants to see you *again* about your child's refusal to participate in gym class. Your goal in reducing stress is to lower the level of distress in your life. Then you can more fully enjoy the eustress!

Mind and Matter

All too often, we think of attitude and pain as a process of mind over matter, as if there's this constant wrangling within your body about which is in control. What a difference it makes when we think in terms of mind *and* matter! You see, it doesn't have to be one or the other. In fact, it can't. Your mind and your body are an inseparable pair.

This mind/body duality has been at the center of Eastern cultures for centuries. In our Western culture, we tend to view the concept more as *psychosomatic*—and as such, something somehow shameful. That our thoughts and feelings can influence such physical sensations as pain implies that all we need to do is "will" the pain away. If only it could be so simple!

There is probably no connection more complex than that which links mind and body. Recent research implies the process may be even more complicated. In an interview with Bill Moyers for his book, *Healing and the Mind* (Doubleday, 1993), neuroscientist Candace Pert, Ph.D., discusses the body's "psychosomatic communication network." In this system, she says, *neuropeptides* are to the body's physical responses what emotions are to the mind's.

In fact, Pert and other researchers believe there's compelling evidence that these molecules are actually biochemical messengers that communicate emotion. They might trigger anger or sadness just as, for example, a rising blood sugar level triggers your pancreas to release insulin. Such a concept has tremendous implications for conditions like chronic back pain. You probably won't ever be able to "will away" the problems that cause your back to hurt. But what if you could use your mind to tell your body to release more of its natural painkillers, endorphins? You could have the relief you need, when you need it, without potentially harmful side effects. An amazing creation, this body of yours!

> **Back Basics**
>
> **Psychosomatic** means "mind and body." **Neuropeptides** are biochemical substances found in your brain cells as well as in many other kinds of cells throughout your body. They influence how you feel.

The Power of Perception

You've probably seen those mind-teaser images, either at shopping-mall art shows or in psychology books. Some high-tech versions, like those you see as posters or even as collections in coffee-table books, look like pointless geometric patterns until you let your focus slacken and suddenly a three-dimensional picture pops out. Others are simpler, like those you see in materials dealing with how humans perceive the world around them. Often just black-and-white drawings, these images shift from an old to a young woman or a vase to two faces. What you see depends on, well, what you choose to see.

How your back hurts differs depending on where you choose to focus, too. Do you feel every little twinge and ache, maybe see in your mind's eye hundreds of nerve endings on fire? You're focusing on one small area of your back, your body, your life. What happens if you loosen your focus to see a different picture, as you would when looking at an image that appears to be just a myriad of geometric shapes? Let your inner vision relax, and "see" perhaps a nearby shoulder that feels fine. Shifting your point of view changes your perspective. While looking at your pain differently may not make it go away, you can bump it from center stage.

Back Talk

According to insurance industry statistics, only one in four workers returns to work after one year off if the cause of the year-long absence was back problems. Among those who are off for two years, virtually none end up returning to work. Fortunately, about 85 percent of people with back pain feel better and return to work within a two or three weeks.

Understanding the "Cycle of Sickness"

Something happens to you when you're hurting. Apart from whatever causes your pain, when that pain becomes chronic, it traps you in a "cycle of sickness." You hurt, therefore you're doomed to hurt. You move and your back hurts, so you avoid movement. Others respect your pain and treat you like you hurt, getting things for you and changing what they expect from you. This all reinforces your perspective that you do, indeed, hurt. What else can you do but hurt and be hurt?

But this isn't Jumanji, the legendary, mystical game where once you start playing you have to play forever and each move leads to an adventure more terrifying than the one before. You're free to leave this game that is your cycle of sickness, whenever you choose. Doing so takes some concentration and effort, but it's easier than you think.

Breaking Free

Make changes one at a time, and start small. Choose one back-healthy activity from this book and add it to your life. For example, get into and out of bed with movements that protect, rather than agitate, your back (take another look at Chapter 5, "Posture Perfect," if you can't remember how to do this). Do this one thing for a week. Next week, add another back-healthy activity—perhaps a daily walk. And so on, until your back pain is nothing more than an aspect of your life you notice only occasionally.

Creating Your Own "Cycle of Wellness"

You may not recognize at first that each back-healthy activity replaces a link in the cycle of sickness. It's a natural and unavoidable effect—you have to stop getting in and out of bed awkwardly, for example, in order to do so smoothly and gently. Every 30 minutes you spend walking is 30 minutes you're not sitting or lying on the couch. Before long, you'll be living a "cycle of wellness" instead.

Keep this cycle alive and well by continuing to focus on what you *can* do instead of what you can't do. You may not end your back pain entirely, but you will change the way you feel about it, and the extent to which it governs your life.

Slow Down, Be Happy: Lower Your Stress Level

Ours is a rush-around culture. We hurry here and hurry there, trying to squeeze more minutes from every hour, more hours from every day. (There are even those of us who think we can do eight days' worth of living in each week.) Why? We don't actually get more done. In fact, we probably do less when we rush because we forget things or do them halfway, so we end up doing them again.

All this rushing generates tremendous stress. Your body responds by gearing up its resources—your pulse races, your heart pounds, your breathing quickens. Even though you might know there's no good reason for this, your body can't help it. Somewhere along the evolutionary path, progress overlooked a key detail—you don't fight saber-toothed tigers anymore. So when it feels stress, your body reacts by getting you ready to fight or flee. Problem is, of course, you're not going to do either—unless you count weaving through traffic to make your dental appointment.

Stress feeds the "cycle of sickness" by tensing your muscles, which in turn intensifies your pain. When you hurt, you feel stressed, and your muscles get even more tense. Instead of a bit of a backache, you may feel like you hurt all over. Though you need some stress in your life (just as a guitar string needs a certain amount of tension), too much stress can damage your sense of well-being as well as your body.

Back Off!

Stress causes your muscles to tense and feeds pain. Pain makes your muscles more tense, which makes them hurt even more. If you're feeling tense and uptight, take a few minutes to relax and regain control. Once the stress-tension-pain cycle starts, it's hard to break.

How Stressed Are You? A Self-Quiz

Yeah, okay, my life has stress, you concede. But do you know just how stressed you are? Here's a quick self-quiz to give you a little insight.

1. It's 10 p.m. You've just settled into your favorite chair for a half-hour of reading before bed when you 14-year-old son pops in to tell you that oh, by the way, he forgot to tell you he's supposed to bring a vegetable tray for tomorrow's surprise birthday party for his homeroom teacher. You…

    a) Get dressed, go to the store to buy vegetables, and spend the next hour slicing and dicing.

    b) Cover your face with your book and sob.

    c) Tell your son you're sorry his forgetfulness will mean he won't be able to meet his obligation.

2. Your day started with the discovery that you washed your entire wallet and now have to replace everything that was in it, and ended with the boss chewing you out at the staff meeting for missing an assignment you didn't know was yours. When you get home, you…

    a) Pop a cold one and crash on the couch.

    b) Replay the events of the day over and over in your head.

    c) Stand in a hot shower and let your tension and anger go down the drain with the water.

3. It's 2 a.m. and everyone else in your house is sound asleep. You're…

    a) Sitting at the kitchen table balancing your checkbook.

    b) Still awake, thinking about all that you have to do tomorrow and wondering if you remembered to turn off the office copier.

    c) Dreaming.

4. You're coming around the dairy aisle at the grocery store with a carton of milk in your hand when—blam! Someone crashes into you from the other direction, sending your milk carton splashing to the floor. You…

    a) Start screaming "How could you be such an idiot!" at the other person.

    b) Cry.

    c) Check to be sure the other person's okay, then ask the checkout clerk to have someone clean up the mess.

5. Your stomach feels like its turned inside out, your mouth is so dry you couldn't lick a stamp though your palms are sweaty enough to take over that task should the need arise, and your heart's pounding so hard you can see your chest move. You're…

    a) Waiting outside your boss's office for your performance appraisal.

    b) Pulled off the side of the road after barely escaping a collision with a dump truck.

    c) Just about to drop 110 feet straight down on the world's wildest roller coaster.

6. Your mother's coming from out of state for her first visit with you since you've been married. The morning she's due to arrive, you're…

a) Scrubbing the inside of the dishwasher.

b) Rearranging the guest room.

c) Reading the newspaper and enjoying a bagel and a glass of fresh-squeezed orange juice.

7. It's starting to get dark, but you're not finished painting the back of your house. You...

a) Pull the car around back and turn on the headlights to finish up.

b) Brush faster.

c) Clean everything up and go in for dinner.

Give yourself 5 points for every A, 3 points for every B, and 1 point for every C. If your score is 12 or lower, you're doing a pretty good job managing the stress in your life. If your score is between 13 and 25, consider adding some stress-relief techniques to your daily activities. And if you scored 26 or higher, look out—you're ready to blow! Your lifestyle could well be the death of you if you don't get rid of some pressure.

Back to Nature

Not very satisfied with your life right now? Try this exercise: On one side of your paper, write down three things that make you unhappy. On the other side, write down what you could do to turn those dissatisfactions into satisfactions. Then make it happen!

Five Things You Can Do to Lower Your Stress Level

No matter how stressed you are, there are quick and easy actions you can take to lower the load on your body and mind (not to mention your poor back). Here are five things you can do to lower your stress level—right now, or anytime, anyplace.

1. **Breathe.** Not that panicky, half-hyperventilation stuff that hits you when you're stressed, but the yoga-style focused breathing. Take a slow, deep breath in, hold it for 10 seconds, and let your breath out, slowly. Repeat five or six times.

2. **Prioritize.** What's the most important thing you have to do among the six or so tasks you're struggling to juggle? If you don't know because they all seem equally important, get a pencil and a piece of paper. Draw two lines down the center of the page. Label the left side "task," the center "what will happen if I don't do it," and the right side "Do/Delegate/Delete." Now fill in your chart. If you and only you can do the task, mark it "do." If someone else could do the task, mark it "delegate." And if it really doesn't matter whether the task gets done, or the consequences of not doing it right now are minimal, mark it "delete." (What you delete from today's list you can move to another day when you have more time.)

3. **Slow down.** How fast do you drive on familiar roads? Be honest—you don't have to say it out loud. Most people routinely travel faster than the posted speed limit,

usually because they're running late. But you don't save that much time by speeding, and you generate great risks for yourself and others. Driving 45 miles an hour in a 35 mph zone, for example, gets you to your destination 10 miles away only four minutes faster than driving the speed limit. (And if there are traffic lights along your route, it could take you longer to get to where you're going—lights are synchronized for the posted speed limit.) Yet you're more likely to get a ticket, get in an accident, and if you're in an accident, be seriously injured.

4. **Visualize.** What do you see when you think of yourself in ideal circumstances? Visualize the things you want to do. Capture this image in your mind's eye, and consciously focus on it throughout the day. See yourself making small steps toward turning this vision into reality, and reward yourself for progress (though in this case, progress is its' own reward!).

5. **Say no.** Can't, you say? Sure you can! Try it right now—NO! Sorry to break it to you, but no one is indispensable. Ask family members to pitch in with housework and yard work. Delegate tasks to appropriate coworkers, and ask for additional help with special projects. Let other parents volunteer for bake sales and field trips once in a while. Amazingly, things get done even when you don't do them.

Of course, you'll still have days with more to do than time to do it all. The key is to use these stress busters in combination to ease as much of your load as possible. You might even get a little time just for you!

Today's Priorities—Example

Task	What Will Happen If I Don't Do It?	Do/Delegate/Delete
1. Drive kids to school	They walk; it's a beautiful day, and school is less than a mile away	Delete
2. Wash kitchen floor	Floor looks dirty; no one home tonight but me	Delegate or delete
3. Morning marketing presentation to We Be Big, Inc.	Company loses bid; I lose job	Do
4. Pick up Ruth at airport	Someone else has to do it	Delegate
5. Lunch meeting with VP, Accounting	Could lose department share of budget surplus	Do

My Priorities Today

Task	What Will Happen If I Don't Do It?	Do/Delegate/Delete
1.		
2.		
3.		
4.		
5.		

If You Think It, It Can Be: Meditation

People new to meditation often have an image of an old man with a long gray beard sitting cross-legged on a floor mat, eyes closed and hands outstretched, his mind completely blank. In reality, people of all ages use meditation to relax and relieve stress. You can adopt a yoga position for meditation if that suits you, or sit any way and anywhere that you can let your body relax. And it's not that you have nothing on your mind— you still have plenty going on inside your brain.

During meditation, you may focus on one particular thought to the exclusion of all others. Or you might hold a peaceful, restful image in your mind's eye. Some people quietly chant a *mantra* while they meditate, to help them stay focused. Others appear to be asleep. How you meditate is less important than that you do it. A few minutes of meditation every day is more useful than an hour once a week. Try meditating at the same time each day, to get yourself in the habit.

> **Back Basics**
>
> **Mantra** comes from Sanskrit words that mean "free from constant thought." Repeating a mantra helps you focus and get in touch with your inner self.

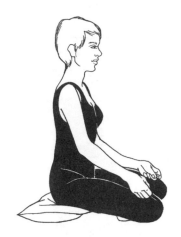

Meditate in a sitting position that's comfortable for you and allows you to sit with the best posture. Placing a folded towel or pillow under your tailbone can help make a classic cross-legged meditation pose feel like nirvana, no matter how flexible you are.

Envision Your Back Pain Free: Guided Imagery

What if you could travel to nirvana any time you wanted? Right there in the middle of that sales meeting, you could take off for the most wonderful place imaginable? You already have your ticket, and you don't need luggage!

Guided imagery is a powerful tool for stress and pain relief. You can do it just about anywhere, anytime (though we'd suggest you stay in reality when driving, even if your back hurts). The concept is simple—you imagine yourself someplace pleasant, and let your mind take you there.

Back Basics

Biofeedback is a process of consciously affecting body activities that usually happen without conscious intervention, such as muscle tenseness and pain perception. Some people can use biofeedback to influence brain waves and even heart rate, allowing them to induce a state of relaxation.

Close your eyes and imagine you're sitting on a cloud high above the world. You're floating just a little, almost weightless, so there's no pressure on your back. A warm breeze touches you softly, and takes away the tension you feel. It comes back again and again, until you're completely relaxed. Without tension, the pain is gone from your back. You feel comfortable and stress free.

Nice little interlude, isn't it? When it's time to return to reality, be gentle with yourself. Let the cloud lower you gently back to Earth. Keep the warm breeze with you for a while, if you like, to keep blowing away the tension as you get back to the activities of living.

You don't have to go to the clouds, of course. You can go anywhere you like. If guided imagery sounds a little "out there" to you, it's really not so esoteric. Everyone daydreams—think of guided imagery as a directed daydream with a mission.

A Little Back Talk Can Go a Long Way: Biofeedback

Biofeedback teaches you to listen to what your body tells you, and to "talk" back. Some techniques use machinery to measure body activities such as your pulse rate. By watching a monitor, you see the effects of your efforts. Other techniques emphasize conscious awareness of how your body feels and acts, so you can learn to manipulate its sensations.

Biofeedback takes training and time to master. You'll probably want to work with a health care professional who specializes in it to learn the basic techniques. Once you get it down, however, biofeedback can be an effective way to lower stress and reduce your perception of pain.

With a Little Help from Your Mind: Hypnosis

They're uproarious entertainment—audience volunteers who come up on stage to be hypnotized. Once they're under, the hypnotist plants suggestions. "When I clap my hands three times, you'll squat down on the floor, flap your arms like wings, and quack like a duck." Sure enough, the hypnotist gives three sharp claps and her volunteers are right down there on the floor ducking it up.

Real hypnotherapy isn't quite so dramatic or entertaining. A licensed, professional hypnotherapist will start by talking with you about your problems and concerns. What do you expect hypnosis to accomplish for you? How do you feel about being hypnotized? Since not everyone responds to hypnosis, the hypnotherapist may ask you to answer some questions that don't seem related to your issues.

The trance-like state you enter when undergoing hypnosis is somewhere between wakefulness and deep sleep in terms of consciousness. When you're in this state, you respond to your surroundings, though you aren't consciously aware of what happens. The hypnotherapist uses this particularly receptive state of mind to plant ideas and suggestions about how you can respond to certain circumstances when you're fully conscious.

Back Care

Choose a hypnotherapist carefully. Ask for, and verify, credentials and references. It's important for you to trust your hypnotherapist, so you have confidence in her ability to help you. And don't worry—you won't do anything under hypnosis or by posthypnotic suggestion that goes against the core values by which you live your life.

Back Basics

A **posthypnotic suggestion** is an idea the hypnotherapist suggests to your mind when you're in a hypnotic state that will trigger a response or reaction when you're fully conscious.

For example, she might suggest that when you feel your back begin to tense and tighten, you'll stop what you're doing and do a few relaxation or stretching exercises to turn the tenseness back. Or when your back starts to ache, you'll look at something white and feel your muscles relax. These *posthypnotic suggestions* are intended to increase your awareness of what's going on with your body and your back, so you can respond and react before the pain takes control.

It's also possible for a hypnotherapist to teach you how to put yourself into a trance-like state for relaxation and as a way of getting away from your back pain for a little while. Hypnosis is very relaxing, and many people "awaken" from a session feeling as though they've had the best night's sleep ever.

The Least You Need to Know

➤ A little stress is healthy; too much stress can make back pain more difficult to deal with and compromise your well-being.

➤ Stress creates tension, and tension feeds pain. When you relieve stress, you relieve tension and pain as well.

➤ Which relaxation techniques you use aren't as important as doing something on a regular basis to control stress and its effects on your body and your life.

➤ You can't always make your back pain go away, but you can change the way you feel about it and how much you let it interfere with the rest of your life.

Part 4
Cut to the Fix

Surgeons must be very careful
When they take the knife!
—Emily Dickinson, American poet (1830–1886)

If your back pain won't go away, can you cut it out? It's tempting to look to surgery as the "fix." Surgery is a good choice, and sometimes the only choice, for certain back problems. For other back problems, however, surgery won't help much—and can even make things worse.

The chapters in Part 4 take a look at which back problems surgery can help, and what you can expect if you choose surgery to help yours.

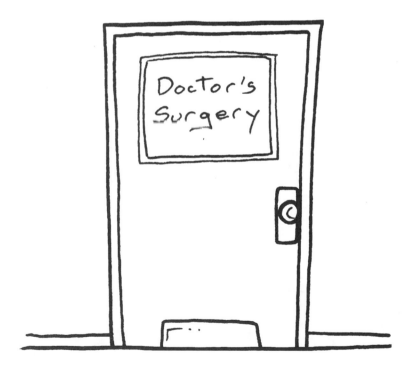

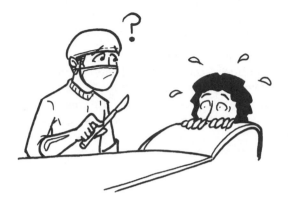

Chapter 15

To Operate or Not?

In This Chapter

➤ Making the decision to have surgery

➤ How to choose a surgeon

➤ Health habits to improve your recovery

➤ Preparing yourself for surgery

October 16 may not be an especially memorable date on your calendar, but it stands as a milestone in medical history. On that date in 1846, a young dentist named William T.G. Morton dripped ether into a breathing apparatus placed over the mouth and nose of a patient about to have a large tumor removed from his tongue. The straps binding the patient tightly to the operating table were completely unnecessary, and the surgeons removed the tumor without a sound or twitch from their patient. The event demonstrated a discovery that changed the practice of medicine—anesthesia.

Today, 250,000 Americans undergo surgery for low back problems each year. How do you know whether you should be among them? Don't leave this important decision to your doctor alone. After all, it's your back, your health, and your life. The more you know about your condition and the options available for treating it, the better prepared you are to make the decision that's right for you.

When Is Surgery the Best Choice?

We've come to view surgery as a "quick fix" for much of what ails us. In America, which leads the Western world in the number of surgeries performed, the individual whose body remains in original condition is as much an oddity as a Dalmatian without spots. We willingly—even eagerly—give up an inflamed appendix, a gall bladder blocked with stones, organs infiltrated by cancer. We exchange an eye lens clouded by cataracts, and repair hearts that can no longer keep pace. We even let surgery reshape our faces, bust lines, bellies, and tushes. Why, then, can't surgery fix this aching back?

Surgery can't fix what the surgeon can't see. Most back pain lacks a clear, precise origin. One minute you're fine and the next you hurt. You're not really sure what happened to set your back afire, and neither is your doctor. With perhaps 85 percent of all back pain rooted in muscle problems of some sort, surgery is seldom the treatment of choice. (Unless you're having bladder or bowel function problems as a result of your back problem, in which case surgery will be first on the options list.) Pain alone, though it may turn your life upside down, is not reason enough to stretch out on the operating table.

The Two-Percent Solution

Even among the 15 percent or so whose back pain involves disks, bones, fractures, or other structural problems, surgery remains a treatment of last resort. Doctors sometimes refer to back surgery as a "2-percent solution"—the answer for only about 2 percent of all back pain situations. The reason? For as much as we like to think of the human body as a biological machine, there's more to it than that. Despite the sophistication of modern medical technology, your body holds many secrets. Just because a technique or procedure works on a computer-generated model, or even the guy whose office is two doors down from yours, doesn't mean it'll work on you.

Don't get us wrong—we're not surgery bashing. Today's back surgery techniques bring relief for thousands of Americans each year, and that's great. If you're among them, that's great, too. But we do want to emphasize that surgery is just one tool. If you only had a chainsaw, you'd be in great shape for trimming trees but in a world of hurt when you wanted to clip a coupon from the newspaper. You have to use the right tool for the job!

Test Results

The most significant indication that your back needs surgery may not be sophisticated tests but the picture your words paint. As we've said, tests like CT scans, MRIs, and even x-rays can show structural abnormalities that have nothing to do with your pain. And certain symptoms don't really need imaging procedures to tell your doctor what's causing them, though surgeons like to pinpoint the problem before they chance surgery.

What if you have sciatica, or tingling and numbness in one leg, and your imaging procedures don't show anything? Odds are high that surgery is not your solution, at least not yet. Today's imaging procedures are incredibly accurate. If an MRI or CT myelogram doesn't show what your doctor expects to see, it's not likely that cutting you open will show much more. Normal test results offer a compelling reason to avoid surgery; abnormal test results are no proof that surgery will fix your aching back.

Understand the Potential Benefits and Risks

Overall, two thirds of back surgeries are successful—those who have surgery find relief from pain and return to their normal lives. Those whose back pain has been a constant companion for years, which is often the case, may feel that surgery gives them a new life. When success is the outcome, the risks seem worthwhile. But when you have to live with an outcome that is less than you and your doctor expected, the price for trying seems steep.

Success varies with the procedure. Surgery that fuses vertebrae together is more likely to have complications than surgery that doesn't involve fusion (simply removing a prolapsed disk). Surgery might relieve your sciatica, for example, but leave you with back pain (either from the surgery or another cause). And as wonderful as surgery is when it can fix your back problem, it can also create new problems. One unavoidable consequence of surgery is scar tissue, which is thicker and less flexible than regular tissue. Scar tissue can itself crunch down on nerves or limit your movement.

Certain factors create greater risk for you, too. Are you overweight? Obesity complicates surgery by making it harder for the surgeon to get to the site of your problem. Fat tissue has a good supply of blood and nerves, which means more bleeding during surgery and more pain afterward. Do you have a chronic condition other than your back problem, such as heart disease, diabetes, or alcoholism? This can affect your body's ability to heal following surgery, as well as which anesthetic agents and pain medications your doctor can use and how you react to them. Your age can become a risk factor, too—in general, if you're over age 60, you face greater risks during surgery than you would if you were younger. This is partly because you're more likely to have other medical problems and partly because your body just isn't as efficient as it used to be.

> **Back Off!**
>
> Beware the "wonder cut" testimonial. This is where a person writes or talks about how wonderful he or she feels after having undergone Dr. Doesgood's patented miracle procedure. Surgery success depends on many variables, few of which have much to do with the procedure itself. As a matter of ethics, few doctors would keep a promising new procedure a secret from other doctors.

Will Surgery Help *Your* Back?

In general, if your main complaint is back pain, however excruciating, you're less likely to find relief from surgery than if you have leg pain. Pain, numbness, and tingling down your leg to your foot are signs that something is pressing against the nerves leaving your spinal cord—a something that often turns out to be a prolapsed disk or spinal stenosis. Spondylolisthesis, in which one vertebra slips forward over the one beneath it, also creates pressure on the nerves and sometimes on the spinal cord. Surgery is often a successful solution for these conditions. Remember, though, that many back problems, such as worn disks and arthritis, come about as a result of the normal degeneration that occurs as we grow older. Unfortunately, there's no cure for this, surgical or otherwise.

For the majority of people, back surgery is an option—known as "elective" in the medical world. Consider this option carefully, even if it appears to be the choice that makes the most sense. Try conservative approaches first. Though surgery has never been safer, it still carries risks both during and after. If something other than surgery can help your back, these are risks you don't have to face.

Back Talk

French barber-surgeon Ambroise Pare (1510–1590), viewed as the father of modern surgery, learned his trade in a Paris hospital as an apprentice treating war casualties. Pare was a quick study, not afraid to blend the learnings of ancient healers with his own observations. Pare's preference for wound dressings made of egg whites and rose oil over the contemporary practice of pouring boiling oil into a wound earned him the gratitude of his patients and a reputation as a skilled healer.

Could Back Surgery Help You? A Self-Quiz

You're reading this book because you have, or have had in the past, back pain serious enough to make you willing to invest in ways to make the pain go away. No doubt you've wondered if maybe, just maybe, you might be a "2-percenter" for whom back surgery can mean a new life. No book can replace the judgment and recommendations of your health care providers. But these five questions can give you a snapshot of how your doctor sees your situation.

1. Do you have numbness or weakness down one or both legs? Yes _____ No _____

2. Do you have a fracture or spondylolisthesis that is putting pressure on your spinal cord or nerves? Yes _____ No _____

3. Have you tried conservative care for at least three months without any relief of your symptoms? Yes _____ No _____

4. Do imaging procedure results show abnormalities that are known to cause the symptoms you have? Yes _____ No _____

5. Do two or more specialists agree on a surgical solution for your problem? Yes _____ No _____

If you can't answer "yes" to at least three of these questions, hold off on surgery. You more likely have a problem that surgery can't fix.

Choosing a Surgeon

For several centuries, choosing a surgeon was fairly simple. You walked down the main street of any town or city and looked for a red and white striped pole. It was the same way you found a haircut—the master of the razor was both barber and surgeon. A popular barber was worth the wait, whichever service you needed. Not surprisingly, no one went looking for a surgeon unless there was no other alternative.

Between the battlefield and the laboratory, surgical methods slowly improved. Advances in anesthesia made surgery more tolerable for patients, and the discovery of antibiotics dramatically improved outcomes. Surgery today is a sophisticated specialty requiring several years of training. Many surgeons sub-specialize in particular areas, such as those most likely to perform back surgery—orthopedics (bone) or neurosurgery (brain and nerves).

Orthopedic Surgeon or Neurosurgeon?

Your spine is a bundle of nerves and bone. Should a bone specialist or a nerve specialist operate on it? Maybe both. An *orthopedic surgeon* looks at your back from the perspective of its bone and cartilage structure. What can surgery do to improve the structure? A *neurosurgeon*, on the other hand, views your back as a network of nerves. What can surgery do to restore the network's function to normal? The answers to these questions often straddle the line between the two specialties. A bone or cartilage problem interferes with a nerve's function. Fix the former, and you fix the latter. For this reason, the surgical team that operates on your back may include both an orthopedic surgeon and a neurosurgeon.

Back Basics

An **orthopedic surgeon** specializes in treating problems of your body's skeletal structure. This includes bones and connective tissue. A **neurosurgeon** specializes in treating problems related to your brain, spinal cord, and nervous system.

Measuring Up

More important than which specialty your surgeon represents are his qualifications to practice in that specialty. Look for a surgeon who is *board certified* in his specialty. Surgeons complete five to seven years of specialized training after completing medical school, at the end of which they apply for board certification as evidence of their expertise. Board certification requires doctors to take a series of rigorous tests to demonstrate their knowledge and competence in their chosen specialties. Different organizations certify different specialties. Orthopedic surgeons, for example, receive board certification through the American Board of Orthopedic Surgery (ABOS) and are designated as "diplomates" when they achieve board certification.

While board certification is a key qualifying factor, it's not the only one. How many times has your surgeon performed the procedure she recommends for you? Is the procedure standard or experimental? How often does the procedure succeed? Does your surgeon teach other doctors how to do the procedure, or write about it for medical journals? This is not always easy information to obtain, but it can make a difference (most surgeons will tell you if you ask). And don't be afraid to use your subjective judgment. How do you feel about this surgeon? Are you comfortable putting your back and your life in her hands? You want similar information about the hospital where you'll have your surgery. Does your surgeon do your kind of surgery there often? Do other surgeons? If so, the hospital's surgical team is familiar with your surgeon's routines, which makes for smoother interaction. The hospital's nursing team is also familiar with postoperative care for your kind of surgery. Your care is a team effort, and it helps when the team members are experienced. Practice may not make them perfect, but it sure makes them better at what they do.

Back Basics

A physician who is **board certified** has completed extensive additional training and passed a series of rigorous tests in his chosen specialty. A physician who is board eligible has completed the training necessary to take the board examinations.

Only Fools Rush In

Unless you stand to lose the use of your legs, back surgery isn't likely to be an emergency. (Some fractures, spinal tumors, and severe sciatica that affects bowel or bladder function can be emergencies.) Nonsurgical treatment is almost always an option, so take enough time to gather the information you need to make a decision based on knowledge, not just on pain or the promise of relief.

Do You Need Another Opinion?

Put yourself in this situation. Your car's been making strange noises lately, and you finally got worried enough to take it in to the mechanic for a checkup. The news is not good—the mechanic says you need a new transmission. It'll take a week in the shop and cost about $1,000. What do you do? Another mechanic might have a totally different perspective, suggesting that you change your transmission fluid and filter, then drive the car for a while and see how it behaves. And a third mechanic might say the problem's not your transmission at all, but a faulty computer chip. Each diagnosis and recommendation has different costs and levels of inconvenience.

If you got three such diverse opinions, you might just want to trade your car for a bicycle! At the very least, you'd probably go to the library to read up on transmissions. The point is, even something that should be straightforward and mechanical often isn't. Your back may have its mechanical tendencies, but it's far from straightforward. And unfortunately, as we've mentioned, back surgery is not always successful.

Back surgery is a major undertaking. Given its risks, and the high percentage of surgeries that fail to accomplish what they set out to do, it's to your advantage to get another opinion. Don't worry about hurting your doctor's feelings—second and even third opinions are very common when considering various treatment options. In fact, when your primary care doctor sends you to a surgeon, he does so to get another opinion.

When you schedule an appointment for another opinion, consider seeing a doctor who specializes in a different area of medicine than the doctor who recommended surgery. If you first saw an orthopedic surgeon, schedule a second opinion appointment with a neurosurgeon. This gives you a different perspective on your situation, and may present alternatives you hadn't previously considered.

Other practitioners can offer still more perspectives, though beware information overload. Which ones might provide useful options for you to consider depends largely on what kind of back problem you have. Weigh your options carefully before making a decision.

What You Don't Know Can Hurt You: Informed Consent

"Informed consent" is a concept with both legal and personal elements. For your doctor and the hospital where you have your surgery, informed consent is a legal document you sign giving your permission for the surgery to take place. Your signature also certifies that your doctor explained the potential benefits and risks of your surgery to you.

From your perspective, informed consent means that you've gathered as much information as possible about your diagnosed condition and the various treatment options available. After careful consideration, you've decided surgery offers the greatest potential.

Back Talk

The Internet's World Wide Web has become an easy and amazing source of information on nearly any topic. With a computer, a modem, and a telephone line, this vast, virtual library is right at your fingertips. Use caution and common sense when evaluating what you find. There is, unfortunately, a lot of misinformation and outright advertising out there, too, and sometimes it's hard to identify. Look for corroborating sources and reputable sites, such as those sponsored by professional organizations.

While doctors and hospitals want you to fully understand your surgery and its possible outcomes, they tend to emphasize the legal elements of informed consent. Take informed consent to heart. Be sure you fully understand all aspects of surgery before agreeing to it. Whether it's the right decision for you is seldom clear-cut, and you may even see specialists whose opinions differ.

Ask lots of questions. Make a list of your questions and go over them until you feel comfortable (most surgeons are happy to share what they know with you). Be sure you fully understand what your surgeon expects the surgery to accomplish. Could you end up worse off than you are now? What is the likelihood of that happening? How soon can you expect to be back to your regular activities? Back to work? Fully recovered?

Preparing for Surgery

Once you make the decision to have surgery, do what you can to be ready. You'll probably have several weeks before your surgery date. Use that time to smooth the way for your recovery.

Give Up the Smokes

If you smoke, you read (or at least see) the warnings every time you tap a cigarette out of the package. You may view your decision to smoke as a lifestyle choice, and we won't argue with that. One of the things that makes our country so great is the tremendous freedom we have to make choices about how we live, no matter how detrimental those choices are. But there are consequences for those choices, and with smoking, one is that you make yourself an undesirable candidate for surgery.

Back Care

Can't count the number of times you've tried to quit smoking? The typical smoker makes three to five unsuccessful attempts before becoming a nonsmoker for good. When you slip, try to identify what triggered the temptation. Put your cigarettes away, and plan in advance three ways you can derail the temptation when it surfaces again. Every time you try to quit, you move closer to success, so hang in there!

You may think of smoking as something that primarily affects your lungs. It does, of course, but smoking affects your whole body from your teeth to your toes. Nicotine, the addictive chemical in tobacco, constricts (narrows) blood vessels throughout your body. Less blood gets through to cells that do all the work living requires, so they get less nutrition and oxygen. Working with limited resources is challenge enough under ordinary circumstances. The call to engage in healing can be more than your straining cells can handle.

Numerous studies show a much higher failure rate in surgeries such as spinal fusions (fusing two or more vertebrae together to stabilize and support your spine) in smokers than in nonsmokers. Smokers also experience more pain after surgery than their nonsmoking counterparts, and get less relief from pain medications. The difference is significant enough that a growing number of back surgeons will not take a smoker to surgery. A smoker's lungs don't do the best job of handling anesthetic, either. Smoking increases other risks of surgery as well, from blood clots and pneumonia to heart attack.

There's even some evidence pointing a finger at smoking as a factor contributing to disk problems. Even under ideal circumstances, intervertebral disks don't exactly have an abundant supply of blood. When smoking shuts down what they do get, disks become almost brittle. This makes them especially vulnerable to herniation and degeneration.

Making a major lifestyle change is hard and requires strong motivation. If you're facing surgery, this is the perfect time to stop smoking. Ask your doctor about the many smoking-cessation aids now available to help you ease free from nicotine's grip. Go ahead, give 'em up. You have nothing to lose and everything to gain.

Eat for Good Health

It's sometimes hard to eat right when you feel bad, so focus on good nutrition while you're waiting for your turn in the operating room. Watch what you eat and try to improve the nutritional value of what passes your lips. Add more fruits and vegetables to each meal and cut back on the sweets and fats. This will both reduce calories and increase your intake of important vitamins and minerals. Fat's not all bad, after all—it is your body's stored energy supply, which could come in handy to meet the extra demands of healing.

Some foods may even alter your body's ability to perceive pain. Red wines, hard cheeses, and chocolate are well known for their ability to trigger migraine headaches. They may do the same for other pain as well. Other foods may help your body release natural pain-relieving substances. People who eat a diet high in yellow and orange vegetables, rice, greens, and noncitrus fruits typically require less pain medication following surgery than those whose diets are low in these foods. Nutrition may play a much more significant role in healing than we know.

Drop a Few of Those Extra Pounds

If your back hurts, the last thing that's on your mind is exercise. If it hurts to lie on the couch, your pain-distorted brain tells you, just imagine what it'll feel like to walk around the block. Well, sit up and change the channel. Sure, it may not feel that great to walk. But we can almost guarantee you won't feel worse than you already do.

Your body needs regular activity to keep it functioning at peak performance—not just your muscles but all body systems. Try taking a deep breath while lying on the couch or sitting in your recliner. Not an easy thing to do, is it? Now stand up (gently and slowly). Stretch your muscles a bit (again, gently and slowly), and take a nice, deep breath. Let it out and take another. Don't you feel

Back Basics

The process by which your cells use energy and clear waste is called **metabolism**. When your metabolic rate is high—during activity and exercise—your cells use more energy and your body burns more calories. When your metabolic rate is low, your body converts more calories to fat.

185

better already? Now imagine how you'll feel walking around the block, taking in deep breaths of fresh air!

Regular activity, even if limited by your pain, revs up your body's *metabolism*. That means you're burning more of the calories you're taking in. (And if you've been lying around on the couch with nothing to do but snarf snacks and channel-surf, you're probably taking in far more calories than your body needs. (Sorry to hit you when you're already hurting, but your clothes don't shrink between doctor appointments.)

Extra weight puts extra stress on all of your body systems, especially the one that supports you. Consider that each leg is roughly 15 percent of your body weight. If you weigh 150 pounds, each leg weighs about 22 pounds (about the same as a two-year-old child). Every time you take a step, your leg and back muscles lift and drop that weight. Remember the pendulum effect? The farther away from your body the weight is, the more strength and energy it takes to move it. So that 22 or so pounds is a pretty hefty load from your back's perspective.

The best time to manage your weight, of course, is before it grows on you. But it's never too late to make changes. Unless your doctor specifically tells you not to, add small doses of physical activity to your daily life. Even a few lost pounds help your back, not to mention better-conditioned muscles.

Prepare Your Body/Mind Connection

If back pain has been your constant companion for some time, you might already be using meditation and relaxation techniques to help relieve stress and pain. Once you know surgery is in your future, you can use these methods to help you relax through the rigors and stresses of surgery.

Back to Nature

It's no joke that laughter is called the best medicine. Laughing boosts your mood and takes your mind off your problems. Rent funny movies to watch while you're recovering, and encourage your friends to share jokes and humorous stories.

You don't have to do anything fancy or formal to meditate. Many people find soothing music helps set the mood (Mozart is a common favorite). You might also prefer to listen to a guided meditation or guided imagery (visualization) tape. What you do is less important than that you do it. (Chapter 14 covers these methods in detail.) Meditation helps you relax and find the calm within, while visualization helps you "see" the outcome you desire in your mind's eye. Prayer is another method for connecting with a source of comfort and healing that is beyond yourself.

Though your meditation and visualization methods may seem worlds away when you're wheeled into the recovery room after surgery, you can still put them to work as your anesthesia wears off.

Prepare Your Home and Your Family

Depending on the kind of surgery you're having, you may need help with basics like dressing and bathing when you return home after surgery. Involve your significant other in some of your doctor's appointments and planning activities, so he or she knows what to expect. Do you have children at home? Explain your surgery to them, and help them understand that you may not feel or look your old self right at first, but that you'll rapidly improve as your back heals. Let them play small roles in your recovery plans to help them feel needed and appreciated. Young children, especially, are frightened by a parent's temporary inability to function normally.

Here are some things you can do in advance to make your after-surgery experience less stressful:

➤ In the two weeks or so before your surgery, package and freeze an individual serving of the meals you prepare. After your surgery, you can just pop one in the microwave for a nutritious, delicious meal.

➤ If your recovery will take some time, consider installing grab bars, raised toilet seats, and a shower or bath chair in your bathroom. There are numerous other assist devices available to make life easier, too—talk with your surgeon about those that might be helpful for you.

➤ The evening before your surgery, pick up throw rugs and other items that you might trip on after surgery.

➤ Set up a "recovery station" for your first few days or so at home following surgery. Have your medications, a glass or pitcher of water, the telephone, and TV or stereo controls within easy reach.

➤ Protect your need to rest, especially for the first few days after your surgery. A few days before your surgery, establish a time (or times) for friends to call or visit, and let them know you won't answer the telephone or door at other times. Then turn off the telephone for a few hours at a time, so you really can rest.

If you'll stay overnight in the hospital, find out when your surgeon is likely to release you and arrange for someone to pick you up. If your surgeon plans to give you prescription pain relievers for the days immediately after your surgery, have the prescription filled and ready for you before you leave the hospital.

Be Sure You're Covered

Since few back surgeries are emergencies, many health insurance policies require authorization before they'll cover the costs. Your doctor may have to fill out a form or send a letter explaining how the planned surgery will improve your condition. Your doctor's office will probably ask you about insurance and may take care of all the necessary arrangements. The hospital, too, will ask about your insurance coverage. However, you're responsible for all the bills in the end, so it's worth your while to give your insurance company or health plan office a call a few days before your surgery just to be sure everything is squared away.

The Least You Need to Know

➤ Surgery is done for about two out of every 100 people who have back pain. Even people with herniated disks usually improve without surgery, though surgery may produce faster relief.

➤ All surgery has risks, and can cause more problems than you started with. Learn as much as you can about your condition, so you can make informed and wise decisions about your care.

➤ What you eat and whether you smoke are lifestyle matters that can have a major influence on how quickly you recover from surgery.

➤ Surgery is most effective for relieving the leg pain associated with herniated disks or spinal stenosis—it is less successful for back pain.

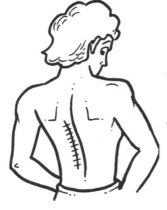

Chapter 16

What to Expect with Surgery

In This Chapter

➤ Presurgery preparations

➤ Different kinds of anesthesia

➤ Common back surgeries

➤ When back surgery fails

No one likes surprises when it comes to surgery. Knowing what to expect can make your surgery experience a more pleasant one. Doctors and hospitals handle hundreds or thousands of surgeries a year, and sometimes lose sight of how things look from the patient's viewpoint. Though each surgeon and hospital has unique procedures, back surgeries share a number of common aspects.

Countdown to Surgery

Once you and your surgeon agree that surgery is your best treatment choice, the surgeon's office schedules operating room time. This sets a series of events in motion to get you ready for surgery. Your surgeon will probably have a handout that outlines the process for you, all the way from scheduling surgery to your postoperative (after surgery) visits.

Though you may view your scheduled surgery date as if it's carved in stone, there are many reasons it can change right up until the time you're wheeled through the operating room doors. One of the most common reasons for changing the date is irregularities in your presurgery tests. There could be an abnormal value in one of your blood tests, for example, or results that your doctor didn't expect. Your doctor will check out any results that vary from normal before taking you to surgery.

And if you have a cold, don't be surprised if it's the anesthesiologist who puts the kibosh on your plans until it clears up. You need strong, healthy lungs to carry you through surgery and recovery, especially if you have a general anesthetic. You also want your immune system in prime condition for fast healing.

Presurgery Workup

About a week before your scheduled surgery, you'll probably have some basic laboratory tests. Your surgeon's office may handle this, or you may go to the hospital where you'll have your surgery. Generally you'll have some blood drawn for tests to measure your blood's cell counts and clotting ability. Unless you have abnormal results, you probably won't hear anything more about these tests. If you're a heavy smoker or have a history of lung problems, your surgeon may request a chest x-ray.

Back to Nature

Is surgery in your future? It won't hurt to increase your intake of vitamin C, which is vital for soft and connective tissue healing. Even though your body can't store vitamin C, increasing your intake helps assure that your body at least gets as much as it needs. One good source of vitamin C is fortified orange juice.

Meeting with the Anesthesiologist or Nurse Anesthetist

You'll meet with an *anesthesiologist* or *nurse anesthetist* before your surgery, usually during your presurgery workup though sometimes the day of your surgery if you're later on the surgery schedule. This is usually, though not always, the anesthesiologist who will be in the operating room with you.

Back Basics

An **anesthesiologist** is a medical doctor with additional training and expertise in the specialty of anesthesia. A **nurse anesthetist** has a nursing degree with special training in the delivery of anesthesia. The word **anesthesia** comes from Greek words meaning "without sensation."

The person who will give your anesthetic will ask you about any allergies you have, medications you take regularly, ongoing health conditions, lifestyle matters such as alcohol consumption and smoking, and what previous experiences you've had with surgery and anesthesia. He or she will listen to your heart and lungs with a stethoscope, and discuss the kinds of anesthetics typically used for your surgery. Some people prefer a block to a general or vice versa, which the anesthesiologist will take into consideration. The anesthesiologist will also tell you what you can eat and drink the night before surgery, and tell you when you need to be NPO (nothing by mouth). Since many anesthetics can cause nausea, the anesthesiologist doesn't want there to be anything in your stomach for you to throw up. Not only is this messy, but it can also cause you to choke or even get pneumonia if you aspirate (get vomit and saliva down into your lungs).

When the Big Day Arrives

Your surgeon's office will tell you when to be at the hospital. It doesn't hurt to get there a little early, in case there are administrative details left to handle or the admitting department is unusually busy. This gives you a chance to relax and get oriented to your surroundings before heading off to the operating room.

You get to wear those snazzy hospital clothes—a gown that ties down the back and those cute little paper booties. If you're lucky, you also get a bonnet to keep your hair in its place (and not flying all over the operating room). Usually a nurse or other health care professional will come in to put in an IV—an intravenous solution to give your body plenty of fluid.

Back Talk

The "sleep apple" of Snow White fame was actually a medieval form of anesthetic. Those who study such things speculate that the formula saturating the apple was a mixture of opium, mandrake, hemlock, and wine, among other substances—all potential poisons. Snow White is fortunate to have awakened at all. Medieval medical texts instructed healers of the time to have their patients inhale the fumes from a sleep apple, not eat it.

Feel No Pain: Anesthesia

It wasn't so long ago that good anesthesia was a strong, well-placed right hook. A surgeon's reputation relied on speed, not necessarily skill. Through the years, surgeons tried other methods with varying though ultimately unsatisfactory results. To reach unconsciousness, patients had to consume so much of substances such as alcohol and opium that they risked dying from overdose.

In 1846, an observant young dentist named William Thomas Green Morton noticed that ether drops applied to a decayed tooth gave not only relief from toothache but also calmed the sufferer enough for the dentist to pull the offending bicuspid. Morton wondered if ether could numb an entire body in the same way it numbed the gums. As was the custom at the time, he tested the theory on a willing subject—himself. On the evening of September 30, 1846, Morton doused his handkerchief with ether, held it to his nose, and took a deep breath. He awakened eight minutes later, aware of nothing since looking at his watch before he took the fateful breath. Two weeks later Morton repeated the demonstration on a real patient before pulling his tooth, launching a new era in surgery.

Despite its anesthetic qualities, ether was far from perfect. Ether is extremely flammable, and the crude apparatus for using it exposed the administrator to the fumes as well. Dosing was imprecise, and the results unpredictable. Today's anesthesiologists have a wide range of anesthetic agents to choose from, most of which are far safer and easier to use (and more pleasant to awaken from).

Nighty-Night: General Anesthesia

General anesthesia is the most common form of anesthesia for many surgeries. The anesthesiologist will first put you under by giving you a medication in your IV (the catheter, or small plastic tube, in your vein) to float you gently off to sleep. For longer surgeries, the anesthesiologist then will insert a tube through your mouth into your trachea (windpipe) to help you breathe and deliver controlled amounts of anesthetic gas to your lungs. For shorter surgeries, you may also be given oxygen and anesthetic through a mask. Inhaled anesthetic agents induce a deep sleep similar to the level of unconsciousness of a coma. Unlike a coma, however, the sleep is controlled and you awaken as the anesthesiologist lightens or stops the amount of anesthesia you're breathing.

The most significant risk of general anesthesia—a reaction to the anesthetic agent—is rare. General anesthesia does have a tendency to make patients nauseated; the anesthesiologist generally gives you an injection before you fully awaken to help decrease the nausea. You might also have a sore throat from the tube in your throat.

No Sensation: Blocks and Locals

For surgery on your lower back, your doctor may offer you an *epidural* block or even a local anesthetic, depending on your procedure. For a local anesthetic, the anesthesiologist or surgeon injects your skin and the tissues around the surgery site with a drug that numbs the area. You'll feel the pressure of your surgeon's actions, but very little discomfort. Many minimally invasive procedures are done under a local anesthetic. The anesthetic gradually wears off over a period of several hours.

Back Basics

Epidural means "around the hard." The tough casing protecting the brain and spinal cord is called the dura mater ("hard mother"). An epidural anesthetic is injected between the dura mater and the bony spinal canal.

An epidural block is a little more involved. After numbing the skin, the anesthesiologist inserts a needle between the dura and the bony or spinal canal, into a space called the epidural space. He then threads a tiny, flexible tube called a catheter through the needle and removes the needle, leaving the catheter in place. During your surgery, the anesthesiologist can continue to inject enough anesthetic drug through the catheter to keep you comfortable. The catheter can remain in place after surgery as well, to administer medications for postoperative pain relief.

The drug works by numbing the nerve roots as they leave your spinal cord, blocking them from transmitting pain signals (which is why the method is called a "block"). Body parts along the nerve routes lose sensation and the ability to move. As with a local anesthetic, with an epidural block you'll feel the pressure of your surgeon's actions but little or no pain. An epidural block lasts longer than a local—up to several hours depending on the anesthetic drug used. It takes several hours to completely wear off as well.

Though you're awake during a procedure done under a local or a block, the anesthesiologist usually can, if you wish, give you an intravenous sedative to relax you. You may fall asleep, though not into the deep sleep of a general anesthetic.

The one potential drawback to an epidural block is that you can get a monster headache afterward. This happens when the needle nicks the dura, allowing spinal fluid to leak out. Though this is uncommon with an epidural, it does occasionally happen, and is more common with a spinal block. Lying down flat helps prevent a headache after an epidural or spinal block. A "spinal" headache can last for a few hours to several days. The usual treatment is lying flat in bed until the headache goes away.

Back Talk

In the early 1800s, German chemist Friedrich W.A. Sertürner (1783–1841) isolated the chemical ingredients in opium. He noticed that one of them had the ability to relieve pain and produce a deep, euphoric sleep. The substance, which he named "morphine" after the Greek god of sleep, Morpheus, gave doctors the ability to precisely control both dosage and effect. While it is possible to synthetically re-create morphine, the process is long and complicated. Today, manufacturers still produce morphine from opium poppy extract.

Analgesia: Pain Management Immediately After Surgery

You'll usually get an injection of pain medication before you leave the operating room if you've had a general anesthetic, and as your anesthetic begins wearing off if you've had a block or a local. Again, this depends largely on your procedure. Laser surgery and other minimally invasive procedures (surgeries that require very small incisions) are such a limited intrusion into your body that pain after surgery is often minimal as well.

While you're in the recovery room, the nurses who monitor your progress as you emerge from anesthesia may offer you pain medication when you awaken. It's a good idea to take the offer. Pain during the first 24 to 72 hours after surgery is normal. Many hospitals now use PCA (patient controlled analgesia), which allows you to release a measured amount of pain medication into your IV at regular intervals (usually every 10 minutes or less).

Minimally Invasive Procedures

Technology now offers the prospect of new alternatives in surgery. Thanks to the *arthroscope*, in some situations surgeons no longer have to slice you from stem to stern to work on your back. A small incision allows the surgeon to insert the arthroscope into the surgical site. *Fiber optics* light the way, giving the surgeon an excellent view. A channel on the outside of the arthroscope permits the surgeon to insert specially designed flexible surgical instruments that the surgeon operates remotely. These tools can include scalpels (small, razor-sharp knives) for precision cutting, rotating blades for shaving small segments of cartilage and bone, and even laser instruments.

Some minimally invasive procedures can be done under local anesthetic, and patients can walk out of the hospital hours after surgery with minimal discomfort. The nature of your back problem and any complicating factors determine whether a minimally invasive procedure will work for you. Because these procedures are relatively new, they are still considered more experimental than standard. Not all surgeons are qualified, or willing, to perform them.

Back Basics

In a minimally invasive procedure, the surgeon usually uses a special lighted, flexible tube called an **arthroscope** to view the surgical site and carry out the surgery. Endoscopes rely on **fiber optics**, bundles of hair-like glass threads that transmit light at its full strength from the light source to the end of the tube.

Back Talk

The word "laser" is actually an acronym that stands for "light application by simulated emission of radiation." While the light from an ordinary light bulb contains many different wavelengths, a laser sends out a beam of light that is compressed into a single wavelength. An infrared laser uses a low-frequency wavelength that generates heat as it cuts. An ultraviolet laser (called an eximer laser when used for medical purposes) uses a high-frequency wavelength that penetrates without generating any heat. The beam cuts by breaking the chemical bonds that hold cells together. This gives the surgeon very precise control.

Radiofrequency Thermocoagulation

Radiofreqency thermocoagulation, also called radiofrequency ablation, uses electrical impulses to burn away very small amounts of selected tissue. For back pain, surgeons often use this procedure to shrink an inflamed joint lining to reduce swelling. When the lining of a facet joint becomes inflamed, it can put pressure on the root nerves exiting from the spinal cord. Reducing the swelling relieves the pressure and usually the pain. Surgeons may also use this procedure to destroy certain nerves, such as those feeding facet joints, purely as a last resort pain relief measure.

Radiofrequency thermocoagulation may not relieve pain over the long haul. The same circumstances that set the stage for an inflamed joint lining—normal degenerative processes—are likely to recur, and with them comes the return of the pain. Like minimally invasive surgery, radiofrequency thermocoagulation is more experimental than some other techniques we've discussed here because there isn't yet enough evidence to demonstrate consistent effectiveness.

Percutaneous Procedures

Percutaneous procedures often take place on an outpatient basis with local anesthesia or an epidural block. The surgeon inserts an arthroscope through a small incision in the skin, from which he or she can view the problem disk. Using micro-instruments manipulated from outside the scope, the surgeon can cut away the protruding portions of the disk so there is no longer pressure on the nerves.

Percutaneous procedures remain experimental, largely because there is little evidence to support their effectiveness. In fact, percutaneous laser surgery has proven to be less effective than other surgical procedures. Get another opinion before seriously considering percutaneous surgery.

Back Basics

Percutaneous means "through the skin." In percutaneous surgeries, the surgeon makes a very small incision and inserts an arthroscope through which the surgeon can see and manipulate instruments.

Open Procedures

In an open procedure, your surgeon makes and works through an incision over the trouble spot. She typically cuts through muscle and connective tissue to reach and repair the damaged area. Open procedures are almost always done under general anesthesia, and can take several hours. Some open procedures are same-day surgery, while others require a day or two in the hospital following surgery.

Microdiskectomy

Microdiskectomy is the standard surgery for prolapsed disk problems. In a micro-diskectomy, the surgeon makes an incision (usually two or three inches long) over the involved vertebrae, and cuts through the muscle and connective tissue to expose the bone. Viewing the area through a *surgical binocular microscope*, the surgeon uses conventional instruments to remove the damaged disk. The microscope magnifies the area to give the surgeon a clear view. Microdiskectomy is often an outpatient surgery. If you have a microdiskectomy, plan on spending two to six weeks recovering at home before returning to your regular activities.

Back Basics

A **surgical binocular microscope** is a viewing device with two eyepieces that magnifies the area in which the surgeon is working. The dual eyepieces allow the surgeon to see three-dimensionally. The magnification makes it possible to operate through a much smaller incision.

Back Basics

Laminae are the bony arches of the vertebrae that you can feel when you run your fingers down your spine. One arch is called a lamina. The word is Latin and means "thin plate."

Conventional Laminotomy and Diskectomy

In a laminotomy and diskectomy, the surgeon makes a substantial incision along the top of the spine, cutting through skin, muscle, and connective tissue to expose the vertebrae. The surgeon then removes pieces of the vertebrae, called *laminae*, on either side of the damaged disk. These pieces are the bony arches you can feel when you touch your spine. After removing the laminae, the surgeon can cut the damaged disk away from the nerves and spinal cord.

Conventional laminectomy and diskectomy are major undertakings, typically used only when the surgeon can't get to the herniation through a less invasive procedure. Most patients spend about five days recuperating in the hospital, and another three to six weeks recovering at home before being able to return to regular activities. Though the surgery leaves a significant scar, it has a success rate of about 96 percent, with a 7 percent recurrence rate. This means that most people experience relief from their disk problems and pain following surgery, though a few will have back problems again in the future.

Spinal Fusion

Surgeons perform spinal fusion surgery to permanently join two or more vertebrae. The procedure requires the surgeon to craft supporting structures from bone (usually taken from your hip) or from synthetic materials. Generally, rods, plates, hooks, and screws temporarily hold the fusion in place until it fully heals (about six months). A second surgery removes the hardware when the fusion is stable.

Spinal fusions are sometimes necessary to correct spondylolisthesis, spinal stenosis, and scoliosis. The procedure can also stabilize your spine when you have severe osteoarthritis, dislocated facet joints (as might occur in a motor vehicle accident), or a tumor removed. Most spinal fusions are done as open surgeries, since there is often significant damage to repair. However, some fusions can be done through percutaneous endoscopic surgery.

Recovery from spinal fusion surgery can be extensive. The typical patient spends five to seven days in the hospital, then goes home for six to eight weeks of limited activity. This may be changing, however. A recent research study had some patients follow the traditional recovery strategy while some other patients went back to work and regular activities after just two weeks or less of rest at home. The study coordinators found that those patients who got right back to living healed faster and felt better about the whole experience.

Though spinal fusion may fix one problem, it may create others. Permanently fusing vertebrae alters your spine's natural mobility. Reduced mobility can put pressure on other disks and vertebrae, resulting in aches and pains you didn't have before.

Will Once Be Enough?

For 70 to 80 percent of those who have back surgery, once will do it. For the remaining 20 to 30 percent, however, back surgery doesn't live up to its expectations. If this seems like a high rate to you, you're not alone—it's the main reason surgery is a last-resort treatment for most back problems. Failed back surgery is so commonplace, in fact, that there's a syndrome for it—read on!

Failed Back Surgery Syndrome (FBSS)

The success rate for your back surgery depends on what kind of surgery it is. Open procedures are the most likely to succeed. Endoscopic, or closed, procedures are much more likely to fail—that is, leave you feeling worse than you did before surgery.

The symptoms of FBSS usually surface within two years of your surgery, and are all too familiar—a recurrence of your pain as well as tingling, numbness, and weakness in your leg on the affected side (and sometimes both sides). You're now in the unenviable position of deciding whether to have another surgery or tough it out with nonsurgical treatment.

Though many people opt for repeat surgery, there is growing evidence that holding out may be the better choice over the long term if your problem is a herniated disk. About 85 percent of all disk problems will heal themselves if allowed enough time, even without surgery (though this can take a year or so). The damaged disk's tissues eventually shrink and recede, relinquishing their stranglehold on your nerves. Once the pressure subsides, the pain soon does, too. The $64,000 question is, can you wait it out? There's no way to tell in advance which approach will work for you.

Though imaging procedures often confirm the presence of scar tissue in and around nerves in FBSS, equally often there's no visible evidence of any physical damage or reason for continued pain. This is particularly frustrating for those who had a clear reason for the pain that took them into surgery (a herniated or prolapsed disk), then end up with pain for which there is no identifiable cause. Some doctors believe that during the healing process following surgery, regenerated nerves get their signals crossed and send messages that your brain interprets as pain.

An experimental procedure called epiduroscopy may bring relief to those who have scar tissue pressing on nerves. During epiduroscopy, the surgeon uses a special endoscope called a myeloscope to view the area of scarring. After loosening the scar tissue (usually with a pressurized stream of saline solution), the surgeon can inject the area with a chemical substance that dissolves the scar tissue and releases the pressure on the nerves. The surgeon may also inject a local anesthetic for longer pain relief and a steroid to further reduce swelling.

Is It Worth a Repeat?

Overall, between 15 and 20 percent of those who have back surgery do it again within two to four years. Whether it's worthwhile for you to repeat a failed back surgery depends on your situation. For continuing pain apparently related to the same problem for which you've already had one surgery, another surgery isn't likely to help and may do even more harm.

The likelihood that you'll improve declines with each surgery for the same problem—from a little over 50 percent for the second surgery to about 25 percent with a fourth or fifth surgery. The flip side is that 45 percent of surgical patients say they are *worse* after a fourth or fifth operation. So the odds are against you. If another disk ruptures, however, or a new problem develops, your odds of success with a second surgery are about the same as if you'd never had back surgery.

Unfortunately, there's no crystal ball to tell surgeons which patients will enjoy success and which will suffer failure with back surgery. You and your doctor may feel that you have little choice but to try surgery again if it doesn't work the first time. Though you may find it hard to believe when yours is prodding and poking your painful back, doctors are compassionate people who don't like to see others suffer. That's why they choose to devote their lives to healing. So if there's a chance another surgery will help you, they're usually willing to support that option. Again, it's up to you to weigh the pros and cons.

What happens if you decide against a repeat surgery? The result is no more certain than if you give the scalpel another shot. Some people gradually get better, learning to adapt to the limitations of a sensitive back. Others continue to experience pain and their search for relief from it. Even if you're in the latter category, don't give up hope. There are many alternative approaches that could help (which we discuss in later chapters).

The Least You Need to Know

➤ There are many options available in anesthesia today to make your surgery experience as comfortable as possible.

➤ Many new techniques in surgery are more experimental than standard.

➤ Though back surgery is great when it accomplishes its intended purpose, it can also create other problems.

➤ About a fourth of all back surgeries fail to achieve their intended purposes. Be sure you understand what your surgeon expects surgery to do for you and what risks you face.

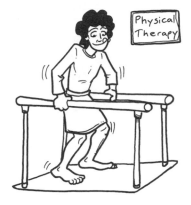

Chapter 17

The Road to Recovery

In This Chapter

➤ Getting your recovery off to a good start

➤ How to manage postoperative pain

➤ Physical therapy and your personal rehabilitation program

➤ Keep the faith—life does get easier!

Though you probably slept through most of the action, your body has been through quite an ordeal. It's been cut, poked, prodded, tugged, and sewed—and it's not especially happy about it. Just after surgery, it hurts. And it will hurt for the first few days, until the swelling goes down and the wound starts to heal. Don't panic—swelling is a normal body response to injury of any sort, even surgery. And you'll be enjoying the activities of your life before you know it.

"Will I Ever Be the Same?"

Surgical pain heals fairly quickly (easy for us to say). You should be pleasantly surprised to discover that you feel better and stronger every day. You may be back to normal in no time.

Surgery offers no guarantees, of course. You and your surgeon both hope you'll feel better after surgery than you did before, and most people do. The kind of surgery you've had determines how close to "before" you'll get when your recovery is complete.

You might start thinking in terms of how you want to be now, rather than comparing your present to your past. After all, you know so much more about back health now that you've had back surgery. You understand the importance of exercise and nutrition. You know that regular exercise keeps your back and body strong and healthy. You may not want to return to the way things were, but to instead focus on moving forward into a life where back pain is but a distant memory. But first things first. Let's get your recovery underway.

Keeping a Lid on Postoperative Pain

Most people feel much better after surgery, even though they may have some *postoperative* pain. Gone is the pain that defined their lives for so long. (A few even feel like dancing for joy right there in the recovery room, though we suggest you hold off until the anesthetic wears off completely and you regain your senses.) Oh, sure, there's some surgery-related pain (which can downright take your breath away with one wrong move). The great thing about surgery pain, though, is that those surgery wounds generally heal very quickly. Postoperative pain just doesn't hang around for long.

For many people, the fear of pain after surgery is far worse than the pain itself. Depending on what kind of surgery you've had, your doctor will prescribe or recommend an analgesic. Many of the over-the-counter NSAIDs are as effective at relieving postoperative pain as mild narcotics are, and have fewer side effects.

Discuss pain relief with your doctor before you leave the hospital, so you're prepared when it's time to walk out the door. If you have drug allergies, or have previously had an unpleasant experience with a pain medication, let your doctor know before your prescription goes to the pharmacy. As excited as you may be to get back home, your body's pretty tired after all it's been through. You don't want to wait around while the nurses try to track down your doctor.

For the first few days after your surgery, you might want to take pain medication on a regular schedule. Maintaining a constant level in your system helps soothe the nerves irritated by surgery, keeping pain at bay. As you start feeling better, switch to taking pain relievers just as you need them. Remember, it takes 30 to 45 minutes for pain medication to make its way into your system.

Wound Care

No matter what kind of surgery you've had, you have a wound that needs care. With a percutaneous procedure, that could mean nothing more than changing a

Back Basics

Postoperative means after the surgery. You may hear it shortened to "postop."

Back Care

Nausea is an unfortunate but common side effect of many pain medications, especially those that contain codeine. Take your medications with a full glass of water and some crackers or bread. This will give your stomach something else to work on so it doesn't get quite as upset. If your pain medication makes you throw up each time you take it, ask your doctor to prescribe or recommend something else.

Band-Aid. For more extensive open surgery, you could have sutures (stitches) or staples and a dressing. You'll receive written instructions for how to care for your surgery site when you leave the hospital.

Dressing Changes

Often, your surgeon will remove any sutures right before you go home, or at your first postoperative visit. Many surgery sites don't need bandages by the time you come home. The exposure to air helps the wound heal, and your clothing keeps the area clean. If your surgeon tells you you'll need dressing supplies, buy them before you have your surgery or have someone buy them for you before you go home. You'll probably need someone to help you remove the old bandages and put on new ones.

Showering and Bathing

You can resume showering or bathing as soon as you feel like doing so following most surgeries. If you have sutures or staples, check with your surgeon about any bathing restrictions.

Taking a bath might be another story. To reduce the risk of infection, don't sit in a tub of water until your surgery wound heals completely. Also, when your incision site stays wet, the edges get soft and can begin to pull apart. The soggy tissues look pretty appealing to infection-causing bacteria, which might drop in and try to make themselves at home.

After showering, allow your back to dry completely before getting dressed. Don't use talc or other after-shower powders on your back until it's completely healed.

Preventing Infection

Surgical wounds are very clean. First, your surgery takes place in a *sterile* environment, with sterile instruments. The surgeon scrubs your skin with an *antiseptic* solution before making a single cut. Second, those cuts the surgeon makes have sharp, even edges. When it's time to close them up, they make a smooth line. It's the kind of wound an infection likes least—there are no ragged nooks for it to gain a foothold.

Within a few days, the wound's edges are firmly sealed and well on their way to healing. After this point, infection is unlikely. To keep it this way, keep the area dry and clean. Unlike your hands, which are out there getting into everything, your back is sheltered. If you have a large incision site, follow your doctor's instructions for dressing changes and protecting the area. Before changing a dressing (yours or a loved one's) wash your hands with antibacterial soap for 15 seconds.

Back Basics

Environments or instruments that are **sterile** are germ free. **Antiseptic** chemicals clean skin and other surfaces, destroying bacteria and microorganisms that could cause disease. An **antibiotic** is a drug that fights bacterial infections.

In the real world, bacteria are everywhere (though not all are bad—many serve useful purposes until they get somewhere they shouldn't be). Bacteria especially like to live where it's warm and moist. If you notice any signs that your incision could be getting infected—such as swelling, redness, or increased pain at the site, or a fever—contact your surgeon's office right away. Your surgeon may want you to take an *antibiotic* to keep any infection from settling in.

Regaining Strength and Function

You've been at less than your best for quite some time now. First the back problems, then the surgery. It's time to get back in shape. It'll take some effort on your part to regain strength and function in your back as well as in other muscle groups that haven't gotten much of a workout since your back problems took you out of action. Be patient! You will make progress, even if it seems like slow going for a while.

Generally, for the first six weeks following your surgery, you can walk, use a stair-climbing machine, and swim (after your stitches are out). Your surgeon may also restrict certain activities, such as lifting, bending, and twisting, for up to 12 weeks (depending on your surgery).

Physical Therapy

If you've had back problems for a long time, as have most people recovering from back surgery, going to physical therapy for postop rehab might be like going to visit old friends. If you've been seeing the same doctors during your back problems, in fact, you're probably going back to the same clinic that worked with you before your surgery. Some of the treatments probably will look and feel familiar, too.

Your physical therapy clinic no doubt works frequently with patients referred by your surgeon, and they know what outcomes your surgeon expects. The clinic has numerous written procedures for various surgeries. Your surgeon knows that the clinic's therapists will take the time to learn about you and your particular situation, and develop a rehab program that integrates the appropriate written procedures with your needs.

Physical therapy aims to restore function and flexibility not just in your back but also in other muscle groups that support your back's activities—arms, legs, and abdomen. Before your surgery, your back pain limited your motion and strength. Now, your surgery has fixed the problem causing that pain.

But during surgery, your surgeon may have cut through muscles and connective tissue to get inside your spine. Your body views the incisions as damage, and treats them like wounds (which, technically, they are). So it protects those muscles while they heal by making it hurt when you use them. Physical therapy has to treat those muscles, too, to get you back in peak operating condition.

Your rehab program may run several weeks to several months, depending on what kind of surgery you've had and how long you've been on the inactive list. The goal of every rehab program is to return you to your regular lifestyle—smarter, stronger, more fit, and confident in your ability to maintain back-healthy habits.

Range of Motion

How far can you lift and extend each arm and leg? How far can you bend forward, backward, and from side to side? These actions—called flexion, extension, abduction, and adduction—give an indication of your flexibility and your range of motion. Flexion is the action of bending, and extension is the action of straightening. Abduction is the action of moving your arms and legs away from your body, and adduction is the action of moving your arms and legs toward your body (laterally, or to the sides). These actions measure in degrees how far and in how many directions you can move.

At first, the physical therapist will support and assist you as you go through a series of stretches and exercises to improve your ability to move through a reasonable range of motion. The therapist may start with a *diathermy* or *ultrasound* treatment to warm your muscles and increase circulation. Depending on your needs and your rate of recovery, your physical therapy may involve a variety of conditioning and strengthening exercises as well. Once you're more comfortable in a routine, you can practice your exercises at home. (Be sure to comply with any restrictions your surgeon has given you for bending or twisting.)

Teaching Your "Old" Body New Tricks

Odds are, you've developed quite a few bad habits through the years. Now is the perfect opportunity to teach your "old" back some new tricks. In addition to working with you on flexibility and mobility, the physical or occupational therapist will help you develop positive posture habits, lifting methods, and back-safe ways to handle the activities of your life.

Exercises You Can Do at Home

Your physical therapist can show you exercises you can do at home that complement your rehab program. Until your rehabilitation is complete, don't do exercises on your own without consulting

Back Basics

Diathermy and **ultrasound** are forms of heat treatment to relax muscles and increase their blood supply. Diathermy generates heat by directing high-frequency electrical currents into body tissues. Ultrasound uses high-frequency sound waves to produce a similar effect. Neither method hurts, though you can feel warmth and sometimes tingling.

Back Care

Be sure to stretch properly before beginning home exercises. Physical therapists recommend a three- to five-minute routine of gentle stretches to ready your muscles for action. Stretch all major muscle groups, even if you plan to exercise only one or two of them.

either your doctor or your physical therapist. The exercises you may have done before surgery will again be helpful for conditioning your back and preventing pain, though your surgery site may need to heal completely before you can do them safely.

Returning to Regular Activities

As soon as you're feeling better, you'll be eager to return to your regular activities—particularly if back pain has long kept you from the experiences you enjoy. For many routine activities, the sooner you return to them, the better, as far as your back is concerned. Some discomfort is normal, especially if you're doing things you haven't done for a long time. Sharp or sudden pain is a warning, however. Stop until the pain goes away, then resume what you were doing slowly. If pain hits again, describe the situation to your physical therapist at your next visit.

Back Talk

A study of Marine recruits who sprained their ankles during boot camp showed that while they were generally able to return to regular activities after six weeks, their injured ankles didn't feel "right" for about six months. To reach 100 percent sometimes you have to get back to living while you're still at less than 100 percent.

Sitting and Standing

Everyone has a beloved chair or sofa that's the perfect place to relax and rest. Take a look at yours with the fresh eyes of one who wants to keep this repaired back in tiptop shape. Is it low to the floor and a bit on the saggy side? Does it suck you in and wrap around you when you sit down, and refuse to give you up without a struggle? As many happy hours as you've shared with those cushions, it might be time to find a new favorite.

The ideal chair provides firm thigh and lower back support. Many recliners do a good job of this, and some even have adjustable back supports. Many sofas and armchairs provide good support, too, and you can always place a lumbar cushion or rolled towel behind your lower back for extra support. Lower yourself onto, and raise yourself up from, a sitting position by using your thighs and arms as much as possible.

When you stand, take care not to lock your knees. This posture tips your pelvis forward, which exaggerates your lumbar curve and throws the rest of your spine out of its natural alignment. Don't stand or sit in the same position for longer than 15 or 20 minutes. Get up and move around to keep your muscles loose and your back flexible.

Stay tuned in to how your body feels during the activities of your life. Do you bend over when you stand at the sink to do dishes or at the counter to prepare dinner? Practice standing tall and upright. Or consider not standing at all, but sitting on a tall stool instead.

Driving

Driving has become such a mainstay of modern living that taking away your wheels takes away your independence. No one likes to rely on others for conveniences like running to the store for milk. Being able to drive again is a return to self-sufficiency, a sure sign that your recovery is nearly complete.

Don't push it. While not being able to drive is a major inconvenience, don't lose sight of the responsibility driving encompasses. When you buckle that seatbelt and turn the key, you must be ready to react to any situation that confronts you—even if you're just going to the store for milk. Quick movements behind the wheel—avoiding a dog in the road or a child whose bicycle is out of control—involve both your reflexes and your responses. You must be fully alert (what are you taking for pain and when did you last take it?) and your muscles must be capable of responding to your brain's frantic "brake and turn the wheel now!" commands, not frozen by unexpected pain.

For a while, your back will be sensitive and vulnerable. This would not be an especially good time to get in a car accident (not that any time ever is). The force of lunging forward and then slamming back in your seat is not much fun even when your back's normal.

Cherish your return to independence—yes. But don't put yourself and others at risk by rushing it. Depending on your surgery, you could return to driving within a few days (most percutaneous endoscopic procedures) or not for several weeks (open surgeries).

Back Off!

DO NOT DRIVE if you are taking narcotic pain medications or muscle relaxants that can make you sleepy. Even if you think you're fine, these substances impair your judgment, timing, and ability to react in an emergency. If you think back surgery was bad, imagine multiple broken bones or worse!

Chores and Household Duties

We won't tell on you if you want to play like you can't do much around the house. But don't play the ailing invalid for too long—the truth is, getting back to your regular activities does wonders for your back and for your mood. Bet you never thought of washing dishes and sweeping the floor as mood elevators! But even these simple tasks can bring you joy (or at least a sense of satisfaction)—especially if your back pain kept you from doing them before your surgery.

Keep strenuous chores—vacuuming, washing floors, scrubbing showers, mowing the lawn, washing the car—on your "don't do" list until your doctor tells you it's okay to resume them. These activities involve a lot of stretching, reaching, and rapid movement that probably won't feel that great anyway.

Work

Most people can return to work two to six weeks following back surgery. Whether it's two, six, or somewhere in between for you depends on many variables. If you had a spinal fusion and you move pianos for a living, it's going to be a while before you return. On the other hand, if you've had a microdiskectomy and your recovery has gone smoothly, you could be back to normal fairly soon.

Moderate physical activity at work won't do your back any harm as long as you take a few precautions:

➤ Protect the surgery area from bumps and knocks. (You have to be careless only once for this caution to engrave itself on your consciousness.)

➤ Avoid lifting until your doctor gives you the go-ahead. This means books, file folders, and paper for the copy machine as well as heavy loads. Also watch the bending (your surgery site will remind you to mind your posture).

➤ Change your position frequently. Whether you mostly sit or stand at your job, switch every so often. If you usually sit, stand for a few minutes every 20 to 30 minutes. If your job involves a lot of standing, try to balance your weight evenly on both legs (don't lock your knees). Take short sitting breaks several times each hour to give your back a break.

➤ Walk as much as you can (though lay off the five-mile hikes for a few weeks), and do simple stretching exercises frequently throughout the day.

You don't have to stop these activities just because you're feeling better. In fact, continuing your back-healthy habits will go a long way toward keeping your back feeling good.

Sleep Positions

Most surgeons recommend you sleep lying on your side with your knees slightly bent, with a single pillow beneath your head and a pillow between your knees if that's more comfortable. Lying on your back puts pressure on your surgery site, and lying on your stomach contorts your spine into unnatural curves.

If you've struggled with back pain for a long time, you've probably tried various mattresses and sleeping surfaces. The best surface for back comfort is firm (not hard) and supportive. Your mattress should allow your spine to rest in its natural alignment.

Back to Nature

Having trouble sleeping? Try a short walk outside, weather permitting, about 45 minutes before you intend to go to bed. Follow your walk with a nice, warm cup of chamomile tea. The walk will stretch and relax your muscles, and stepping outdoors will give you a refreshing change of scenery. Chamomile is an herb reputed to calm and relax—and the warmth of the tea will do the same.

Take care getting in and out of bed. To get into bed, sit on the edge of the bed with your feet still on the floor. Using your pillow-side arm for support, pull your legs, together, up onto the bed. Leaving your knees bent, lay your head on your pillow. Don't twist at the waist. You should now be lying on your side with your knees bent. Slowly straighten your legs. If you want to lie on your back or your other side, rotate your entire body all at once (again, don't twist at the waist). To get out of bed, reverse the process.

Ditch the Heels—Dress for Healing

Pay attention to what you pull out of your closet in the morning—not to make a fashion statement, but to dress for healing. You'll feel more comfortable in sweats and loose-fitting items than in tight waists or high heels (which aren't especially good for your health, anyway). A certain amount of swelling is normal with any surgery, as your body attempts to cope with all that has happened to it. Plus you're likely to be a bit stiff and sore. So for the first few days after surgery, sweats might be all that you can pull on in the morning. Loose-fitting clothing is less likely to irritate your incision. If you have to wear shoes, choose a pair with low or flat heels. Stay comfortable until you're feeling back to normal (and even after, if you get to liking it).

Life Beyond Pain

When you have an injury, pain automatically limits your movement—your body's way of slowing you down so your injury can heal. Some pain is normal in the first days following your operation. This, too, is a natural way for your body to force you to rest and recover. Just don't let the discomfort keep you down.

Yes, we meant to say discomfort, and no, we don't mean to minimize what you feel. Your body's ability to heal is remarkable. A few days after surgery, there's really no need (from your body's perspective) to keep hurting. Pain's role in keeping you still while healing takes place has served its purpose, and it's time to move on. The problem is, it still hurts when you move. This, too, is normal—it's just not the same kind of pain you had before. It's more of an ache and a stiffness; and if your muscles could make noise, they'd be groaning.

Your muscles aren't used to movement. Your pain has kept them in check for so long that they've become quite comfortable doing as little as possible. Now that you're calling on them to get you up and going, they're resisting. They want you to think they still hurt because then they get to rest again. Don't let them get away with it! The longer your back remains inactive, the harder it is to get it into action again. It will hurt to move if you wait too long.

Let the stiffness flow out of your back naturally. When you first get up, sit at the edge of your bed for a minute or two to let your back adjust to an upright position. Do a few gentle stretches while you're waiting—raise one arm slowly over your head and then back down to your side. Repeat with the other arm. Do this several times, then raise both hands above your head at the same time. Feel your back stretch as you do. When you stand, come to your feet slowly, so you don't make any sudden moves that could startle your back. Take smooth steps to avoid jarring your back. And hold yourself upright, as though there was a string attached to the top of your head pulling you up.

Maintain proper posture—it may feel awkward at first, but your back will thank you for helping it support itself.

The most important thing is to keep moving. If your back sends you a sudden, sharp pain, stop for a minute. Take a few deep, slow breaths, then pull yourself into a positive posture. And start over. Your back will get the idea, and before you know it all these little "tricks" will be second nature.

Back to Nature

A little creative visualizing can keep you going when you feel like calling it quits. Make yourself comfortable in a quiet place and close your eyes. Visualize yourself doing the things you want to do. Fix this picture of your active self firmly in your consciousness. Open your eyes, and act like the picture. When the going gets rough, stop and close your eyes for a moment to recall your picture.

Give Yourself Time to Heal

As you embark on your personal road to recovery, be kind to yourself. Remember, no matter how motivated you are, healing takes time. It's a wonderful feeling to take those first steps after surgery and realize that although you hurt from your operation, the back pain that has laid you low for months or years is finally gone. You might as well be walking on air. Then the euphoria wears off, and reality isn't quite so rosy.

Recovery is, at times, hard work. You'll have frustrating days when nothing seems to go right and everything you do hurts. But you'll also have days when you can take a walk around the block on a sunny afternoon, bend down to give your dog a pat on the head, or hug a child—all without pain and maybe without even noticing how special these actions are until you remember how long it's been since you enjoyed them. Cherish these days—they can carry you through the rough times.

The Least You Need to Know

➤ Your back surgery is the perfect opportunity to trade in back-breaking habits for back-healthy ones.

➤ Pain related to your surgery usually fades quickly as your surgery site heals.

➤ Physical therapy helps you return your back and body to working condition.

➤ Getting back to regular activities soon, including housework and even your job, can speed your recovery.

Part 5
A Healing Touch

Touch is the oldest way of healing. Touch is deeply reassuring and nurturing.
—Rachel Naomi Remen, M.D., in Bill Moyers' book Healing and the Mind *(1994)*

Hands-on healing goes back thousands of years, preceding even written record. Ancient healers used touch and manipulation to ease pain and to restore body parts to their rightful positions so healing could take place. These concepts remain valid today, appearing in therapies ranging from acupuncture to physical therapy.

The chapters in Part 5 discuss various methods of relieving back pain and promoting healing through touch.

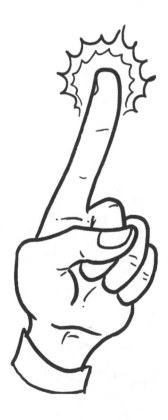

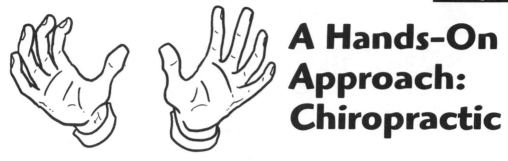

Chapter 18

A Hands-On Approach: Chiropractic

In This Chapter

➤ How chiropractic got started

➤ Common misperceptions about chiropractic

➤ Relieving back pain with chiropractic

➤ How to choose a chiropractor

Roughly 20 million Americans visit chiropractors each year, 68 percent of them for back and neck problems. With more than 70,000 practitioners licensed in the United States, chiropractic is the country's third largest group of health care providers, behind allopathic (conventional) medicine and dentistry.

How Chiropractic Got Its Start

Chiropractic care got its serendipitous start in 1895, when Daniel David Palmer noticed an apparent connection between a janitor's report that he heard his back pop just before he went deaf in the ear on the same side. A self-trained magnetic healer (one who uses energy to heal), Palmer turned his efforts to healing the janitor's condition. When he placed his hands on the man's neck, he felt a slight bulge, as though the bones had shifted.

Believing there to be a relationship between the pressure this was putting on the nerves and the man's hearing loss, Palmer began to massage and manipulate his employee's neck. As Palmer suspected, this restored the bones to their rightful positions, released the pressure on the nerves, and restored the lost hearing. Palmer termed his manipulations *chiropractic* and began using the technique on others. Two years later, Palmer opened the first school to train those who wanted to learn his methods.

Today's chiropractor receives extensive education and training and has an intimate knowledge of how the back's intricate and intertwined elements function. Adjustment and manipulation techniques are gentler and kinder to delicate structures than were the often forceful movements Palmer and early chiropractors used. But the basic premise remains the same—do what you can to remove the obstacles, and the body will heal itself.

Back Talk

Daniel David Palmer (1845–1913), known as the father of chiropractic, was born March 7, 1845, in what was then the "wild Canadian west"—Toronto. As a young man, Palmer studied a popular healing art of the time, magnetic healing. He eventually settled in Davenport, Iowa, where he enjoyed a large practice for nine years before performing the first chiropractic adjustment on a janitor who lost his hearing as the result of a pinched nerve in his neck. The school Palmer started in Davenport in 1897 is today one of America's largest chiropractic colleges, Palmer College of Chiropractic.

Common Misperceptions About Chiropractic: A Self-Quiz

"The trouble with people is not that they don't know but that they know so much that ain't so," wrote Henry Wheeler Shaw, alias Josh Billings, in his 1874 book *Josh Billings' Encyclopedia of Wit and Wisdom* (turns out his words are a little of both). What do you know about chiropractic that just isn't so? Test yourself with this self-quiz!

1. Anyone can be a chiropractor. All you need is an office with a sign out front.

    True _____   False _____

2. Why bother with a chiropractor? You can just crack your back yourself and save a few bucks.

    True _____   False _____

3. Once you start going to a chiropractor, you have to keep going.

    True _____   False _____

4. Better make sure your chiropractor is small, otherwise he or she could break your back.

    True _____   False _____

5. Chiropractic hurts.

   True _____   False _____

6. Hold onto your checkbook—chiropractic is expensive.

   True _____   False _____

7. Chiropractors will try to convince you not to go back to your regular doctor.

   True _____   False _____

8. Chiropractic can cure just about anything that ails you.

   True _____   False _____

Are your perceptions of chiropractic more miss than hit? If you answered "false" to all eight questions, give yourself a pat on the back! Misperceptions and misunderstandings about chiropractic are common. Read on for the straight scoop.

1. To the contrary, chiropractors are trained and certified doctors. They have a minimum five years of postgraduate training and education, and must pass a comprehensive, national board-certification test before they can practice chiropractic. There are 18 colleges of chiropractic medicine in the United States. As well, chiropractors must be licensed in the state where they practice.

2. Well, you *could* crack your own back, though then you'd need a chiropractor for sure! When your chiropractor adjusts your spine, the manipulation and pressure are controlled and very specific. When you crack or pop your back, you're giving your spine a sudden, twisting jerk. If you feel better afterward, it's because you've released or freed stiffened facet joints. You could just as easily give yourself a strain or sprain, or create an area that's weakened because it's too loose (chiropractors call this hypermobility). When your chiropractor does an adjustment, you may indeed hear some popping and cracking. This is an unintentional consequence of moving bones and joints, however, and is not a goal.

3. Once you start going to a chiropractor, you may want to keep going, but that's not the intent. A main focus of chiropractic is patient education—helping you understand how your back functions and what you can do to keep it in good working condition. Often, people come to a chiropractor when they've tried everything else and nothing works. What state do you think your back is in by then?

Back Basics

Chiropractic comes from two Greek words—*chiros*, meaning "of the hand," and *prakticos*, which means "operative." Today, the term identifies the philosophy and practice of the healing method that uses spinal adjustments and manipulations to restore alignment to the spine and related structures.

(No, not Georgia!) It may take some time to realign your spine and retrain your out-of-control muscles. As much as your chiropractor likes you, he or she wants you to become self-sufficient in caring for your back.

4. Chiropractic is about technique, not brute force. No matter what size your chiropractor, it's nearly impossible for him or her to break your back—or any other bones, for that matter. You could be at risk for fractures during mild activity of any kind, of course, if you have severe osteoporosis. Part of your initial examination, before your chiropractor ever puts a hand on you, is a full health history. If you could have osteoporosis, your chiropractor will send you to your regular doctor for care.

5. Chiropractic adjustments don't hurt. If yours do, there's something wrong. Tell your chiropractor right away, so he or she can pinpoint the cause of the pain and avoid repeating it. Though moving bones around sounds pretty aggressive, it's really quite gentle. Chiropractors spend many years in school and in training to learn how to coax, not force, your spine into its proper alignment.

6. A visit to your chiropractor probably costs less than a trip to your hair stylist. In many states, health plans and insurance cover chiropractic care in the same way they cover conventional medical treatment. Most chiropractors are very up-front about their fees, and discuss them at your first visit.

7. A chiropractor's role in the health care continuum is quite clear. Though at times it may overlap with that of your regular doctor, your chiropractor serves you in a different way. If your chiropractor detects a problem that requires medical attention, he or she will refer you to your regular doctor without delay. Most chiropractors welcome the opportunity to provide care that complements conventional medical care, and even to work in tandem with your regular doctor to develop the most effective treatment approach for your back problems.

8. Though it certainly can improve your overall well-being by correcting problems with the structures that form the literal and figurative backbone of your life, chiropractic doesn't actually "cure" anything. The human body, chiropractors believe, is self-healing. The practitioner's mission is to remove obstacles to the body's own mechanisms. (Chiropractors sometimes describe their work as an attempt to prevent "dis-ease"—to keep you free from problems that interfere with your ease of movement and a healthy, enjoyable life.) Spinal adjustments can't (and aren't intended to) treat cancer, ear infections, or diabetes. These conditions, like many others, require conventional medical care. Chiropractors are trained to recognize signs and symptoms of diseases, and to refer people who have them to a physician for prompt medical attention.

> ### Back Talk
>
> What causes your joints to pop and crack? No one knows for sure, though the prevailing theory holds that when joints move, the fluid surrounding them releases tiny bubbles of nitrogen gas. (Nitrogen is a normal substance in your body, just as oxygen is.) The sound you hear comes from these bubbles popping—they apparently get a lot of pop for their size!

Back Out of Whack: Subluxation

Your back hurts. It's stiff and sore, and you really don't like to move in certain directions. Your regular doctor can't find anything wrong, but you feel lousy. You may have a *subluxation*, two or more adjacent vertebrae that no longer function properly together. The situation creates a range of symptoms, from inflammation to nerve compression—and of course, pain.

When conventional (allopathic) doctors typically think of a subluxation, they think of an acute injury—for example, when a blow to the tip of a finger partially dislocates a finger joint. (Ouch!) There's usually some damage to the surrounding tissue that contributes to the pain. Treatment is often an external force to move the two bone ends back into alignment with each other, such as splinting, or taping the injured finger to the healthy one next to it.

Chiropractors view a subluxation as a condition that develops over time. A spinal subluxation results when tissues that are tense or constricted pull the vertebrae out of alignment, but do not damage the surrounding tissues. Maybe you've strained the muscles, causing *adhesions*. Or perhaps other soft-tissue problems are stressing the bones. In any case, a fixation results—the involved vertebrae don't move freely, as they should. Your chiropractor will try to get to the bottom of the problem by releasing the fixations and adhesions through manipulations and adjustments.

> ### Back Basics
>
> *Sub* means "less than," and *luxation* means "dislocation." The term **subluxation** describes a situation in your spine where xyour facet joints are slightly out of alignment. **Adhesions** are abnormal growths of fibrous tissue that connect normally separate body parts.

Because many people often wait until nothing else works, they come to the chiropractor with a variety of problems. It takes time and patience to sort through the mess your body's become—be willing to allow both. And some subluxations stubbornly resist efforts to correct them, especially if they've ruled your back for a long time. Just as you resist altering the route you take to work each morning, your muscles and connective tissues follow the patterns they find comfortable (even if their habits cause you discomfort).

Back Off!

A subluxation that crosses over into spondylolithesis territory and is putting pressure on root nerves or your spinal cord can be a serious medical condition. Mild spondylolithesis responds especially well to chiropractic, often better than allopathic remedies or physical therapy. But severe spondylolithesis could require surgery.

Back to Nature

Ask your chiropractor to show you techniques you can use on your own to help relax and stretch your back. Such gentle exercises can work in concert with your chiropractic treatments to get you back in action faster.

Adjustments for a Better Back

Chiropractic adjustments emphasize gently encouraging subluxated vertebrae to go back where they belong. Chiropractors don't actually "move" bones—after all, your skeletal system is designed to keep its parts firmly in place. Without movement *between* bones, however, you're not going anywhere!

Chiropractors stimulate and manipulate sections and parts of your spine to improve mobility and reduce the pressure surrounding the subluxation. When your connective tissues can move freely, they'll restore themselves to proper placement and function.

The essence of chiropractic is manipulation by hand. Many chiropractors supplement manual adjustments with various tools. One commonly used is called an activator. This small, hand-held device delivers a gentle but rapid percussion that nudges tissues into place. Your chiropractor may use other tools as well. Don't hesitate to ask what the tool does, and how it works.

What a Pain in the Neck (and Shoulders)

When your neck hurts, it's not long before the rest of your back follows. This is because you tend to hold your neck stiffly in whatever position causes the least amount of pain. The rest of your back reacts by altering its curves, which tenses muscles that aren't used to those positions. Relieving your neck pain through chiropractic adjustments brings the rest of your back into alignment as well, so your back feels good all over.

Lower-Back Pain

No part of your body takes more abuse than your lower back. It's a wonder you can have times when it doesn't hurt! Chiropractic attempts to restore alignment to the vertebrae in your lower back, and relax stressed muscles and ligaments. Your chiropractor also may teach you posture exercises to give your lower back more support when you're doing the things you have to do that cause it the greatest grief, like sitting and lifting.

Back Talk

Though chiropractic is a relatively young healing art at just over 100 years old, spinal manipulations for health have been a part of healing for thousands of years. Ancient Chinese cultures used manipulation methods to treat various ailments. Ancient Greek and Egyptian medical writings include descriptions and drawings of treatments involving spinal stretching and alignment.

Treating Back Pain

Several recent studies show that chiropractic care achieves better results than physical therapy or medication when it comes to relieving acute low back pain. Chiropractic relaxes the structures of your back, improves circulation to the injured area, and helps prevent adhesions from forming by keeping connective tissues freely moving.

Treating Nerve Pain

Nerve pain happens when the nerves in a particular area get irritated. This can happen in an injury, where none of the other tissues are very happy, either, or without a precipitating event (what doctors call idiopathic). Chiropractic assumes that nerves send pain signals because something is interfering with their ability to function properly. Chiropractic helps heal nerve pain by removing the obstructions that cause it—subluxation, adhesions, tense muscles, stiff joints. Once the underlying cause goes away, so does the pain.

Back Care

Since most back pain arises from soft-tissue problems, x-rays seldom offer any insight into what's causing your pain. To limit your exposure to unnecessary radiation, ask your chiropractor what he expects x-rays to add to an understanding of your condition or to your therapy. If there's no specific expectation, pass on the pictures.

Adjunctive Therapies

Many chiropractors also use *adjunctive* therapies—treatments that work in harmony with chiropractic approaches. These might include ultrasound and diathermy (deep heat treatments), massage, range of motion exercises, and nutritional counseling. This reflects the generally holistic approach of chiropractic—looking at the health of your whole self, not just at the problems in your back.

Back Basics

Adjunctive means "along with." Adjunctive therapies are those that complement the chiropractic or other care that's the primary treatment.

Body in Balance: Nutrition and Exercise

With so much back pain related to our lifestyles—eating fast food, getting too little exercise, and not getting enough sleep—it makes sense to give back to our bodies the sustenance they need to take care of us. Your chiropractor may suggest regular exercises to strengthen your back as well as improve your overall physical condition. Proper nutrition matters, too. Your body can't work at its best on low-grade fuel, which is what many of us expect it to do with our haphazard eating habits. Your chiropractor may offer you a nutritional evaluation to assess your body's nutritional status and to suggest changes for improvement.

Aligning Mind and Spirit: Psychic Health

No, you're not going to walk out of your chiropractor's office with the ability to read minds and predict the future. Psychic health means taking care of the nonphysical aspects of your existence. Your chiropractor might suggest breathing techniques, biofeedback, meditation, visualization, or imagery to help you reduce the stress in your life, empower and support your body's natural healing abilities, and regain a sense of control over its direction. Once you learn these methods, you can practice them anywhere, anytime.

Choosing a Chiropractor

With so many chiropractors out there, how do you find the one that's best for you? Well, how do you go about finding a conventional doctor or a dentist? Most of us ask our friends and coworkers whom they see, and what they think of the provider as a person and as a health care professional. Technical qualifications are of course important, but few of us have the knowledge to assess them. Instead, we rely on how we feel about the provider. Does he listen first, then talk? Does she explain what she's doing during an examination? After all, as human beings we're relationship-oriented—even if the bond we seek lasts only a few minutes.

It's also important to find a chiropractor who shares your philosophical beliefs about the role chiropractic care plays in your health. If you want to blend nutritional therapy with meditation for stress relief and traditional chiropractic adjustments for your back pain, you need to identify a chiropractor who enthusiastically supports you in your approach.

Chiropractor Qualifications

Your chiropractor should have diplomas and certificates hanging prominently in the office that provide evidence of his or her education, training, and board certification. If you don't see any of these items, ask about them. Chiropractors undergo an extensive education and training regimen. After they're licensed and in practice, they take postgraduate continuing education courses.

Once board certified and state licensed, chiropractors are qualified and permitted to order lab tests and imaging procedures, bill insurance companies, diagnose conditions, and prescribe treatments. Chiropractors don't prescribe medications, and they don't perform surgery. They can, and often do, conduct nutritional counseling and prescribe nutritional supplements.

Different Kinds of Chiropractors

Just as there are different approaches in allopathic or conventional medicine, there are different philosophies and practices within chiropractic. Some chiropractors blend techniques within a personalized approach to chiropractic, drawing from various methods they believe are effective.

➤ **Traditional.** Traditional chiropractic focuses on correcting subluxations by restoring your spine's alignment. Subluxation, in the traditional chiropractic view, interferes with both nerve activity and energy flow. A traditional chiropractor typically uses physical manipulation to mobilize your facet joints and adjust your spine, though she may also use an activator or other tools.

➤ **Nonforce.** Nonforce chiropractors forego traditional adjustments and manipulations of the skeleton in favor of low-impact hand movements. They believe this is less traumatic for your body and produces quicker, often permanent, relief and correction.

➤ **Holistic.** Holistic chiropractors draw from a body of knowledge to supplement traditional chiropractic techniques, including acupuncture, herbology, homeopathy, dance and body movement therapies, vitamin therapies, and others. If you decide to use a holistic chiropractor, make sure you're comfortable with his or her approach and therapies.

Ask a lot of questions, and ask to see printed materials about particular treatments the chiropractor proposes for you. If the chiropractor is reluctant to provide you with additional information, move on.

Back Off!

Don't stop medications your physician has prescribed for you without first checking with him. Your medical condition caused your doctor to believe these medications were necessary, and stopping them could have harmful effects.

And remember, there can be dangerous interactions and side effects between herbal remedies and any allopathic medications you're taking, such as blood pressure pills or thyroid replacement. Make sure you tell your allopathic physician and chiropractor about any herbal remedies and medications you're taking. People taking prescription antidepressants, for example, should not use products containing hypericum (St. John's Wort).

The Chiropractor as Caregiver

Your chiropractor's emphasis on getting out of the way to let your body heal itself makes him or her a natural member of your health care team. Most chiropractors enjoy working in a collaborative manner with other practitioners to provide you with the most effective care for your situation and condition.

Working in Joint with Your Primary Care Physician

To hear the media tell the story, there's nothing but animosity and distrust between chiropractors and allopathic physicians. No doubt there are individuals who just don't get along, either on the basis of philosophical differences or plain, old personality clashes. But for the most part, chiropractors and physicians consider each other as valid practitioners in the continuum of health care.

When your chiropractor and your primary care physician can work harmoniously, you get the best of both worlds. It's worth your effort to seek out practitioners in each to guide your health care needs. If your doctor refers you to your chiropractor, or vice versa, you need look no further. If you're just starting out, ask one for recommendations about the other. Professionals who respect each other's expertise are delighted to have opportunities to work together.

When to Seek Other Care

Quite simply, you should seek other care when you're not seeing the improvement you think you should. Chiropractic is like any other healing method—if it's not working, it's time to make a change. Often, your chiropractor will be the first to recognize that you're not making the expected progress, and to recommend either alternative methods or a visit to your primary care physician.

Most chiropractors are very supportive when you're the one who decides to call it quits. If yours gets angry or threatens that you'll never feel good again if you leave, waste no time getting through the door. This is unethical, unprofessional, and flat out wrong. (We give the same recommendation about other practitioners, including allopathic physicians.) Your health is your responsibility; caregivers are here to help you fulfill it, not take it away from you.

Are There People Who *Shouldn't See a Chiropractor?*

Chiropractic is generally safe for people of all ages with a wide range of conditions. The exceptions are those with moderate to severe osteoporosis. If you have osteoporosis, your bones are weak and maybe even brittle. This makes them susceptible to breaking under stress that wouldn't daunt healthy bones. Chiropractors screen for osteoporosis at the first examination, and most refuse to do alignments or manipulations if you have it.

Other exceptions are those who expect miracles. Chiropractic, like allopathic medicine, can work only with what you bring to it. Miracles happen, of course, but they come from a Greater Source—greater than either your chiropractor or your physician. To get the most from chiropractic, it's important for you to have realistic expectations and a complete understanding of what chiropractic can—and can't—do for you.

The Least You Need to Know

➤ Chiropractic emphasizes removing obstacles so the body can use its own abilities to heal itself.

➤ Chiropractic is an ideal complement to allopathic (conventional) medicine.

➤ Chiropractic is generally safe and useful for people of all ages, though people with moderate or severe osteoporosis should avoid chiropractic adjustments because their weakened bones are especially vulnerable.

➤ When done properly, chiropractic adjustments don't hurt.

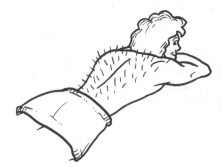

Ancient Chinese Wisdom: Acupuncture

Like yoga, acupuncture dates back thousands of years. Scholars speculate that early healers used acupuncture therapy for pain relief and even surgery at least as long ago as 2500 B.C. and probably even earlier (acupuncture "needles" made of bone have been found dated from this period). Since written forms of language didn't debut until around then, records are skimpy. What we do know for sure is that acupuncture originated in ancient China, and its practice remains fundamentally the same today.

An Ancient Treatment with a Modern Benefit

Early Western visitors to China reported witnessing amazing medicinal uses of *acupuncture*, from anesthesia during surgery to healing bone fractures. Needles sometimes even penetrated internal organs such as the liver in an attempt to heal diseases afflicting them.

Acupuncture migrated to Western cultures primarily as a therapy for pain relief in the mid 1800s when travelers returned with wondrous stories of their headaches and toothaches being needled into oblivion. Chinese immigrants who settled in America and other Western cultures brought their methods with them. French Jesuits also brought acupuncture back to Europe from China. But interest remained limited until the early 1970s, when an American journalist traveling in China got appendicitis. Chinese surgeons removed his inflamed appendix and treated his postoperative pain with acupuncture, and he reported his experiences to the world.

Acupuncture remains an integral aspect of Traditional Chinese Medicine (TCM) today, and exists in most cultures around the world. In the late 1990s, a group of Western physicians visiting Beijing, China, observed a cesarean section (surgical birth) performed with acupuncture as the only anesthesia. The young woman on the operating table was cheerful and talking with her doctors, eager to see her new child, and completely comfortable. Chinese surgeons do many other surgeries using acupuncture anesthesia, too, from removing tonsils to setting fractured bones.

While most Westerners instantly think "needles" when someone says "acupuncture," this ancient therapy is more a philosophy of wellness than a procedure or technique. Though most people in Western cultures seek acupuncture therapy for pain relief, that's often more a side benefit than a goal for the *acupuncturist*. Acupuncture restores your body's balances to a healthy state by manipulating its flow of life energy, or chi. The acupuncturist can insert needles to do this, or use other methods.

Back Basics

Acupuncture means "point puncture." The word describes the ancient Chinese practice of stimulating certain points along the body's energy meridians. An **acupuncturist** has special training and expertise in acupuncture. Most states require acupuncturists to pass a licensing exam, and some states require acupuncturists to also be licensed physicians (M.D.s, D.O.s, or D.C.s).

These Needles Don't Do Shots

If the mere thought of sticking needles into a body that already hurts (yours) makes you break out in a cold sweat, relax. Acupuncture needles are so fine—almost hair-thin—that four of them can fit inside the hypodermic needle through which you typically receive an injection. With needles so thin and flexible, a skilled acupuncturist can often slip them into position without setting off pain reactions in your nerves. The poke is less than a mosquito bite (and leaves no nasty itch or sting).

Back Off!

The standard of practice (and in the U.S., a legal requirement in most states) today is for acupuncturists to use sterile, disposable needles—a fresh set for each acupuncture treatment. Be sure your acupuncturist follows this essential health practice to prevent the spread of infectious diseases such as hepatitis and AIDS.

The acupuncturist selects needles of varying lengths, and inserts them at angles of 15 degrees to 90 degrees depending on the treatment. After insertion, the acupuncturist might activate the needles in some way, or leave them still. Common techniques include rotation, raising and thrusting (moving the needle quickly up and down), and plucking, scraping, or trembling (vibration techniques). A treatment session usually lasts 20 to 45 minutes, during which you often feel deqi—a tingling sensation as the needle is inserted—but no pain or discomfort. Most people feel significantly better after a single treatment, though chronic conditions may need several sessions.

Heat Treatments: Moxibustion and Cupping

Heat sometimes intensifies an acupuncture response. The acupuncturist generally uses one of two methods to heat up an acupuncture point—moxibustion or cupping. Moxibustion is the stimulation of an acupuncture point with heat, either by heating an inserted needle or by burning a cone-shaped herbal mixture, called mugwort or moxa, as it is held near an acupuncture point. Moxibustion often relieves the pain of arthritis and other joint inflammations.

Cupping is another heat therapy in which a cup (made of metal, wood, or glass) is heated and then quickly placed over an acupuncture point. As the air inside the cup cools, it creates a partial vacuum and pressure over the point. Acupuncturists or TCM doctors often use cupping to treat low-back pain, sprains, and soft-tissue injuries. Cupping is well known in other cultures, too, including Eastern Europe and Italy.

Pressuring Pain: Acupressure and Acumassage

Sometimes the acupuncturist will apply steady pressure with the fingertips or a special instrument to an acupressure point instead of inserting a needle, or massage the areas along the relevant meridian. Westerners often view acupressure (the first technique) and acumassage (the second technique) as kinder, gentler forms of acupuncture. They really are "weaker" forms of point stimulation, though are often effective for relieving pain caused by soft-tissue problems.

East Meets West: Old Techniques, New Technologies

Though the basic concepts of acupuncture haven't changed for centuries, modern technology has left its impressions. Some acupuncturists use high-tech methods to enhance the old techniques.

Do the Wave: Sound and Laser Stimulation

Sonopuncture uses high-frequency sound waves and laser stimulation uses low-frequency light waves to

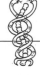

Back Care

As if it's not enough that acupuncture can relieve your back pain (as well as other aches and ailments), it apparently does so with almost no risk. Possible side effects such as infection or minor nerve damage at a needle site are so rare that your odds of negative effects are millions to one. The most significant complaint about acupuncture (and it's also quite uncommon) is that it didn't work as well as expected.

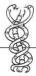

Back Care

Those tissue flaps you call your ears might be useful for more than funneling sound to your eardrums. They're rich in acupuncture points for, among other things, relieving headaches, stopping smoking, and controlling addictions. Don't be surprised if your visit to an acupuncturist for a pain in your back finds you with needles in your ear!

stimulate acupuncture points. These techniques are usually done without needles, using the ultrasound or laser machine to focus a beam of sound or light directly at the acupuncture point. With these procedures, you often get the same deqi sensation that occurs with needle acupuncture, and a similar level of pain relief.

Back to Nature

Acupressure and acumassage are techniques you can sometimes learn to do yourself to relieve pain, either your own or a loved one's. An acupuncturist can show you how to do them and where for the problem or pain you have.

Plug in: Percutaneous Electrical Nerve Stimulation (PENS)

With PENS, the acupuncturist inserts the acupuncture needles, then attaches the ends to electrodes. The electrodes send a mild flow of electrical current through the needles, delivering a stronger stimulation to the points. You may feel mild to moderate tingling, depending on the frequency of the current. Don't worry, you won't get shocked—the voltage is too low to do you any harm.

Back Talk

Though we view PENS as an approach borne of modern technology, Chinese surgeons actually used "electro-acupuncture" for the first time in 1958 during surgery to remove a patient's tonsils. Today, TCM doctors in China routinely add electrical stimulation to acupuncture anesthesia to intensify the effect for major surgeries.

The Eastern View: Channeling Chi for Healing

Back Basics

Metaphysical means "beyond the body." The term is often used to describe events that appear without an apparent or tangible explanation.

From the Eastern perspective, acupuncture works by unblocking the flow of life energy, or chi, in your body. The Western view might consider this a *metaphysical* approach, since you can't use your physical senses to confirm chi's existence. In the Eastern view, this clarification isn't necessary—how could you be here if chi didn't exist? The concept of chi is the foundation of Eastern medical practices. With the flow of energy altered, balance is restored, and healing takes place.

The Meridian Network

Chi, you remember from Chapter 10, flows through unseen channels in the body called meridians. Your body has 12 primary and eight secondary meridians. Though the meridians roughly parallel your body's network of nerves, the two systems (nerves and meridians) are not linked.

Each of the six pairs of primary meridians serves organ systems. Two of the secondary meridians, also called odd or extraordinary, are paired and two are not. The secondary meridians serve various psychological and psychic (spiritual) aspects. Where the meridians come near the skin's surface, acupuncture points give access to them. Ancient Chinese texts identified around 350 points, though contemporary acupuncture uses nearly 2,000.

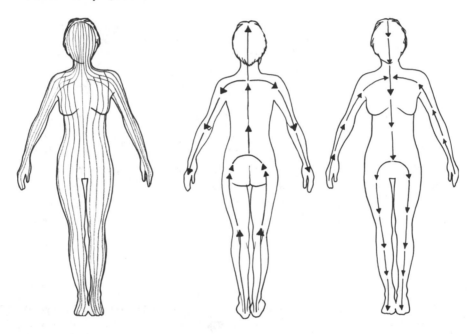

Eastern traditions such as acupuncture, reflexology, and QiGong employ the concept of releasing blockages in the body's zones of natural energy flow to restore health and wellness.

Achieving Balance: Yin and Yang

The concept of pairing is vital to Eastern medicine. Pairing is necessary to achieve balance, or homeostasis, the desired outcome of Eastern therapies. When homeostasis exists, there is health. When it does not, there is "unwellness."

Chi, your life energy, also exists in a pairing. "Yin" is the cold or dark side of chi, represented as feminine or female. (No snide thoughts or comments, now!) Yin is also passive and moist, and moves medially (from outside to inside). Yin's opposite is "yang," represented as masculine or male. Yang is warm, light, active, and dry, and its movement is lateral (from inside to outside) and upward. Homeostasis can exist only when yin and yang are balanced.

Yin and yang.

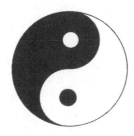

Back Talk

The term "homeostasis" has somewhat different meanings in Eastern and Western medicine. In Eastern medicine, homeostasis means "state of equilibrium," and reflects a balance among body, mind, and spirit as well as between yin and yang (energy forces). Restoring homeostasis is the goal of all healing methods. In Western medicine, homeostasis refers to your human body's efforts to maintain its organ systems in a constant environment, regardless of external influences. Your body automatically adjusts to achieve homeostasis—for example, sweating and shivering are involuntary actions to keep your body's temperature stable.

Unblocking the Flow

When an obstruction blocks a meridian, it alters the flow of chi, creating a yin-yang imbalance. Your symptoms, along with your responses to questions that may seem unrelated to your back pain, tell the acupuncturist where your blockages are. When the acupuncturist applies a therapy (such as needling) to the relevant points, it releases the blockage and restores the balance of yin and yang.

From an Eastern perspective, back pain, even when it results from a known injury, is present not because of the injury but because there's an imbalance in your chi. Yes, you may have strained your back trying to lift that box of books. But other obstructions are at work as well, or you wouldn't have gotten injured in the first place.

There's not always a logical relationship between the acupuncture points the acupuncturist uses and the location of your symptoms. Your acupuncturist may choose points at the area of your back pain, for example, and also others that are along the meridians governing that area. It's in this mix-and-match that the acupuncturist's knowledge and experience make a difference.

> ### Back Talk
>
> Following a lengthy study of acupuncture, the National Institutes of Health (NIH) concluded in November 1997 that "there is clear evidence" that acupuncture therapies are effective for a many ailments. NIH specifically identified fibromyalgia and low-back pain as conditions that respond well to acupuncture.

The Western View: Electrochemical Interference

The Western view of acupuncture shifts from chi to nerve impulses. Acupuncture works because it interferes with your nervous system's ability to transport pain messages or because it stimulates cells to release endorphins, your body's natural pain relievers. There is some scientific evidence supporting each of these explanations, though none that is conclusive.

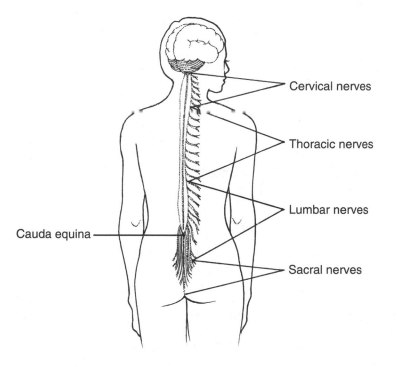

The spinal cord and major nerves.

Cervical nerves

Thoracic nerves

Lumbar nerves

Cauda equina

Sacral nerves

The Nerve Network

Your nervous system, as you know, is the core of your body's functions. Nothing takes place, not even a breath, without an instruction from your neurological command center, the brain. Most of these instructions pass through your nervous system without an inkling of knowledge on your part, sort of like the myriad of signals your personal computer processes in the background when you sit down to write a letter.

The "intrabody" expressway of this network is your spinal cord, with the root nerves branching from it serving as major highways to get signals to and from various organ systems and body parts. Smaller nerves branch from those, threading to every cell in your body.

At certain places, key nerves pass close to the surface of your skin. These nerves are often the target of therapies such as TENS (transcutaneous electrical nerve stimulation) that attempt to disrupt signal transmission along the nerve route. Others are deeper, accessible only by drugs, injections, or surgery.

Back Basics

Endorphins are natural painkilling substances your body produces. They work by stimulating special cells, called opiate receptors. The term is short for "endogenous morphines," or morphine-like chemicals the body produces. **Enkephalins** are similar to endorphins, though they are produced and released by different cells in your brain and nerves.

Activating Your Body's Natural Painkillers

East and West agree on one aspect of acupuncture—it stimulates the body's own healing systems. How it does so is where the two cultures part ways. While Eastern medicine holds the view that acupuncture therapies stimulate and alter the flow of chi, one explanation Western medicine offers is that the stimulation is biochemical.

Back Talk

Approximately 10,000 licensed acupuncturists practice in the United States. About 4,000 physicians (M.D.s, D.O.s, or D.C.s) are also trained in acupuncture. They're a busy group, treating more than one million Americans and handling 12 million visits a year.

Your brain controls thousands of different chemicals your body needs for various functions. Most are held in reserve until the time of need. Adrenaline, for example, floods your system when it's time for fight-or-flight. *Endorphins* and *enkephalins* are two substances your nervous system (brain and certain nerve cells) produce and release only under certain circumstances, such as an injury. Other events that affect cell activity also can trigger the release of endorphins, such as intense physical exercise ("runner's high") and acupuncture. Acupuncture is known to release other messenger hormones that have regulatory functions in the body, including ACTH (adreno-cortico-trophic hormone) and LH (luteinizing hormone).

Choosing an Acupuncturist

Who you choose as an acupuncturist depends on what you're looking for in terms of approach and philosophy. Acupuncturists can be conventional physicians (M.D.s or D.O.s), chiropractors (D.C.s), and, in some states, podiatrists (D.P.M.s) who do acupuncture. Acupuncturists can also be trained in Traditional Oriental Medicine (TOM) or Traditional Chinese Medicine (TCM).

Some conventional physicians who practice acupuncture are equally comfortable with Eastern and Western perspectives, while others prefer the more scientific approach popularized by Western medicine. One is not necessarily better than another; what matters is that you connect with an acupuncturist who is comfortable and compatible with your approach and expectations.

Acupuncture Qualifications

Acupuncture qualifications vary among countries and from state to state in the U.S. In some states, only licensed physicians (M.D.s and D.O.s) can practice acupuncture, though they need no special training to do so. Other states recognize practitioners who are not physicians, such as TOM or TCM acupuncturists, and have standardized testing and licensing procedures in place. A few states don't regulate acupuncturists at all.

Most acupuncturists who practice TOM or TCM acupuncture have completed three or more years of intense, specialized training that includes many subjects besides acupuncture. They're also trained in anatomy and physiology, diagnostic procedures (predominantly Eastern with some Western thrown in), herbal therapies, and other relevant areas.

Conventional physicians (M.D.s and D.O.s) who also practice acupuncture may or may not have TOM or TCM training. It seems you'd want someone who's had more than a weekend's worth of training—which is all some states require (if that). The most common training program for physicians includes 220 hours of training plus a supervised practice period. Acupuncture, whether you lean to the East or to the West, is a complex system. There are acupuncture programs that provide solid training from a Western perspective for physicians.

> **Back Care**
>
> You should feel comfortable when you're with your acupuncturist. He should explain treatments and point selections and answer your questions in language you understand.

The bottom line? Find out what your state or location requires in terms of both education and licensing. Then ask the acupuncturist you're considering about his or her training, experience, philosophy, and interests.

The Acupuncturist as Caregiver

Acupuncturists who are conventional or TOM or TCM physicians are natural choices for primary caregivers. If you're lucky enough to link up with one, you'll get the best of both worlds.

If your acupuncturist is not a physician, be sure to maintain a relationship with a doctor who can oversee your general health needs. You'll want to be sure your conventional doctor is open to complementary medicine.

When to Seek Other Care

It's time to seek other care when your condition fails to improve within a reasonable amount of time, or if it gets worse. Risks associated with acupuncture are very rare, especially if you've verified that your acupuncturist follows accepted practices for cleanliness and infection control (clean office environment, sterile, single-use needles).

As helpful as acupuncture is for a wide range of ailments, let common sense frame your expectations. Nothing, as we've said before, cures everything. Acupuncture may appear to do this since it can relieve pain and other symptoms for so many health problems. But remember, it's relieving the symptoms, not necessarily curing the underlying condition. Symptoms that keep coming back require a conventional medical evaluation.

The Least You Need to Know

➤ From the Eastern perspective, acupuncture redirects the flow of chi, or life energy.

➤ From the Western perspective, acupuncture redirects the impulses your nerves transmit and releases messenger hormones like endorphins.

➤ Many acupuncturists are also physicians who can oversee your general health care needs as well.

➤ Contemporary acupuncture practices often blend modern technology with ancient techniques.

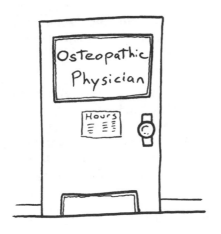

Chapter 20

Focus on Function: Osteopathy

In This Chapter

➤ The development of osteopathy

➤ Viewing the body as a unified whole

➤ Osteopathic manipulations for back pain

➤ The osteopathic physician as a primary caregiver

In nineteenth-century America, doctors didn't have a whole lot to offer patients in many circumstances, beyond a potion and a prayer. If you survived the treatment, you'd survive the disease. Potions were often just this side of poison—a line hard to see and easy to cross when it came to the finer points of dosing. As Thomas Edison was working in his laboratory to produce a practical light bulb, a physician named Andrew Still was developing a new philosophy in the practice of medicine.

The Self-Healing Process

Disenchanted with the ineffectiveness of what he could offer his patients, Dr. Still looked back in history to the teachings of the world's most famous man of medicine, Hippocrates. Dr. Still drew from the ancient Greek belief that the body was a unified entity fully capable of healing itself if the physician would support its self-healing instead of intervening by trying to take over the healing process. From this core philosophy evolved the form of medical care he called, and we still know today as, *osteopathy*.

Dr. Still deviated from the teachings of Hippocrates in one important and defining way. In his new medicine, osteopathy, he defined the musculoskeletal system as the largest access point to restore the body's health and function, surmising that the body's dysfunctions reflected in the bones, muscles, and fascia.

Back Basics

Osteopathy is a form of medicine that views the human body as a unified organism, at the core of which is the musculoskeletal system. It comes from the Greek words *osteo*, meaning "of the bones," and *pathos*, meaning "disease," a reference to the musculoskeletal system's role and influence in the body's health.

Contemporary osteopathic medicine places high importance on the value of the musculoskeletal system. In addition to conventional training similar to that which allopathic physicians receive, future osteopathic physicians also learn osteopathic manipulation and holistic approaches to healing. Four tenets, or principles, guide today's osteopathic physician:

1. The body is a unit; the person is a unit of body, mind, and spirit.

2. The body is capable of self-regulation, self-healing, and health maintenance.

3. Structure and function are reciprocally inter-related.

4. Rational treatment is based upon an understanding of the basic principles of body unity, self-regulation, and the interrelationship of structure and function.

Back Talk

Andrew Taylor Still, M.D. (1828–1917), practiced medicine in what was in his time the frontier of Kansas and Missouri. During service as a physician in the U.S. Army during the Civil War, he was distressed at how little the medical practices of the day could do to help soldiers wounded in battle. Many of them died, it seemed to him, from attempts to treat them rather than from their injuries. He observed that when he let the body's natural healing process remain in control, soldiers were more likely to recover. These observations became the foundation for a new kind of medicine, osteopathy, that Still started practicing when he returned to civilian life.

All for One and One for All: The Body Unified

In the osteopathic view, your body is a collection of systems that work together. Somewhat like a chain of dominoes, what affects one system affects all. Unlike dominoes, however, the cause and effect is sometimes difficult to see. Referred pain is a good illustration of how this works—you hurt in one place because of a problem in another. While we've come to easily identify some of these less direct connections—kidney problems and mid-back pain, for example—we have trouble finding others.

Your Back: The Center of Your Health

Collectively, bones and muscle account for about 60 percent of your body's mass. At the center of this collection is your back. Everything hangs from your spine in some way—your arms connect across the top, your legs attach at the bottom, and your head tops it off. You can't move even your little toe without involving your back—or triggering an amazingly intricate series of events that starts in your brain and continues through numerous bodily systems.

Palpating the Source of Pain: OMT

Osteopathic physicians receive extensive training in using their hands to palpate, or feel, for musculoskeletal problems. A *D.O.* (doctor of osteopathy) may gently probe and move your aching back and other areas of your body to determine what limitations exist. This tactile evaluation might be different from what you're used to, particularly if this is your first visit to a D.O. It's an important part of the osteopathic approach, however.

In osteopathic medicine, this approach is the first step in what is known as *osteopathic manipulation therapy*, or OMT. Next comes diagnosis—determining what the problem is and what underlying causes might exist—and treatment recommendations. Treatment emphasizes relieving your pain, correcting the cause, and restoring mobility to prevent the problem from coming back. For back pain, a D.O. may combine conventional treatments such as anti-inflammatory medication with osteopathic manipulations. A D.O. may also treat your back pain by treating other areas of your body.

Back Basics

Osteopathic manipulation therapy, or OMT, is the essence of osteopathy. It encompasses the process of evaluation, diagnosis, and treatment.

Relieving Pain: Everything in Its Rightful Place

If contemporary osteopathy has a motto, it might be "function follows form." When the structures of your body are properly maintained, they will work smoothly and painlessly. From the osteopathic perspective, healing relies on restoring your body's natural balance. Often the imbalance appears physical (such as low-back pain) yet has other connections (such as stress). Relieving the pain requires identifying and relieving the underlying cause.

Say, for example, you played 18 holes of golf over the weekend, and by Monday morning the twinge you felt at the eleventh hole has become a twisted knot of pain just above your hip. You strained a muscle. A D.O. would of course examine the injury, and consider the apparent cause. Then he or she also might check your posture, weight, and muscle strength, looking for preexisting, interrelated tissue imbalances that might have set the stage for your injury. Perhaps your abdominal muscles are weak, or you hunch your shoulders when you stand, throwing your lumbar curve out of whack. Or perhaps it's something much more complex.

A D.O. would suggest ways to correct the underlying problem as well, perhaps recommending a series of exercises to improve muscle strength and flexibility, and nutritional changes to give your body the fuel it needs to function at peak performance. (Or maybe you just have a bad swing, in which case you need the assistance of a golf pro, not a doctor.)

The Osteopathic Examination

The osteopathic philosophy that the body's systems are inseparably intertwined guides the D.O.'s examination when you arrive for your appointment. In addition to checking out the reason for your visit, a D.O. will ask questions about any other medical conditions and your general well-being, and look for signs of other problems that could be related to your condition.

Especially if you're seeking care for back pain, a D.O. will examine your posture—standing, sitting, and walking—and muscular functions. He or she will also ask about your nutrition and other lifestyle matters, viewing your condition in a holistic way. While the focus of any therapy will be on treating the problem that brought you to the doctor, the D.O. will also offer suggestions to prevent the problem from happening again.

Back Talk

Many people view osteopathy and chiropractic as close cousins. This is accurate in the sense that both use manipulations to restore function, strength, and flexibility. Both also view the spine as crucial to your body's health and well-being. But the two approaches differ in philosophy as well as practitioner education, training, and scope of practice. Depending on their training, D.O.s are qualified to treat a wide range of illnesses and injuries both medically and surgically, while chiropractors specialize in treating the spine and neurological problems that arise from it only, and cannot perform surgery or prescribe medicine.

Strain-Counterstrain (Indirect Technique)

Strain-counterstrain is a unique technique for healing muscle strains and pulls. After identifying the involved muscles, the D.O. creates a situation of complete relaxation in those muscles by manipulating (moving) relevant body parts. Treating low-back strain, for example, might involve manipulating the hip and leg on the affected side while monitoring a tender point, to achieve complete relaxation in the hurting muscles.

The premise of strain-counterstrain is that sometimes muscles get stuck in a stretching mode and are unable to relax. This causes pain. Releasing the stretch relieves the pain. Strain-counterstrain is the exact opposite of stretching, and is aimed at relieving pain from muscle spasms. This is an *indirect technique*.

Osteoarticular Manipulation (Direct Technique)

Sometimes the D.O. determines the cause of your back pain is a reduction of motion of bones as they connect at a joint. Using a procedure called osteoarticular manipulation, the D.O. precisely moves the musculoskeletal structures to help the joint return to its proper functioning. Once proper function is restored, the joint regains mobility and the muscles can function normally. This is a *direct technique*.

Back Basics

In osteopathic medicine, **direct techniques** move the involved area or tissue *toward* the barrier to its normal motion. **Indirect techniques** move the affected area or tissue *away from* the barrier to its normal motion.

Myofascial Release

Myofascial release is a form of deep manipulation that stretches myofascial tissue, the thin, membrane-like covering over muscles and other connective tissues. This technique uses a combination of pressure and massage-like movements to increase circulation to the area and release tightness in the myofascia. Myofascial release is especially effective in situations of injury where there has been trauma to the muscles and connective tissues. Myofascial release can be either direct or indirect.

Back Care

Do you have myofascial pain syndrome or fibromyalgia? Osteopathic myofascial release may be effective for relieving pain in chronic pain syndromes such as these.

Muscle Energy Techniques

Some D.O.s use various muscle energy techniques in an attempt to restore normal function to bones, muscle groups, and connective tissue. With *isometric contraction*, the D.O. holds a joint in place and instructs you to contract certain muscles. This encourages the connective tissues to return the joint to its correct position.

In *isokinetic contraction*, you contract specified muscles against resistance to strengthen the muscle fibers.

Choosing an Osteopathic Physician

There are nearly 40,000 licensed osteopathic physicians practicing in the United States, roughly 6 percent of all physicians. They provide care for more than 38 million Americans.

Many are in family practice, internal medicine, and pediatrics—the primary care specialties—though D.O.s can specialize in any area of medicine they choose. D.O.s typically practice side by side with M.D.s in physician groups, clinics, and hospitals.

Back Basics

Isometric contraction is an osteopathic technique that encourages connective tissue to restore a joint to its normal function. **Isokinetic contraction** strengthens muscle fibers through contraction against resistance.

Osteopathic Physician Qualifications

Following graduation from an undergraduate college or university, future osteopathic physicians enter one of the 19 accredited schools of osteopathic medicine in the United States. There, they complete a comprehensive and extensive course of training—5,000 hours over four years, comparable to conventional medical school.

Before being eligible to practice, osteopathic doctors also complete an additional three to five years of internship and residency training and must pass a series of rigorous board examinations to demonstrate their knowledge and proficiency (again, the same as conventional physicians). Lastly, an osteopathic physician must obtain a license to practice in the state of his or her choice.

Back Talk

In the United States, osteopathic physicians have the same practice rights and responsibilities as their allopathic counterparts. They provide general and specialty care in more than 60 areas of medicine, from family practice to surgery. In Europe and Canada, licensing and practice requirements for doctors of osteopathy (D.O.s) are different from those that regulate medical doctors (M.D.s), and vary among countries or provinces.

The Osteopathic Physician as Caregiver

On the surface, you may not notice any difference between an M.D. and a D.O. Depending on their post-graduate specialty training, both can diagnose and treat adults and children, prescribe medications, perform surgery, and deliver babies. The osteopathic emphasis on the unity of body systems gives D.O.s a natural orientation toward holistic health care and prevention.

The comprehensive nature of a D.O.'s training means that he or she can recognize when your back problem requires interventions such as medication or even surgery (some D.O.s specialize in orthopedic surgery). If osteopathic manipulation interests you, seek care from an osteopathic physician who is a member of the American Academy of Osteopathy.

Sports Medicine and Your Back

Sports medicine is a natural specialty for D.O.s, particularly because it provides the ideal opportunity to blend conventional medicine and osteopathic practices. The vast majority of sports injuries involve muscles, ligaments, tendons, and bones. Those who are drawn to the philosophy of osteopathic medicine generally have a strong interest in the musculoskeletal system. Professional sports teams and college athletic departments often have team doctors who are osteopathic physicians.

Preventing Sports Injuries

There's no question that certain sports carry more risk of back problems than others. You're far more likely to strain your back golfing or playing squash than by walking or bicycling. This doesn't mean these activities are bad—indeed, they're very good for you as long as you don't get hurt.

While you often can't prevent injuries, you can take precautions to reduce your risks. If your favorite activities encourage or require protective gear, use it. Follow a regular exercise routine to keep your back and abdominal muscles, as well as the rest of you, in good shape. Warm up before beginning a sports activity, and "warm down" afterward. And maintain the body weight recommended for your height, so your back doesn't have to work overtime when you hit the court, diamond, lane, green, road, slopes, track, or field.

Back Care

Are your muscles ready for the exercise they're about to receive? Warm them up with gentle stretching, and move through a few paces of your activity or sport before getting started. Take a few swings if you're playing tennis or baseball, a few shots if you're shooting hoops, a short spin if you're going in-line skating. This gets your muscles ready for action.

Can't Give Up Skiing?

You don't have to give up skiing, golfing, or any other sport that puts fun in your life. While these sports can put great stress on your back, there's no reason to stop what

Back Off!

In skiing and other sports where speed is part of the thrill, coming to a sudden stop could cause serious problems. A hard fall in which you land on your back could fracture vertebrae. If you feel pain in your back as well as tingling or numbness in your arms or legs, have a doctor check you over.

you enjoy "just in case." But do yourself a favor: Invest in lessons. You'll learn how to protect your back, knees, and other vital body parts. And you'll improve your performance.

If you do hurt while you're playing, stop. Take a brief rest. Does the pain go away? If so, resume your activity and see what happens. If you hurt again, in the same place, or you still hurt after a few minutes of rest, stop for the day. Ice the area as soon as possible and a few times over the next 24 hours.

Treating Injuries with Care

Did you overdo it this weekend? Push the envelope, exceed your limits, crash and burn, hit the wall? Whatever your sport calls it, it doesn't feel very good the next day. Treat your body with extra kindness as it recuperates.

Remember, sooner is better than later when it comes to strains and sprains. The sooner you start treating your injury, the faster you'll return to your favorite activities. Carry a couple chemical cold packs in your car, so you can slap some ice on sore muscles on the ride home. Follow the guidelines for self-care in earlier chapters to give yourself the best chance at a rapid recovery.

The Least You Need to Know

➤ Osteopathic doctors, often called D.O.s, function in the same capacity as medical doctors (M.D.s) in the United States.

➤ Osteopathy views the human body holistically, as an integrated, unified organism. When there is a problem in one area, it affects all other areas of the body in some way.

➤ Osteopathic manipulations are specialized techniques to restore the normal position and function of joints and other components of your musculoskeletal system.

➤ Their comprehensive training in the musculoskeletal system gives D.O.s an ideal foundation for specializing in sports medicine.

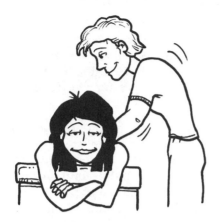

Chapter 21

Hands-On Healing: Therapeutic Massage and Physical Therapy

In This Chapter

➤ The healing power of touch

➤ What kind of massage should you try?

➤ Adding an Eastern touch

➤ Physical therapy techniques for back problems

There's nothing like a soothing, relaxing backrub to take your mind off your pain. No doubt about it, massage feels good. A massage that makes you feel good all over is often called a holistic massage—there's no particular problem areas, you're just getting all your muscles relaxed. Therapeutic massage, on the other hand, uses hand pressure and movements to relieve specific symptoms such as low-back pain. Massage focuses on this area in particular, and uses certain techniques depending on the nature of the problem.

The Therapeutic Benefits of Massage

It's easy to argue that any massage is therapeutic, since it makes you feel better. But what distinguishes therapeutic massage from "feel good" massage is its ability to relieve your pain and help the underlying problem to heal. There are dozens of different kinds of therapeutic massage; those we discuss in this chapter are the most common.

Not the Country, the Technique: Swedish Massage

When most of us think of massage, it's Swedish massage that comes to mind. The name has little to do with the country of Sweden except that the practitioner who developed most of the movements happened to be Swedish. Per Henrik Ling took a trip to China in the early 1900s and brought back with him knowledge and techniques of massage.

Back to Nature

One reason massage is so therapeutic, say holistic health care providers, is that it stimulates a natural soothing response. From the time we're born, we love to be touched. Touching relaxes and comforts. The rubbing and pressing movements of massage also increase blood circulation to aching muscles, further relaxing them. When tight muscles relax, they stop hurting.

Swedish massage is the most popular form of massage in the United States. It's what you'll find at most spas and health clubs that offer massage. It features a variety of movements, from long strokes to tight kneading. In Swedish massage, the practitioner uses oil or powder on your skin to make the movements smooth and friction free (unless friction is the intent). During the massage, you're generally unclothed with a sheet or blanket covering the parts of your body not being massaged.

Swedish massage is very relaxing; done well, it may put you to sleep. Though generally considered a holistic approach as a whole-body procedure, Swedish massage can be very effective in reducing specific muscle pain such as a strain or spasm.

Back Talk

In ancient China, massage was exclusively the territory of the blind. They performed a style of massage called amma (which means "massage" in Chinese). Amma called on the practitioner to use hands, fingers, elbows, and even knees to massage the entire body. In addition to relaxing and stretching muscles, amma stimulated acupuncture points to release blocked chi, or energy. Amma is still done in China today.

Freeing the Flow of Energy: Shiatsu, Tuina, and QiGong

Shiatsu (pronounced *she-AHT-soo*) is an Eastern form of massage that emphasizes stimulating your body's energy channels (meridians) and energy (chi). The practitioner uses pressing motions at acupuncture points to release blocked chi and restore your body to its natural balance. You get to keep all your clothes on for shiatsu. Though this form of massage arises from a holistic view of health, like acupuncture, it's generally done for therapeutic reasons such as back pain.

Tuina is also Eastern, a form of massage and bodywork practiced in China for more than 2,000 years. Practitioners use a combination of massage techniques and manipulation to relieve pain and restore function. As with shiatsu, unblocking chi is an important component of this therapy. Treatment sessions are usually short (30 minutes) and narrowly focused on the area or part of your body that hurts.

QiGong (pronounced *chee-goong* and sometimes spelled in different ways) is another form of chi stimulation in which the practitioner uses light touch over the relevant acupuncture points as well as the area of pain. This releases blocked chi and allows painful muscles and connective tissues to return to their positions and functions.

Back to Nature

Some massage practitioners bring the therapy to you. Portable massage chairs make it possible for you to receive a relaxing or therapeutic massage in just 15 or 20 minutes. Practitioners often use a form of tuina, and concentrate on the upper back and shoulders.

Delving Deep: Rolfing

Rolfing is a technique for deep connective tissue massage. Named after its developer, Ida Rolf, Ph.D., rolfing emphasizes balance and support for the body's normal structures and positions. The procedure is similar to myosfascial massage, although it is more intense. Some people absolutely cannot tolerate rolfing, while others find pain relief and restored function. During a rolfing session, most people feel a tingling, burning sensation in the skin over the area being rolfed. Rolfing practitioners say this is the releasing of tightened tissues. Rolfing seems most effective in chronic pain syndromes involving connective tissues, such as fibromyalgia. Rolfing is sometimes called structural integration massage.

Massage Strokes Your Back Will Love

One reason massage feels so good is that it feels so good. We humans like being stroked and touched. It helps us relax mentally as well as physically, and to enjoy a sense of comfort and well-being at least for a little while. Massage is more than patting and rubbing, though. There are hundreds, possibly thousands, of specific techniques and procedures that extend massage from "feels good" to effective and therapeutic.

Effleurage and Petrissage

Effleurage and *petrissage* are French terms for the two massage strokes most familiar to Americans. The long, smooth, strokes of effleurage are ideal for large areas such as your back. They bring relaxation and increased circulation to your muscles. Petrissage allows the massage practitioner to focus on a particular, and usually small, area. Using fingertips, the sides of hands, or thumb and finger, the practitioner isolates a muscle or tendon (often the site of greatest soreness) to knead and roll. This focused attention brings greater relaxation to the involved tissue.

243

Compression and Percussion

Compression and percussion are massage methods that exert gentle pressure on muscle tissues. Compression techniques push and roll muscles against deeper tissues and bones. Upon release, the massaged muscles stretch and expand. With percussion movements, the massage practitioner uses rapid chopping actions with the sides of the hands or sharp taps with the fingertips to stimulate and awaken your muscles. These techniques aren't as brutal as they sound—though there is a lot of practitioner action, the moves are quick and relatively gentle.

Friction and Vibration

Friction and vibration techniques generate heat (warmth) and deeper penetration of the massage's relaxing effects. The massage practitioner may knead and press sore muscles to encourage them to relax and loosen up. Rubbing your skin in such a way as to produce heat helps the treatment to reach deeper tissues.

Back Basics

Effleurage is a series of long, stroking movements that massage larger body areas. **Petrissage** is a series of small, kneading movements that massage a specific muscle or tendon.

Massage Your Range of Motion

Massage can work wonders for your range of motion, too. Muscles that are relaxed and stretched are more flexible, allowing your joints to move more fully. It's often useful to follow a massage with movements or manipulations to encourage flexibility and mobility while your muscles are still lulled into feeling good.

Improving your range of motion is especially helpful with conditions such as osteoarthritis and ankylosing spondylitis, where your bones are trying to fuse themselves together. Fused bones (either as a process of nature or surgery) limit your ability to twist, turn, and bend—the common measures of range of motion. Giving you greater range of motion both decreases your pain and postpones vertebral fusion.

Back Off!

While massage is generally very safe, there are some precautions you should take. First, never apply pressure to the front of your neck (throat). When massaging your arms and legs, rub toward your heart, not away, to work with the veins returning blood to the heart (they have valves in them to keep the blood from going the wrong way). And don't massage bruises, which are caused by small blood vessels bursting.

Muscle in on Back Pain

Most back pain, as you know by now, resides in your muscles. Therapeutic massage is a wonderful way to encourage it to move on. Your muscles love nothing more than being rubbed and kneaded. This relaxes them, increases circulation through them, and encourages a good nutrient/waste exchange.

Massage Yourself

You don't have to have someone else available every time you feel like a good massage. You can do it yourself. Of course, there are some places you won't be able to reach. But there are many you can—with astonishing results.

Self-massage techniques generally use fingertip pressure to rub sore muscles. Use firm, steady movements to knead and press the area. Your neck and your lower back are especially good locations for self-massage.

Don't Forget Your Neck and Shoulders

When your lower back hurts, it's easy to focus on it and forget about other parts of your back. Remember, what happens in one area of your back affects other areas. Tenseness in your neck and shoulders, though it seems a separate issue, can aggravate low-back pain. As your back tightens in response, the curves of your spine change. This creates tenseness in other areas, and before you know it, your back hurts all over. So tend to that neck and shoulders, often the first place to show tenseness and pain, to both feel better and keep the problem from spreading.

Back Talk

Though Hippocrates is reputed to have recommended a daily massage with fragrant oils as a means of staving off ill health, the ancient Greek physician Erasistratus (310–250 B.C.) was one of the first Westerners to document massage as a therapeutic technique. Erasistratus believed that much illness resulted from stagnant blood. Frequent massage and hot baths, he believed, were effective ways to get the blood moving again. Unfortunately, he also believed that binding an affected limb tightly enough to prevent any circulation at all also released the stagnation—not a good idea!

The Therapeutic Touch of Physical Therapy

Doctors sometimes refer people with back problems to physical therapy, especially to aid with rehabilitation after back surgery. The combination of mobility and flexibility movements, massage, strengthening exercises, and hot/cold therapies can help you feel better during the time your back takes to heal.

Physical therapy is oriented toward restoring your body to its normal functions. It's pure mechanics—looking at how your back is supposed to work, and attempting to return it to reasonable operating condition. One of its most important aspects is movement—if you're in physical therapy, your muscles are getting a workout. This is good for your back, which more than just about anything likes to be active.

245

The physical therapist may give you exercises and movements to do at home in-between treatments. This "homework" complements your physical therapy, and also gives you greater participation in your healing process.

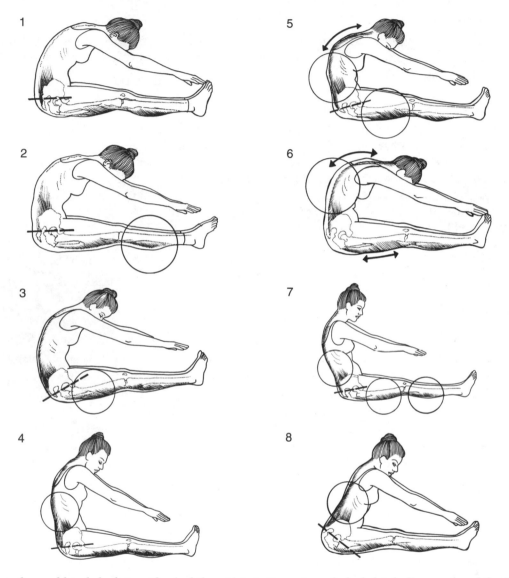

How forward bends look to a physical therapist: 1. Correct muskuloskeletal alignment and flexibility. 2. Correct hip alignment, but tight calf muscles. 3. Incorrect hip alignment, tight hamstrings. 4. Correct hip alignment, but tight lower-back muscles. 5. Overcompensation for tight hamstrings and lower-back muscles causes over rounding of the upper back. 6. Here the leg muscles are flexible, but the tightness in the lower back leads to overcompensation by rounding the upper back. 7. Extremely tight muscles in both the legs and lower back. 8. Back muscles are hyperextended, hip alignment is incorrect (compare this to the correct alignment of figure 1).

The Heat Treatment

Heat feels good. It's soothing and relaxing, bringing a sense of general comfort as well as pain relief. The physical therapist can apply heat to your back in several ways—heating pad, hot packs, ultrasound (using ultra-high-frequency sound waves), or diathermy (using gentle electrical current). Some physical therapists believe ultrasound and diathermy provide greater penetration to deep tissues, though the evidence for this isn't conclusive.

Heat packs come in various sizes and shapes that can conform to your problem area. Many are chemically activated (breaking an activator inside the pack initiates a chemical reaction that causes heat) and can stay warm for 30 minutes or longer. They're usually intended for one-time use.

Heating pads can use dry or moist heat. Moist heat penetrates more evenly and effectively in many situations. Heating pads are flexible, so they can wrap around or shape to fit sore body parts.

Chill Out

Sometimes those aching muscles are getting a little too much circulation, stimulating the nerves and reminding them that you hurt. Ice packs placed against the painful places helps shut down the blood supply, reducing swelling and pain. Practitioners sometimes use ice before stretching movements and myofascial massage, to lower the area's sensitivity. Don't leave ice on for more than 20 minutes or beyond the time your skin feels numb. You could end up with mild (but still unpleasant) frostbite.

Water, Water Everywhere: Hydrotherapy

If you like the water, you'll love hydrotherapy. This rehabilitative treatment approach uses water in several ways to relieve your hurting back. Warm whirlpool baths gently relax and stimulate sore muscles while the water's buoyancy supports your body. Heated exercise pools offer a sense of suspension, taking the pull out of gravity to let you move around with less resistance than you encounter on land. And cool baths or showers can take the sting out of swollen muscles.

Back Off!

That heat may feel good, but don't overdo it. Don't use a heating pad for longer than 20 minutes, and remove it right away if your skin becomes discolored. Don't lie on a heating pad, which can intensify its effect to the point where it burns your skin. And be especially careful in a hot tub or whirlpool bath—you don't want to fall asleep in the water.

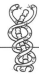

Back Care

Doctor tell you to ice that painful back? Try putting crushed ice in a sealed plastic bag, then lying on it. (Or you can use a bag of frozen peas—just don't eat them afterward!) The pressure of your weight helps the cold penetrate more deeply than if you laid on your stomach and put the ice pack on top of your back.

247

Let's Have a Ball!

A popular physical therapy treatment is the therapeutic ball. If you're recovering from back problems and have been to physical therapy, this is probably already familiar. Therapeutic balls come in various sizes, though most are large enough for an adult to sit on. And that's just what you do—you sit on it. The physical therapist will instruct you in a routine of exercises to do while you're sitting there trying not to bounce.

Though this looks more like fun than therapy, it's actually strengthening and stabilizing your back.

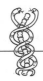

Back Care

Occupational therapy often incorporates activities from your daily routine, to help you regain and improve your functional skills. Do you have special hobbies or other activities you like to do? Ask your occupational therapist about using them in your therapy regimen.

Returning to Normal Function: Occupational Therapy

Occupational therapy is not job training, though it may help you prepare for a return to work if your back problem has taken you out of circulation for a while. Occupational therapy focuses on restoring function in the activities of daily living (sometimes referred to as ADLs), and sometimes specifically for your job or occupation. Occupational therapists use a variety of techniques to improve mobility and flexibility as well as functions such as stretching and lifting. Occupational and physical therapy often go hand in hand.

Practitioner Qualifications

Qualifications for massage and therapy practitioners vary depending on the practice and, sometimes, the location.

Massage Therapists

To qualify for state licensing, massage therapists must complete an accredited massage therapy program, usually 12 months long, and pass a written and demonstration examination. Licensed massage therapists can put the letters "L.M.T." after their names. L.M.T.s often work in physical therapy clinics, sports medicine clinics, private practices, and hospitals. They can perform therapeutic massages with or without a physician's referral.

Physical and Occupational Therapists

Physical therapists and occupational therapists undergo at least four years of education and training through an accredited college program. Before they can practice in most states, physical therapists must then pass registration examinations in the states in which they practice; occupational therapists must pass licensing examinations. The main difference between registered and licensed is terminology. A registered physical therapist puts the letters "R.P.T." or "P.T." after his or her name; a licensed occupational therapist puts the designation "L/O.T." or "O.T." after his or her name (varies from state to state).

Physical and occupational therapists often work in clinics and departments affiliated with hospitals. They provide the services a physician orders; they cannot initiate treatment without written instructions, like a prescription, from a physician.

Other Bodywork Practitioners

Training and qualifications for other bodywork practitioners vary. Those who specialize in Eastern methods, such as shiatsu and tuina, are often trained in Traditional Chinese Medicine. Some jurisdictions (states and cities) have specific licensing requirements for massage practitioners.

The Least You Need to Know

➤ Physical therapy, therapeutic massage, and other forms of bodywork focus on relaxing sore muscles and increasing circulation to them.

➤ Eastern forms of therapeutic massage also incorporate energy manipulation, focused on freeing blocks in the body's meridians to release chi (life energy).

➤ Learning self-massage techniques puts you in greater control of your back problems, giving you another tool to manage and reduce pain.

➤ Practitioner qualifications vary depending on the type of practitioner and the state in which he or she practices.

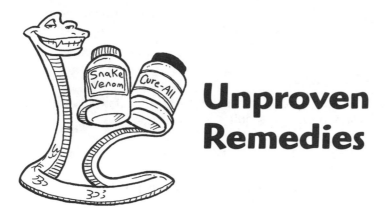

Chapter 22

Unproven Remedies

In This Chapter

➤ What's a sham and what's safe? A fun self-quiz

➤ How to evaluate treatment options

➤ How to cut through the hype when a treatment seems too good to be true

➤ Unproven treatments can do more harm than good

Every medical treatment that's successful today was once unproven and experimental. But for every treatment that's become commonplace, hundreds and even thousands have tumbled into oblivion, unable to prove their hopes and claims.

It's the nature of human beings to question and resist new ideas. Every schoolchild learns, with some amazement, that scientists and citizens alike once not only believed but had "proof" of the Earth's flatness. Venture near the edge, and you would fall off (though to where was never very clear). Curious sailors who questioned this assessment and who often failed to return from their explorations supplied much of the supporting "evidence."

Of course, ship travel was extraordinarily dangerous in times when ocean storms crushed the frail, wooden, wind-powered vessels that dared traverse their borders. But a few ships here and there managed to return to ports of civilization, and rumors spread that the Earth kept going beyond its edges. Explorers like Christopher Columbus confirmed the reports, and today children watch the globe that is their world from the cameras of space shuttles flying high above.

On the other hand, it's also a feature of human nature to believe in promises of quick cures and fast fixes—no matter how unproven or outlandish the claims. Nowhere are we more vulnerable to this apparent contradiction in beliefs than with our health. And always there are those willing to cash in by selling those promises—from magic beads to sophisticated gadgetry.

Fake or Real? A Self-Quiz

So how do you know what's a fraud and what's the real deal? It isn't always easy. See if you can separate fake from fact in this quick quiz!

1. Kiss a frog, cure a sore throat.

   Real _____   Fake _____

2. Sweating and cathartics (heavy-duty laxatives) can cure many diseases by purging the body.

   Real _____   Fake _____

3. The sea might contain the next generation of bone graft materials for surgeries such as spinal fusion.

   Real _____   Fake _____

4. Electricity generates a charge that cures.

   Real _____   Fake _____

5. Eating certain foods and avoiding others can prevent osteoarthritis.

   Real _____   Fake _____

6. Tobacco leaves can cure cancer.

   Real _____   Fake _____

7. Rubbing the sap from certain evergreen trees onto your aching back can relieve your pain.

   Real _____   Fake _____

Five of these statements are fact. How many of them did you get?

1. *Real* (though not an approach we recommend). Researchers have discovered that the skin of certain frogs contains a substance called magainin, which seems to fight infection and speed healing. Don't go licking just any frog, though. Not all frog skin contains magainin, and it takes quite a bit to have an effect. You're not likely to see this product on the market until researchers figure out how to create it in a laboratory.

2. *Fake.* When ancient healers noticed that profuse sweating often bathed a person right before a fever broke, they leaped to the wrong conclusion. The body sweats in response to elevated temperature as a way to cool itself. Creating sweat doesn't "cook" the disease out of you. Likewise, the profuse diarrhea that often precedes the end of a gastrointestinal virus is not purging the body of toxins, as it might

appear. Rather, the diarrhea results from the intestine's inability to function properly because of the toxins (usually in the form of a virus or bacterial food poisoning) that attack it. Once the body's immune system contains the infection (which today might happen with the aid of antibiotics), the intestine's function returns to normal. Causing diarrhea accomplishes little that's therapeutic and can create serious dehydration and other problems.

3. *Real.* The skeletal remains of sea creatures that we know as coral show great promise as a bone replacement in surgeries such as spinal fusion. Coral's porous structure gives body tissues (including new bone growth) a good grip. Though light in weight, coral is strong and doesn't shrink or swell when wet—an important consideration for items implanted into a body that's 65 percent water.

4. *Real.* Now don't go sticking your finger into a light socket or anything like that! We're talking low-level, controlled charges here. The TENS unit, which uses electricity to stimulate nerve endings, is one of many examples (though researchers disagree about its effectiveness). Heart defibrillators, which deliver a powerful jolt of electricity, are another. That electricity has turned out to have valid medicinal uses wasn't always apparent, however. For several decades after the discovery of electricity, electric gizmos and gadgets of all designs and shapes flooded the rapid remedy market. Most made wild, unsubstantiated claims— "Squeeze the handles and feel afflictions of any sort flee from your body." Not until the 1950s and 1960s did scientific research begin to demonstrate the ways in which electricity could—and could not—aid healing.

5. *Fake.* Osteoarthritis occurs when joint tissues degenerate, usually as a function of aging. Unfortunately, there is no known way to prevent this process. There are numerous ways to minimize the discomfort you feel from osteoarthritis, however, including avoiding foods such as corn, citrus fruits, and coffee (caffeine). Some people report cayenne pepper, either in capsules or added to foods, relieves arthritis pain (supported by scientific research of cayenne pepper's active ingredient, capsaicin, as a potent pain reliever—see Chapter 11, "Rx: Medical Approaches to Back Relief"). And according to recent studies, soup stock made from chicken or beef bones with cartilage attached may send glycosaminoglycons (GAGs) to repair your own damaged cartilage.

6. *Real.* Though in the ways we conventionally use them—smoking or chewing— tobacco leaves *cause* cancer, scientists have found ways to use living tobacco plants to produce genetically engineered substances that fight cancer. Hard as it is to imagine, this plant, so notorious for its cancer-*causing* abilities, could now do the opposite. The research results are very promising. Tobacco plants grow rapidly and are easy to control, making them ideal botanical factories.

7. *Real.* The camphor laurel tree is the source of natural camphor, the smelly compound contained in many liniments. Camphor is a mild pain reliever when

applied to the skin. A trip to your local drugstore would be a faster way to get a camphor product, unless you're planning a trip to China, Taiwan, or Japan, where the camphor laurel tree grows.

The Risks of Unproven Treatments

Sometimes the tonic that's supposed to heal does more harm than good. People in pain, especially chronic pain, are easy targets for unscrupulous gimmicks and miracle cures. With Americans spending billions of dollars a year on all sorts of drugs, devices, and treatments for back problems, it's not surprising that enterprising entrepreneurs see a gold mine in your suffering. Beware! At best, sham treatments steal your money. At worst, they can leave you, well, flat on your back (which, as you know, is no position to be in when your back bothers you)—or even kill you.

Do No Harm

Famed Greek healer Hippocrates (460–361 B.C.) taught his students to "first, do no harm." It was far more effective to aid the body in healing itself, Hippocrates lectured his students, than to interfere by using strong treatments and potions. Of course, many of the medicines used in his time were actually low doses of poisonous substances such as mandrake and belladonna (both members of the deadly nightshade family).

Your human body comes equipped with some powerful self-healing abilities, however. Hippocrates' warning is worth heeding even more so today, when it's so easy to reach for the medicine cabinet at the slightest sign of discomfort. Remember that any product you take to help you has potential side effects—be sure the possible benefits are worthwhile.

Back Talk

Hippocrates and physicians of his time believed that health was a state of balance among the four humors that governed the human body—blood, phlegm, black bile, and yellow bile. Healing was a matter of restoring harmony. The fortunate found relief in simple dietary changes; others endured concoctions containing ground beetle bodies and minerals like copper. Bleeding and purging were also favorite approaches.

Deadly Doses

Even "friendly" substances can turn deadly when you take too much. Acetaminophen and aspirin, for example, are extraordinarily toxic when taken in large quantities.

Overdoses of these common drugs are often fatal because they cause permanent and severe liver and kidney damage. Many unconventional treatments use known substances for purposes other than intended (or add substances that aren't identified on the label). Just because a product works well to suppress your cough doesn't mean another form of it will cure your fibromyalgia, for example. Such "off label" use is risky because you're always at risk for side effects. If you hear or read about a new treatment approach, talk with your doctor before you try it. Your doctor has access to information on the latest research and drug manufacturer recommendations.

Check It Out

When you go to the grocery store, how do you buy tomatoes? Do you just toss a few in a bag and head for the cash register? Or do you pick one up, examine it for soft spots and bruises, and maybe even give it a quick sniff before putting it down and reaching for a better one? Yet how do you buy an over-the-counter pain reliever? Some people read labels and compare ingredients, but most buy the brands their friends use or they see advertised. Sometimes we're more selective buying produce than we are in choosing new treatments for back pain!

Ask Your Health Care Provider

Your primary health care provider is your best source for information about treatment options and new approaches. This professional has been caring for you and knows your back problems. She also receives the latest information from research studies and other professional sources that are not always available to the average person. If you find something intriguing, ask your doctor to help you check it out. Remember, though, that your doctor has a busy schedule and may take a few days to a week or so to get back to you. Patience! It's worth your wait to get the straight scoop.

Independent Evidence

There's no question the World Wide Web has caused a sea of change in how we find information. This library at your fingertips puts you in touch with a vast array of materials about every imaginable subject. While Web sites contain much useful information, there's also a lot of nonsense and even outright fraud. Verify what you find through reliable sources such as official associations and printed materials at the traditional library. (Though just because it's in print doesn't make it true, either.)

Try to locate the source of a report that catches your interest, to find out who's releasing the information. And look for evidence supported more by scientific research methods than by anecdotal stories. You can't be too careful when it comes to your health.

If It Sounds Too Good to Be True...

You've heard it before, and we're saying it again—if a treatment sounds too good to be true, it is. Think for just a minute about your doctors. Under the white coats and behind the stethoscopes, your doctors are caring people who want to end your back pain just as much as you do. Why would they hide from you the one treatment that could do just that? They'd be the heroes for "curing" you!

Back Off!

There are certain telltale words that identify questionable products. If the label or the advertisement boasts of "secret ingredients," "overnight success," "proven by millions of people just like you," or "break-through cure," get out your hip waders and shovel. Odds are, by the time you dig through all the hyperbole, you won't find much substance to the claims.

You haven't heard about Hurt-No-More Ultra Back Cream from your doctors because it's not a reputable product, not because they want to prolong your agony. If you have any doubts, just ask them—they'll gladly explain why they haven't recommended or prescribed this product. And if there's a chance Hurt-No-More Ultra Back Cream could help your pain, your doctors will tell you that, too.

Nothing Cures Everything

Check a product's claims. If it can handle everything from bunions to styes (and hemorrhoids, too), odds are, the product is taking credit for Mother Nature's work that will take place regardless. Remember, 85 percent of all back pain goes away in six to eight weeks, whether you treat it or not. A handy situation for the purveyor of the cure-all—after all, who can argue with the product's effectiveness if you get better when you use it? (Never mind that you'd get better if you didn't use it, too.)

"Amazing" Testimonials

"I was so miserable I couldn't even turn on the TV. It was like my back was frozen in pain. Then I tried Pain-B-Gone, and I feel like a kid again! Last week I ran in the Boston Marathon, and next week I start a bicycle tour through Australia. Pain-B-Gone is truly a miracle!"

Nothing is more compelling than the smiling face of someone who's found relief and wants to share his story. Not to begrudge him his joy, but there's no way to know what, if anything, the miracle product had to do with his "miraculous" recovery. Products that rely on personal testimonials seldom have any objective evidence to support their claims—evidence that others can reliably reproduce.

Modern advertising often uses the testimonial, too, with a professional-looking actor or famous athlete touting the benefits of the latest and greatest, clinically proven, fast-acting pain reliever. Ten minutes later, a real-life person (portrayed, of course, by an actor) may praise the same product.

Often the product does what the ads say it does, and there are clinical research findings that support the claims. But usually so do dozens of other products that contain similar ingredients. Read labels and compare prices. Your back doesn't know if you paid $15 or $5 for your pain reliever.

And remember, relief is relative. How well a product relieves your pain, and how quickly, is related to such factors as whether you're at work or at home, the time of day you take it, and what you expect it to do, in addition to the product's actual capabilities.

Back Talk

A good many medical conventions start out scorned by traditional wisdom and end up changing the practice of medicine. For example, a few observant obstetricians first proposed the idea in the 1760s that childbirth or puerperal fever (an often deadly infection following childbirth) was infectious and doctors themselves carried it from one patient to another. Not until the 1890s did doctors wash their hands before, instead of after, delivering a baby. Today, of course, doctors and nurses scrub fastidiously before donning sterile gowns and gloves.

Popular but Unproven Treatments

Scientific research is a long and complex process. Success requires repeatable results, which of course means numerous tests by different researchers. Miracles don't happen overnight; progress occurs over years and sometimes decades. Sometimes procedures and products show great promise in controlled studies, then falter when they move into real-world use. Sometimes they work as expected for years, then develop problems researchers didn't anticipate.

Unproven treatments are not necessarily harmful or useless. Often, there isn't enough demand to conduct full-scale research on a particular idea or approach. There might already be proven, effective treatments available, or only a few individuals who would benefit. Occasionally, extensive study doesn't arrive at any conclusions. Perhaps the *control group* responds just as well to a *placebo* as the *study group* responds to a new medication or device. Or the product works exceptionally well when it works, but it doesn't work in very many people. (We'll talk more about placebos in just a bit.)

The U.S. federal government regulates all medicines, and all medicines must receive federal approval before they can be sold in the United States.

Back Basics

Research studies usually have a **study group** and a **control group**, each containing similar numbers of people with similar symptoms or conditions. The study group receives the item being tested. The control group receives a standard treatment or a **placebo**, which is a pretend version of the tested item. This allows researchers to measure and compare results.

Back Care

Many insurance companies and health plans will not cover treatments or medications that the general medical community considers experimental. If your doctor proposes an unproven treatment, find out who will pay for it and who will take care of you and any additional costs if something goes wrong.

Approved medicines have passed strict testing procedures that evaluate claimed effectiveness as well as possible adverse effects (bad side effects). Devices and procedures (including many kinds of surgery) are not subject to this approval process, however.

This often leaves doctors to decide whether a particular device or procedure will benefit a patient (like you). More and more often, doctors are requiring rigorous testing to help them with these decisions. If your health care provider suggests an unproven treatment, be sure you fully understand why he thinks it would benefit you, and how it differs from conventional (accepted) treatments. Also be sure you know all of the potential side effects.

Chemonucleolysis

When chemonucleolysis made its debut in the early 1960s, it looked like the cure-all for painful herniated disks. In this treatment, the doctor injects a damaged intervertebral disk with a solution of chymopapain, a natural enzyme derived from papaya. The enzyme dissolves the nucleus, or core, of the disk, shrinking the disk and relieving the pressure it placed on the spinal cord or nerves. Optimistic orthopedists and patients alike hoped that at last there was a treatment that could avoid surgery.

After nearly 40 years of practical use, few American physicians view chemonucleolysis as even a viable treatment alternative for most patients. While one study reported that 80 percent of nearly 17,000 patients obtained relief after treatment, other studies had less impressive results. In many people, chemonucleolysis creates reactions ranging from more pain (just what you need when you already hurt) to no change at all. Where the doctor puts the needle is critical; off just a bit, and the chymopapain squirts into nearby tissues and misses its mark entirely.

For some people, though, chemonucleolysis with chymopapain appears to work well. And the procedure is widely used in Europe and in Australia. In multiple studies, researchers have found chymopapain injections to be more effective than a placebo but less effective than conventional surgery. It's important to recognize, too, that surgeons in the United States perform far more back surgeries than surgeons in other countries.

Prolotherapy

Like chemonucleolysis, prolotherapy seems to work in some people. This treatment involves injecting a substance (such as a mixture of dextrose and morruhate sodium) directly into spinal ligaments. The injected mixture causes irritation to the tissues, which in theory then causes the body to generate new connective tissue that stabilizes the joint over time.

Though prolotherapy has been around since 1939, it's failed to gain widespread support either in practice or in research. It's not a pleasant treatment—the injected area remains inflamed and sore for several days to a week, and treatment usually requires at least three and sometimes six or more injections.

In several studies, people in the study group felt no better than people in the control group—and often felt worse because of the treatment's abrasive approach. Most often, doctors use prolotherapy in conjunction with other therapies such as spinal manipulation, exercise, and even steroid injections. This makes it especially hard to determine whether it's prolotherapy or the other treatments that do the most to relieve pain.

DMSO

In use as an industrial solvent since the 1940s, DMSO (short for dimethyl sulfoxide) gained popularity as a wonder drug in the 1970s when researchers discovered it had the unique ability to carry substances into the bloodstream after being applied to the skin. DMSO also seemed to act on its own as a pain reliever when applied to aching joints, sprains, and strains. Regulatory agencies in the United States approved DMSO for limited and specific use as an experimental agent. Despite serious concerns about possible eye and kidney damage, DMSO gathered momentum as a folk remedy for arthritis, multiple sclerosis, and a host of other conditions.

The greatest danger DMSO seems to present is that it often contains impurities that enter your system as well. These may be in the product or from substances you may have on your skin. At this time, limited research continues to study possible benefits of DMSO, though there are no recognized medicinal uses for the substance. This is truly a "use at your own risk" product with unknown side effects.

Snake and Bee Venom

Some people claim to receive relief from arthritis pain from injections of bee venom (also called apitherapy) or snake venom. There's no scientific research to support this, though there are studies underway to examine the actions of certain proteins in bee and snake venoms. Most venoms have an anticoagulant effect—they interfere with your blood's clotting ability, especially at the point of the sting or bite. There's some evidence that the proteins responsible—chemically separated from the toxins in the venom—might help stroke patients, for example. However, this research is still young.

Some apitherapy practitioners have live bees sting around the painful joints; others use a needle and syringe to inject bee venom. Bee venom is particularly dangerous as an allergen—a substance that triggers allergic reactions. Since allergies tend to develop over time, it's possible to suddenly be allergic to bee stings when you weren't before.

Actual snake venom is hazardous under any circumstances. Though practitioners of snake venom treatment say the amounts of poison that enter your system are very small, you're still putting poison into your body. Neither bee venom nor snake venom therapies are recognized medical treatments in the United States.

Back Talk

"Snake oil" was a popular remedy for whatever ailed Americans as the nineteenth century transitioned into the twentieth. Often sold by hucksters with dubious credentials who rode from town to town in horse-drawn buggies, snake oil had very little to do with either snakes or oil. Though formulations varied widely, most contained alcohol or opium. Little wonder they "cured" everything! In the lingo of the times, these cure-alls were called patent medicines. Few disclosed their contents, and trademarks protected most.

High Doses of Vitamins

Many people view vitamins as an insurance policy of sorts for their bodies. You know you don't always eat right, and may not provide your body the nutrients it needs. While most adults probably don't need a general vitamin supplement, they won't do any harm by taking one, either. Your body uses what it needs, and passes out what it doesn't. Like other helpful substances, however, too much of a good thing can hurt. Some vitamins are dangerous in high doses because your body stores them instead of eliminating them. These are often the *fat-soluble vitamins*—A, D, E, and K. But instead of "insuring" your body's needs, extra supplies of them can interfere with regular body functions.

Back Basics

Fat-soluble vitamins come from foods that contain fats and oils, and your body processes and stores them as it does other dietary fats. **Water-soluble vitamins** come from other food sources. Your body takes what it needs from what comes in, and excretes (passes out) any extra.

There is strong evidence that extra supplies of *water-soluble vitamins*—B complex and C—help at times when your body needs more. For example, extra vitamin B greatly lowers the risk of certain birth defects (including spina bifida) when taken just before and in the early stages of pregnancy. There is also evidence that extra vitamin C boosts your immune system's ability to fight infections such as colds. Your body still just takes only what it needs in these situations—it just needs more. Giving it more than that is, well, throwing your money away. And if you're taking extra amounts of fat-soluble vitamins, you could build up toxic levels that can cause serious illness and even death.

Many vitamin compounds, especially multivitamins, also contain minerals such as iodine, iron, and zinc. While your body needs these essential elements for cell activity, it needs only miniscule amounts. The border between enough and too much is measured in fractions of milligrams—sort of like putting angels on the head of a pin. Your body stores minerals in the same way it keeps reserves of fat-soluble vitamins. An iron overdose can easily be fatal; overdoses of other minerals cause serious health problems as well.

"Feel Good" Remedies

There are countless remedies that claim to help you feel good and relieve your back pain in the process. Typically, these are noninvasive—nothing enters your body, so there's little likelihood that the remedy could hurt you. These include aromatherapy, reflexology, polarity therapy, reiki, spiritual healing, and others. You may in fact feel better with these remedies—most emphasize relaxation and calming. However, there is no scientific evidence they do anything to help your back. The risk to you is mostly economic—you could spend a lot of money on "treatments" that really don't do anything.

If you haven't had a doctor (allopathic, osteopathic, or chiropractic) evaluate back pain that you've had for longer than two months, consider doing so before you try un-proven remedies. While it's true that modern medicine often has little to offer for routine back pain, delaying needed medical care for an underlying condition because an unproven remedy makes you feel better could complicate your situation. After all, this is your back, and you're stuck with it for the long haul!

If It's No Good, Why Does It Work?

So why do so many smart, sincere people receive relief from products that have no verifiable benefits? Generally, because there are other healing factors at work.

If I Think It, It Will Be: The Placebo Effect

There are powerful connections between your body and your mind. Researchers have shown over and over again that study participants who receive a placebo often report an improvement in their symptoms. The placebo effect is science's term for the power of positive thinking.

"Psychosomatic" has gotten a bad rap in Western cultures, where we tend to view this mind (psycho) and body (somatic) relationship as something shameful or at least negative. But think of the power this gives you to manage the discomforts of your body! Wouldn't it be the ultimate healing experience to use your mind and your thoughts to influence and change your body?

Back to Nature

Attitude may be the most powerful medicine of all. A positive mindset puts you in control—not necessarily of your condition, but of how it affects you and your life.

261

Life Cycles: All Things Eventually Come to an End

Many back problems are what doctors call "self-limiting"—they'll heal on their own, in time. Remember, 85 percent of back problems go away within eight weeks, whether you do anything to help them or not (and often in spite of your efforts). It's easy and common to credit whatever you're taking or doing. Traditional treatment generally focuses on relieving the symptoms (pain) until that healing takes place. An unproven treatment may make you feel better because you believe it will (the placebo effect). During the time you use or take either traditional or unproven approaches, your back heals itself, but you credit the treatment.

The Least You Need to Know

➤ You're especially vulnerable when you hurt, and there are unfortunately all too many unscrupulous remedies that do nothing but lighten your wallet.

➤ Some unproven treatments are harmful. The key is to explore all the options and consequences before making a decision to try one.

➤ Most accepted treatment practices have undergone extensive research and testing. While this doesn't necessarily make them 100 percent safe (nearly all treatments have possible side effects), it does provide sound information to examine as you consider your options.

➤ The placebo effect is a powerful reminder of the strong connection between the mind and the body.

Part 6
Back-Healthy Living

The doctor of the future will give no medicine but will interest his patients in the care of the human frame, in diet, and in the cause and prevention of disease.
—Thomas A. Edison, American inventor (1847–1931)

Your back health is in your hands. Or feet, as the case may be. Regular activity is the key to keeping your back strong and flexible, so it can take on the burdens of your daily life without complaint or damage.

The chapters in Part 6 offer tips and suggestions for back-healthy—and happy—living, from childhood through old age.

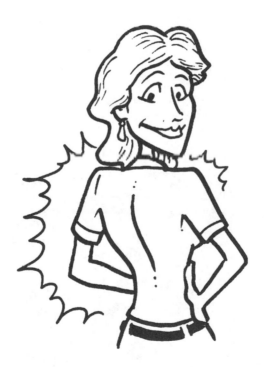

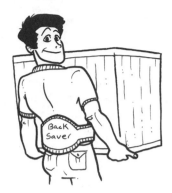

Chapter 23

Back to Work

In This Chapter

➤ Does your work environment support your back?

➤ Simple changes can make a big difference

➤ Activity is the key to back health no matter how ergonomic your workplace

➤ Special needs and risks for home-based offices

Where do you spend most of your time? If you guessed in bed, you're right! But if you work from age 21 to age 65, you spend most of your waking hours at work. Though we look at this as a modern phenomenon, it really isn't. Just a few generations ago, work was the way of life for nearly everyone age 12 and older. Americans continue to enjoy a slight decrease each decade in the amount of hours spent at work (though we lag behind our European counterparts by 8 to 10 hours a week in leisure time).

So what're you doing during those 35 or so hours each week the U.S. Department of Labor's Bureau of Labor Statistics says you're on the job? Odds are, you're sitting or standing.

How Ergonomic Is Your Workplace?

As the human experience has shifted from the wilds of prehistoric times to the containment of modern living, how we interact with our environment has made a tremendous shift. We no longer sit on terra firma to rest when we're tired. We plop our anatomies onto chairs that seem to be either attractive or functional but not especially comfortable. Squatting on the ground, we'd simply get up and move when the position became tiring. In today's office, we often remain in the same position for hours on end. Sometimes, of course, this is unavoidable. For whatever reason, your personal comfort is not your job's top priority.

Ergonomics—the study of how people interact with their environments—aims to integrate your comfort with your productivity. Though in most environments we have a long way to go, we've made considerable progress over the past few decades. Chairs contour more to the human body. Computer keyboards split and curve to allow your hands to fall naturally into place. Shock-absorbing mats give your feet a break when your job is to stand all day. The innovations in ergonomics are too numerous to mention, but do you know how many of them make your workplace a more back-friendly place to spend your time?

Back Talk

OSHA (the Occupational Safety and Health Administration, an agency of the U.S. Department of Labor) issues comprehensive standards for workplace well-being. Most industries now have OSHA ergonomic standards that establish guidelines for worker safety and comfort on the job. Ergonomic standards cover a wide range of workplace environment factors, from devices to protect against injury (such as lumbar supports) to recommendations for preventing repetitive-motion injuries. Your employer's human resources or personnel department should have a copy of the standards that apply to your industry.

Back Care

In the interest of promoting workplace wellness, many employers hire outside consultants to evaluate the company's ergonomics. This provides an objective assessment of the good, the bad, and the ugly—what works, what can be altered to work better, and what can't be changed. Urban areas often have companies that specialize in ergonomic assessments. In other areas, physical therapy groups often offer such a service.

Furniture

If you work in an office, you spend a lot of time sitting behind a desk. How do you feel after 20 minutes? After two hours? At the end of the day? If you routinely leave work with more aches and pains than you brought with you, it's time to evaluate your furnishings.

Your chair should be height adjustable, so you can sit in it with your feet flat on the floor and your thighs relatively parallel to the floor. If you can't achieve this adjustment, get a small footstool to put under your desk to accommodate your height (or lack thereof). Do you hunch your shoulders when you write at your desk? Your chair is too low. Do you bend over? Then your chair is too high. A good reference point is your navel (otherwise known as your belly button), which should be even with the top of your desk.

Do you spend a lot of time in the employee lounge? (Not slacking, of course, because we know you take only your legitimate breaks.) Often the furnishings (this being a generous use of the word) there are castoffs from other uses. Some employee lounges have just folding chairs and long tables. This may have the desired effect of keeping you from overstaying your break time, but it also doesn't allow you to relax and unwind. You're probably better off taking a short walk on your 10-minute break than sitting on a metal folding chair.

The ergonomic workplace.

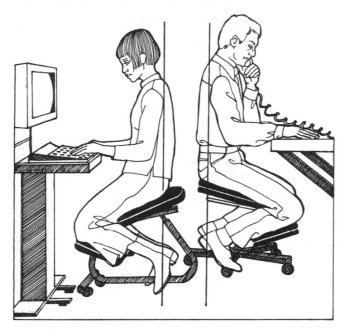

Computers

Do you use a computer in your job? How high and far away is the monitor from where you sit? Do you tilt your head up or slouch to get a better view? When you use the keyboard, are your forearms parallel with the ground? If you rest your hands on your computer keyboard when you type, you could be interfering with their ability to fall naturally on the keys. This causes a tenseness that makes its way up your arms, into your shoulders and neck, and down your back. Try one of those padded wrist rests (say that three times in a row!) to help keep your hands straight when your fingers strike the keys.

Though we say, with a mixture of pride and awe, that the personal computer has altered life like no other device before it, we don't often recognize the full ramifications of the observation. Computers allow you to stay longer in one position without moving because they process information so quickly, you don't have time to rest. It's incredibly easy to sit in front of a computer for hours—unless you create a time for a break, your computer just keeps spinning its disks (dragging you along with it).

Walking and Standing Surfaces

Are you on your feet all day? Do you stand or walk on floors made of wood or concrete? Carpeted or not? Hard surfaces send all the shock of each footstep you take back through your body. Carpet helps, especially if there's a good pad underneath it.

If you're on your feet all day and your back hurts, check your shoes. Are they well padded? Do they offer good arch and heel support? Adding an inexpensive pair of gel inserts can make you feel like you're walking on air. If your back continues to bother you, consider visiting a *podiatrist* to see if custom *orthotics* might give your back a break.

Job Functions

Just what do you do all day, anyway? If you sit at a desk, do you work on a computer or write on paper? Do you spend a lot of time on the telephone? Do you try to fix problems for people who are angry? What you spend your time doing can be as important for your back's health as where you spend it. Stress and tension seem to play key roles in how often and how badly your back hurts. Just as some people may go home from work with a tension headache, others leave with a tension backache.

Some jobs require you to wear a lot of weight around your waist. Police officers, for example, wear gear that weighs in at 20 pounds or more. A carpenter's tool belt can weigh as much or more. This extra weight isn't especially good for your back. Many belt systems now come with shoulder harness options, helping to distribute the load more evenly.

Back Basics

A **podiatrist** is a health care provider (Doctor of Podiatric Medicine, or D.P.M.) who specializes in foot care. **Orthotics** are devices, usually custom-made for your feet, that fit into your shoes to alter the way you walk and stand.

Back to Nature

If yours is a high-stress job, learn a few relaxation techniques that you can do anywhere, any time. Deep, slow breathing is an easy one that can make a remarkable difference in your stress level. Give yourself a mental break once in a while, too—step outside and watch the birds or look at the flowers.

Avoid Back-Breaking Loads

Don't load your back with more than it can bear. It's tempting, we know. After all, you probably don't have helpers who run eagerly to your car when you arrive at work, willing to take all your "stuff" and carry it to your office for you. (If you did, they'd no doubt have back problems, too!) So take it easy. Rather than loading up for one trip, make two reasonable trips. Hold items close to your body to make them easier to carry. If you throw a bag over one shoulder, carry something in the opposite arm that's of equal weight to balance your burden.

Educate Yourself

The most important thing you can do for your back is learn how to protect it. All the ergonomic designs in the world won't help you if you don't know how to use them correctly. If your back is a problem, take a field trip to a store specializing in back-care or ergonomic products. You don't have to buy anything (though you certainly can if the desire strikes you).

Just look around at what's available and how it's used. See how the store sets up sample workstations. Would any of their ideas work in your office or job site? Some stores will let you try out an ergonomic workstation or chair for a few days (with your employer's approval, of course).

Educate yourself about your back, too. You've taken a great step in that direction by buying and reading this book. Try some of our suggestions, and see if they make a difference for you. If not, try something else. Not everything works for everybody. You can't learn what works for you if you don't look around and try various approaches.

Lifting

How did lifting get to be such a problem for us? After all, our ancestors lifted everything from the day's hunt to bales of hay, all in a good day's work. We bend down to pick up a stack of file folders and ppffttt! there goes the back. Have we become weaklings? Partly, yes. Those ancestors who routinely hefted heavy loads did it all the time. Their muscles and bodies were strong and well conditioned. They also knew their limits, and worked out ways to carry items efficiently, since they often had to travel great distances with them. Hunters shared the load of the hunt. We seem to think if we can get our arms around it, we should be able to pick it up. Never mind how heavy or awkward!

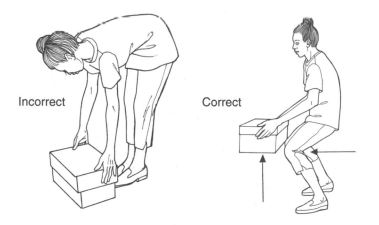

Incorrect

Correct

The incorrect and correct ways to lift heavy objects.

When you lift, use both hands. Bend from the knees, not the waist. Keep the item close to your body, for balance and to reduce the strain it puts on your back. Pivot your whole body if you have to turn (don't twist at the waist)—follow your toes. If the

269

thought that flashes through your mind is, "Aw, I can carry that!" go get someone to help you—you can't. And whenever possible, use wheels, even if your load's not that heavy. Carts, dollies, and hand trucks can make your life so much easier.

Carrying

What do you carry during the day? If your first response is "nothing much," stop and think. Most of us carry far more than we realize—we're so used to our regular loads, we don't notice them. Many women carry purses—if you're one of them, how much does yours weight? More than you think, we'd bet! When that weight's slung over one shoulder, it creates an imbalance that your back has to accommodate by shifting its curvature. By now, you know there must be a way to make life better for your back.

Whatever you carry—book bag, briefcase, tool box—try to balance your load. If you wear your book bag on your back, be sure it has two straps and use them both (one over each shoulder). Remember, the farther from your body your load is, the heavier it feels to your back. If you have young children, consider using a stroller whenever possible, or a backpack made especially to carry toddlers. And remember, carrying some weight correctly might actually increase bone density, not to mention muscle strength.

Lumbar Supports

A lumbar support (sometimes called a back belt) is a wide, belt-like device with shoulder straps. It fastens snugly around your waist and lower back, with strong straps that go over your shoulders and cross or connect across the center of your back. The idea is that when you're wearing a lumbar support, it provides extra support and stability for your lower back. This is particularly helpful when you're bending or lifting.

Back Talk

Many companies require employees whose jobs involve lifting to wear lumbar supports to prevent lower-back injuries. Do they help? Recent research suggests not. The National Institute for Occupational Safety and Health (NIOSH) has concluded there is no evidence that wearing a lumbar support reduces the risk of back injury in a healthy worker. If you already have a back problem, however, a lumbar support gives your lower back extra stability during bending and lifting. Just don't be lulled into thinking you're "safe" because you're wearing a lumbar support. You still need to use proper lifting techniques to reduce the risk of hurting your back.

Get Off Your Duff, You Couch Potato!

What do you do when you get home from work? Your back hurts, so you crash on the couch? Sit up and pay attention! Lying around is about the worst thing you can do for your back (following at a close second is sitting around). You have to get up and get moving to keep your back happy.

Plan to Be Active

Don't just wait for opportunities for activity to present themselves. Plan them! Do you work in an urban or suburban area? Look for a health club nearby that's open early in the morning, late in the evening, and during lunch time. Join it, and schedule time on your calendar to use it. Plan to take a walk at lunch, don't just think you'll do it if you have enough time.

Buy a timer (one that doesn't tick or alarm with an obnoxious sound, if you share workspace with others), and set it to alert you every 30 minutes. When it rings, stop what you're doing, if safely possible, and take a quick stretch break. If your boss or coworkers view this with suspicion, turn it into a productive moment—walk to the supply closet to get some paperclips, or drop your pencil on the floor and stand and bend to pick it up (a nice stretching exercise for your back). Before long, these little diversions will become part of your everyday ritual, and you won't need a timer to remind you.

Question Your Choices

Even if you feel like a cog in a machine by the end of the day, you're no automaton. You're a living, breathing, thinking human being who can make wise decisions by considering factors and consequences. Don't sink into the sofa the minute you walk through the front door until you think about what you're doing and what else you could do. Could you walk to the end of the driveway to check the mail? What about taking the dog for a walk while you're at it? Ask yourself: What is the worst that could happen if I do this, and if I don't? More often than not, your answer will provide your decision.

If Your Back Gives You Problems

Sometimes no amount of ergonomic changes can make your body 100 percent happy. Sometimes there are limits on what can be done in the workplace. And sometimes your back will give you problems, either as a direct or indirect result of your job tasks or work environment.

Just remember—your back isn't in charge, you are. And you now know how to go through your day in a way that protects but doesn't pamper your aching back. You now know that even when it hurts, your back prefers to be active and moving rather than still and immobile.

Do what you can to make your work environment and your job tasks more back-friendly. Think about your work day, and plan times and places to do a few stretches, exercises, or yoga postures. There may never be an ideal job or an ideal workplace as far as your back is concerned, so you'll have to create the best environment you can.

Part Time and Light Duty

Most mid-size and large companies offer some sort of part-time or light-duty option for people returning to work after an injury or illness. If you hurt your back on the job, in most situations your employer is required to accommodate your temporary needs to help you get back in the workforce again.

Light duty generally consists of tasks that require little physical effort. A police officer returning to work on light duty might sit at a desk at the police station, answering telephones and assisting citizens who come in. This is "light" compared to the regular duties of chasing bad guys. Sometimes, however, light duty isn't all that much better for your back than regular duty.

If you've been off work with a back injury, returning to a position where you sit all day is not going to help you much, however, unless you have plenty of opportunities to stand, stretch, and walk. (Though of course, lounging on the couch in front of the TV at home is no better.) As much as possible, discuss your light-duty responsibilities with your supervisor to be sure they help, not hinder, your recovery process.

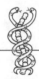

Back Care

Are you returning to light or regular duty that involves a lot of time on the telephone? Use a headset. Whether yours is a basic device with an earpiece and a microphone attached to a band you wear over your head or a high-tech model that fits over your ear like a Star Trek communications device, a headset keeps you from cradling the phone receiver on your shoulder (and cramping your neck) while trying to talk and take notes at the same time.

A return to your regular job duties on a part-time basis is another way to ease back to work. You do your usual job tasks, just not for as long as if you returned to work full-time. Your employer may permit you to work mornings instead of all day, or three days a week instead of five.

Sometimes partial days are easier to accommodate than a shortened work week, both for your back and for your employer, depending on your job's staffing needs and other aspects of your lifestyle. Perhaps you can arrange to work during peak hours, for example from 10 a.m. to 2 p.m., which gives your employer some flexibility in covering other needs.

Work in cooperation with your supervisor to make your return smooth and efficient for you and your coworkers. Keep your attitude and your tone positive. Even if your boss seems uncooperative, he or she is not likely being mean just for the sake of meanness (if this is the case, see the later section on considering a career change). Look for ways that your needs and wishes can benefit others, too. This draws your supervisor and your co-workers into collaboration with you, resulting in less stress for everyone, including you.

Ergonomic Aids and Devices

There are a wide variety of ergonomic aids and devices available for today's workplace, from lumbar support belts to pads that raise your wrists when you type. If these are available to you, try them. Some work, and some don't make a noticeable difference. Many people find relief in simple devices, such as lumbar support pillows to cushion and support the lower back and a short footstool for variation in foot position when standing or sitting for long periods of time.

Most ergonomic aids are designed to maintain your body in proper posture during the activities of your job. Ergonomic chairs, for example, adjust up and down for height and feature adjustable support for your lower back. But no device, however ergonomic, takes the place of regular movement to keep your back from getting stiff and sore in the first place. If your workstation is so ergonomic it could win an award, you still need to leave it once in a while to stretch and relax.

Back to Nature

One of the most effective ergonomic devices you can invest in is a mirror. All too often, you slump into back-hostile positions without realizing you've done so. Your shoulders slope forward, then your back sags—before you know it, everything hurts. Hang a small mirror where you can see yourself when you glance at it. This helps you see your posture, so you can catch that slump before it slides into pain. Don't sit ramrod straight, though—that will also hurt. And remember to move around frequently, to give your muscles a chance to stretch.

Back Talk

Back problems are no laughing matter. They cost American industry more than $50 billion each year in lost time and medical expenses, and are the leading cause of disability in Americans under age 45. About 2 percent of the American workforce—nearly half a million people—miss work because of back problems each year.

Consider a Career Change

We don't mean to sound cavalier, but if your job has become a regular pain in the back, maybe it's time to find a new line of work. Do you love your job, wake up eager to get there, leave with a sense of reluctance? If you do, your situation sounds like the American dream come true—don't let a little thing like back pain shut you out. If your present job doesn't place on your list of favorite ways to spend time, however, you might want to consider making a change.

You certainly won't be alone. Unlike earlier generations who worked a lifetime for the same employer, the typical American today holds jobs in as many as five or more different career fields. There is greater flexibility in job changes than ever before. What would you like to do? What keeps you from doing it? Often, just clarifying the obstacles you perceive to stand between you and your dream job is enough to start you on your way to it.

Don't feel like your back problems need to chase you out of your job, though. Moving *from* something is seldom as satisfying as moving *to* something. Maybe your back gets the process rolling, but in the end you make choices and changes for a variety of reasons.

If you do decide to make a career or job change, pay attention to ergonomic elements in your prospective working environment as you go for interviews. You know now what to look for; don't hesitate to ask to see where you'll be working if you join the new company. Will you have your own workspace that you can customize to meet your needs? Will you have ample opportunity to get up and move around during the workday, to stretch your muscles and relax your back?

When Your Office Is in Your Home

For years, home-based businesses had little to choose from when it came to office furniture. You could buy the same items your former employer purchased—but most small businesses have small budgets. And besides, aren't you working in a home-based business at least partly because you wanted to get away from the corporate environment? You can use home furnishings to create a comfortable setting—but a kitchen table doesn't work as well for typing or computer work as it does for serving meals. And after all, you have to maintain some sense of professionalism.

As the numbers of home-based businesses and work-at-home options grow, so is the home-office furnishings industry. New lines of desks and chairs blend the function of office with the comfort of home. Shop carefully for your home-office furnishings—you'll probably spend more time using them than you did the items in your old office.

Shop around and try things out. Draw out the dimensions of your home-office space on a piece of graph paper, so you know how big your desk can be. Take a tape measure with you when you go shopping, so you know immediately whether the one that catches your eye will fit. Sketch it into your layout to see if you like it.

Back Off!

Beware of lifting hazards in your home-based office. It's tempting to pick up items you know are too heavy just because you want to move them and there's no one to help you. Weigh out how much time you'll save by attempting the lift yourself against how much time you'll lose if you hurt your back. If you're so busy you can't wait to move these boxes of books, what's going to happen when you can't even move yourself?

Create a "Back–Friendly" Environment

No matter where you work, you can improve your environment to be more back friendly. Sometimes it's little things, like raising your computer monitor a few inches. Sometimes it's bigger things, like asking your employer to install shock-absorbing mats where you walk and stand.

Even if workplace adjustments are impractical, you can often make changes in the way you approach your work. If you can't get shock-absorbing mats installed, wear shoes with extra padding and inserts.

Above all, take time for your back. Spend a few minutes every hour doing stretches to relax your muscles and relaxation techniques to refresh your mind and your attitude.

The Least You Need to Know

➤ The only place where you spend more of your life than in bed is at work.

➤ Making ergonomically sound changes doesn't usually require major expenditures. Much of what you can do to improve your working environment is simple and inexpensive.

➤ No matter how ergonomic your workplace, you still need to move around to keep your back healthy. Staying in the same position too long is hard on your back, no matter what that position is.

➤ Limit what you carry on your back and in your arms.

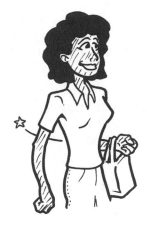

Living with Back Problems

There's a lot about life that isn't fair. Back pain falls into this category. It's not fair that you have back problems. But if you do, you need to learn how to live with it and around it.

You can decide to take charge. You can decide that you will make decisions about your life and the way you want to live it, rather than let your back problem dictate your actions.

Manage Your Pain

You can't always change the situation responsible for your back pain. Sometimes the underlying cause isn't clear; other times, such as with osteoarthritis, there just isn't a way to remove it. So how do you manage your pain so it doesn't take over your life? You might have to go through a little trial and error to find the right combination of approaches for you. Be persistent—relief is out there.

Take Medications as Prescribed

If your doctor has suggested or prescribed medication for your pain, take it, and take it as directed. When you first start taking a new medicine, ask your doctor if you should take it regularly or prn (medical shorthand for "as you need it"). NSAIDs and prescription anti-inflammatory medications are most effective when you take them regularly. Don't wait until you can't stand the pain; martyrs aren't especially entertaining in this day and age.

Don't just decide to stop taking your medications. At the very least, first talk with the doctor who recommended or prescribed them. Discuss your concerns. Is there something about the particular drugs you're taking that worries you, or are you just fed up with this whole medication routine? Sometimes just talking through your concerns puts an end to them.

Use Relaxation and Stress-Reduction Techniques

Relaxation and stress-reduction techniques are easy to take with you wherever you go and to use whenever you want. Perhaps none is as simple or effective as controlled breathing (see Chapter 14, "Imagine a Healthy, Pain-Free Back"). Try guided imagery or visualization to leave your back pain behind.

Back Care

If you're regularly taking NSAIDs for your back pain, ask your doctor about also taking antacids. NSAIDs increase your risk of stomach ulcers, and antacid medications can help protect your stomach.

Research studies show a strong connection between stress and many physical problems, including back pain. Research also shows a strong correlation between the sense of control people feel they have in their lives and their jobs and their levels of pain and disability. Most people who can reduce the stress also reduce the pain. These techniques also give you a greater sense of control over your life and the role your back problem plays in it. Once you see that you can control something you previously had not viewed as within your control—for example, your breathing—you have entirely new possibilities available to you.

Try Chiropractic or Therapeutic Massage

Bodywork is often helpful with back pain. Chiropractic and therapeutic massage can relax sore muscles and release tension. If you're more holistically oriented, you might find relief in shiatsu or tuina (see Chapter 21, "Hands-On Healing: Therapeutic Massage and Physical Therapy").

Nutrition to the Rescue

Can you eat your way to a healthy back? Well, you can certainly eat your way to an *un*healthy back, so it makes sense that the reverse is true!

Too much eating and not enough exercise leads to excess body weight. Obesity is very hard on your back, which already carries quite a burden. When you add extra weight, something has to give and often it's your back. Switching to a more healthful diet—one low in fat—can help you start whittling unneeded calories from your daily intake.

Nutrition isn't just about weight loss, though. Nutrition has do with how your body processes, or metabolizes, the substances you feed to it. Do certain foods have healing powers? There are many diets specific for certain diseases and conditions.

Can You Eat Your Way to a Healthy Back?

Fish oils are acquiring quite a reputation as medicinal foods. Omega-3 fatty oils, found in fish such as salmon, are believed to lower blood cholesterol levels. Now researchers are looking at fish oil as a natural way to control pain due to osteoarthritis. Foods high in calcium are also great for preventing osteoporosis.

Other food substances are finding their way into treatment recommendations, as well. Ginger, cloves, and turmeric are spices that appear to have anti-inflammatory properties. Ginger works by blocking prostaglandins—the same way NSAIDs relieve pain. Some researchers believe garlic has similar properties, though this hasn't been conclusively demonstrated.

Should you take ginger or even garlic to help relieve your back pain? Not without first discussing your interest in doing so with your doctor. Taking what are promoted as therapeutic doses of ginger or garlic could interfere with medications you're taking, either for your back problem or for other reasons.

What Foods Should You Avoid?

Common sense is your best guide when it comes to avoiding certain foods. Clearly, diet plays an important role in many medical conditions, including heart disease and some forms of cancer.

Some studies point to caffeine (found in coffee, tea, cola drinks, and chocolate) as a calcium thief, accusing it of interfering with your body's ability to absorb calcium from your diet. A diet high in salt seems to have a similar effect. Whether these studies are borne out remains to be seen. In any case, you won't go wrong by reducing the amounts of caffeine and salt that you consume. High caffeine levels and salt intake are linked with high blood pressure and other health problems, making it a prudent move to lower your use of these substances.

The Power of Daily Exercise

Nothing gets you going like a brisk morning workout. An early stretching and warm-up session followed by a brisk run or bicycle ride—your body's going to think heaven's come to Earth for the day.

More Activity Means Less Pain

As we've said throughout this book, more is less when it comes to activity and your back pain. The more exercise you get (within reason, of course), the less pain you'll experience. The reasons are probably a combination of biochemical and mechanical.

Exercise stretches and mobilizes muscles. This gets them ready for action. Exercise also releases endorphins, your body's natural painkillers. The combination is irresistible for your back pain.

Automatic Weight Control

Can you walk two miles in half an hour? If so, it's worth 150 to 200 calories of burned energy to your body. So is 30 minutes of in-line skating, bicycling at the comfortable pace of eight miles per hour, and dozens of other activities that are both fun and useful. Regular exercise also boosts the rate of your metabolism, meaning your body burns more energy even when you're not doing anything physical.

Stress Relief

Regular exercise is an automatic stress reducer. Researchers theorize that exercise affects the level of endorphins (natural pain relievers) your body releases, and may affect your brain's release of seratonin (a chemical substance that influences your mood).

Sometimes we spend too much time looking for scientific explanations, however. The bottom line seems simple. How can anything that gives you a respite from reality fail to relieve your stress? Just a thought…

Lifestyle Matters

The human species has an astonishing amount of control over lifestyle matters that no other species on the planet comes close to. When was the last time you saw a wolf breezing down the freeway behind the wheel (steering!) of a brand-new car—not wearing a seat belt? It just doesn't happen.

We, on the other hand, the ones with all the brain cells, are able to choose to do just that, without regard for the peril it puts us and others in. We're free to indulge in a wide range of behaviors that run counter to good health—and many of us choose them without conscious thought for future consequences.

Snuff the Smokes!

There is no other product in America quite like cigarettes. They offer no known health benefits, yet cause or contribute to thousands of deaths every year. What's up with that?

In addition to the damage cigarette smoking does to your cardiovascular system, it's none too kind to your back, either. Within seconds of the time you inhale that

Back Off!

Smokeless tobacco is no better or safer for you than cigarettes. Though you don't get all the inhaled particles, you still get the full chemical load of the processed tobacco, which includes nicotine and more than a thousand known cancer-causing substances. It's the nicotine that causes your peripheral blood vessels to constrict.

smoke into your lungs, your body begins shutting down your peripheral (distant) blood vessels. This decreases the supply of blood and the nutrients it carries—including oxygen and glucose, a form of sugar your cells need to function properly.

Your intervertebral disks don't have the most extensive supply of blood in the first place. Your body's master planner didn't anticipate the potential harm you might voluntarily do to yourself, like smoking. There's no backup system to serve your disks. When you light up that cigarette, you can almost hear your back cry.

The Influence of Drugs and Alcohol

In addition to hiding your judgment and sensibility, alcohol and illicit drugs affect your body in ways even researchers don't yet understand. Combining drugs (prescription, over-the-counter, or illicit) and alcohol is a particularly risky habit—it's easy to cross the threshold of toxicity without even knowing it.

Prolonged substance abuse interferes with nearly every aspect of your body's functions, from the way nerve impulses travel to how your intestines digest food. Misusing drugs or alcohol also can affect any legitimate treatment you're using for your back pain, from medication to massage therapy. Your body just doesn't respond the same when it's under the influence. In fact, muscle strength decreases measurably at three to four drinks a day. Over time, alcohol abuse alters your body in ways that extend beyond intoxication—excessive alcohol use damages your liver, for example, which then affects how your body metabolizes medications.

> **Back Off!**
>
> The first time you use cocaine could be your last. Cocaine can interfere with your heart's electrical rhythms, stopping it from pumping. Though this has little to do with your back, it's a warning worth emphasizing in any discussion of substance abuse.

Emotional and Personal Problems

People show emotional and personal stress in different ways. Some cry, some laugh. Some get headaches, some get backaches. If you don't resolve your personal problems, they're going to show up somewhere, somehow, in your body. Then you have no choice but to handle them.

Numerous studies demonstrate that people with back pain are significantly less likely to file a disability claim if they're satisfied with their lives and like their coworkers and boss. This is yet another reflection of how interconnected our bodies and minds really are.

Psychotherapy, counseling, and even talking honestly from your heart with a trusted friend, mentor, teacher, or religious guide may be valuable in helping you sort out painful problems or to get an objective view on your issues.

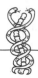

Sleeplessness and Depression

Does your back pain keep you awake nights? It's hard to feel rested in the morning when you spent the entire night tossing and turning. Good-quality sleep is important, both for your emotional well-being and for your body's healing processes to function properly.

Sometimes it's not your back problem that keeps you awake nights but a coexisting problem called depression. This is not your down-in-the-dumps, gee-I-feel-blue sort of thing. Depression is a very real, and sometimes dangerous, condition that may need medical treatment if it interferes with your life.

Many people with depression don't look or act unhappy. Yet deep inside, they're miserable. Depression can be dangerous if it leads to thoughts of suicide. People with chronic conditions and chronic pain often end up with depression.

Back Care

Are you gloomy and uninterested in life much of the time? Are you having trouble enjoying things you usually like, and feeling like nothing is fun any more? Do you have trouble sleeping, and no appetite? Is this a change from the "real" you? You could have depression. Only your doctor can tell you for sure. There are a variety of drugs available today that successfully treat depression.

Your Back and Your Weight

As varied as our bodies are, they spring from the same blueprint. They're designed and built to function in a certain way. As long as we maintain our bodies in compliance with their operating specifications, they'll serve us well. Start to deviate from the specs, however, and performance falters a bit. Some of these deviations are inevitable, the consequences of the aging process. Others we initiate, like gaining weight. This is a change your back notices long before you see it in the mirror because it has to pick up the extra load.

The Pervasive Presence of Excess Body Fat

Your back prefers the trim and fit look not because it's fashionable, but because it makes everyday activities so much easier. Your back is behind every move your body makes—and the more body there is to move, the harder your back works. Excess body fat hampers the muscles in your back and elsewhere in your body in other ways, too.

Body fat doesn't just sit right under your skin in a nice, neat layer. It infiltrates nearly every tissue in your body, padding around organs and muscles. Since excess body fat doesn't have much purpose except to sit there (unless you're saving up for a long, cold winter's hibernation), it gets in the way, restricting and hampering movement. Imagine trying to play tennis or basketball wearing a snowmobile suit!

Restricted muscles can't function as effectively and efficiently as they're designed to do. They sometimes can't extend or contract fully, limiting their lifting and pulling power. They often don't let your joints move freely, either, limiting your flexibility.

Regular exercise can help overcome these problems, restoring and maintaining the freedom of movement your back needs to get you through your day.

How you carry extra weight affects how your back feels about it, too. Many men and some women carry excess body fat across their abdomens. The resulting protruding belly alters your body's center of gravity, and in response your back's lumbar curve deepens. This affects your entire spine, and can cause lower-back pain.

Exercise and Weight Control

One endearing quality of exercise in today's image-conscious world is its ability to keep you not just fit and healthy, but also slim and trim (we're not talking ultra-thin here—just within the weight guidelines for your height). If you regularly get the recommended level of aerobic exercise—30 to 60 minutes at a time, three or four times a week—it's worth about a half a pound a week, without even changing your diet. That may not seem like much, but it adds up quickly—four pounds a month, nearly 50 pounds a year.

Most people achieve a balance between diet and exercise that, unless they're intentionally trying to lose weight, allows them to steer a steady course on the scales. To drop a few pounds, you have to tip the balance so your body uses more calories than you feed it. The most effective way to do this is to both cut back a bit on what you eat (and eat more nutritiously) and increase your activity level.

Dieting alone (without adding exercise) is often counterproductive—the less you eat, the slower your body functions. Your body views a sudden drop in intake as its cue to shift into "prevent starvation" mode, so it slows your metabolism to conserve stored fat for future needs. Increasing your level of activity offsets this effect and encourages your body to burn fat to meet the extra energy needs of exercise.

You'll start to see the effects of your efforts in about two weeks, as your body settles into its new routine. Once you reach your desired weight, maintain your exercise routine and nutritious eating habits to keep it there. Your body likes the new you just as much as you do! The following height and weight tables for women and men will give you some guidelines to follow. The weight takes into consideration wearing indoor clothes and one-inch heels.

Desired Weights of Women Aged Twenty-Five and Over

Height	Small Frame	Medium Frame	Large Frame
4'10"	102–111	109–121	118–131
4'11"	103–113	111–123	120–134
5'0"	104–115	113–126	122–137
5'1"	106–118	115–129	125–140
5'2"	108–121	118–132	128–143

continues

Desired Weights of Women Aged Twenty-Five and Over (continued)

Height	Small Frame	Medium Frame	Large Frame
5'3"	111–124	121–135	131–147
5'4"	114–127	124–138	134–151
5'5"	117–130	127–141	137–155
5'6"	120–133	130–144	140–159
5'7"	123–136	133–147	143–163
5'8"	126–139	136–150	146–167
5'9"	129–142	139–153	149–170
5'10"	132–145	142–156	152–173
5'11"	135–148	145–159	155–176
6'0"	138–151	148–162	158–179

Reprinted with permission of Metropolitan Life Insurance Company, Statistical Bulletin.

*Women between the ages of 18 and 25 should subtract one pound for each year under 25.

Desired Weights of Men Aged Twenty-Five and Over

Height	Small Frame	Medium Frame	Large Frame
5'2"	128–134	131–141	138–150
5'3"	130–136	133–143	140–153
5'4"	132–138	135–145	142–156
5'5"	134–140	137–148	144–160
5'6"	136–142	139–151	146–164
5'7"	138–145	142–154	149–168
5'8"	140–148	145–157	152–172
5'9"	142–151	148–160	155–176
5'10"	144–154	151–163	158–180
5'11"	146–157	154–166	161–184
6'0"	149–160	157–170	164–188
6'1"	152–164	160–174	168–192
6'2"	155–168	164–178	172–197
6'3"	158–172	167–182	176–202
6'4"	162–176	171–187	181–207

Reprinted with permission of Metropolitan Life Insurance Company, Statistical Bulletin.

Get a Life!

The worst part about a bad back (aside from the pain, of course) is that it takes over your life. Don't let it! Reclaim your life by doing the things you want to do. Can't do the things you used to do? Not to sound heartless, but so what? Move on! Life changes, whether you have back problems or not.

Of course, change isn't always easy. In fact, most of us find change, however minor, a disrupting and confusing experience. This is normal—ride it out. Expect minor bumps and small setbacks. Recognize that no matter how you fill your life, your back might still hurt. But when you're busy, you have less time to think about your back pain—and less opportunity to let it rule your life.

Learn Something New

There's no time like the present to expand your horizons. Think you're too old? Well, guess what? You won't get any older if you *don't* try something than you'll get if you do. Time passes, no matter how you fill it. Now is probably not the time to take up skydiving (those landings can be a bit rough on your back), but is there something else you've always wanted to do? So do it!

More often than not, all you have to do is get out of your own way. Let yourself do some of those things you've pushed aside. Sign up for those watercolor lessons! Haul your oboe out of the attic, take up classical guitar, or learn to play the violin. Volunteer at a local senior center or elementary school. Collect stamps or coins or sports cards.

Do whatever makes you happy—just start doing! Learning occupies your mind and gives you something to think about besides your aching back. It makes you a productive, satisfied human being. And it introduces you to new acquaintances, broadening your interests and your circle of friends. (Aren't you getting a bit tired of meeting the "woe is me" gang at the pharmacy every Tuesday?)

Take Time for Yourself

Most of us spend our adult lives wrapped up in our jobs and our families. Not that there's anything wrong with such dedication, but it doesn't leave you much time for yourself. Learn to *make* time just for you, time that has no purpose other than to bring you joy. If this coincides with new interests or activities, great. But it doesn't have to. What you do for yourself might be as simple as actually smelling the roses in your garden or at the park.

Nurturing Your Body/Mind Connection

As you're about to head off to a new life where you're in control of your pain and your lifestyle, remember to nurture your body/mind connection. Try yoga or meditation, and nurture your interests that bring your body and your mind closer together.

The Least You Need to Know

➤ Exercise brings both fitness and pain relief.

➤ Cigarettes, alcohol, and drugs are not only damaging to your back but also harmful to your health and well-being.

➤ Being overweight puts a heavy load on your back.

➤ It's important to take time for yourself.

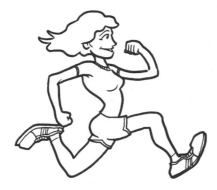

Chapter 25

Women and Back Pain

In This Chapter

➤ How hormones affect your back

➤ Ways to relieve back pain during menstruation

➤ Taking care of your back when you're pregnant

➤ The special needs of your back after menopause

There's a lot of "woman stuff" in this chapter, though certainly no secrets (okay, maybe a few things you didn't know before). But it's not for women, only. Men, we welcome and encourage you to read along, too—especially if there's a woman in your life.

Hormones and Body Design

Women's bodies differ from men's bodies, which we're sure is no surprise to you. There are the obvious distinctions—breasts rather than beards, ovaries instead of testicles. Hormones bear full responsibility for these and many other gender differences. As they shape a woman's body, hormones have but a single biological mission: childbearing. Every design element of a woman's body supports this mission.

To carry out their purpose, a woman's hormones guide her through three linked events in her life. The first is menstruation, the biological rite of passage from girl to woman that begins sometime between ages 11 and 14. During this monthly cycle, the lining of the uterus thickens in preparation for pregnancy and the ovary releases an egg. If pregnancy doesn't occur, the uterus bleeds away its extra tissue and the cycle starts again. The second, for about two thirds of American women, is pregnancy and childbirth. The third, menopause, brings the childbearing mission to closure in midlife (ages 45 to 55).

The Hormones That Rule the Female Body

Hormone	Role	Where Produced
Estrogen	Causes sex organs to develop; plays a role in menstruation; keeps bone calcium levels (incidentally) high; when production ceases, menopause occurs	Ovaries
Luteinizing	Stimulates ovaries to ovulate (release an egg)	Pituitary hormone gland
Oxytocin	Starts and continues contractions during labor	Pituitary gland
Progesterone	Regulates menstrual cycles and maintains pregnancy	Ovaries
Prolactin	Regulates milk production after childbirth	Pituitary gland
Testosterone	Affects sex drive	Ovaries*

*Produced in the testes in men.

The glands that manufacture hormones make up the endocrine system. Hormones play a key role in women's reproductive cycles.

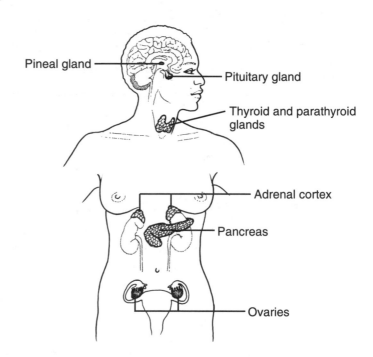

The Female Back

Most hormonal handiwork is pretty obvious, even to the casual observer. Among the more subtle differences hormones sculpt, however, are those that appear in the lower back. If you're a woman, you have a broader, flatter sacrum (those five fused bones below your lumbar spine) and a wider pelvis. Your pelvis also tilts forward a few degrees more than a man's, which gives you a more pronounced lumbar curve. These features come in handy when your body carries and gives birth to a child.

Whether you curse or praise them, the hormones that regulate your menstrual cycle do more than trigger your periods every month. They also cause biochemical changes in your body that soften your tendons and ligaments, giving them greater flexibility. Though you feel this effect most during pregnancy, it happens every month and can cause minor aches and pains in your "pelvic girdle" (the circle of bones, including your sacrum, that forms your pelvis) and in your back. Interestingly, this effect (some associated increase in backache probably due to ligament softening) has also been reported by some women who take hormone replacement therapy after menopause...but before you stop taking your estrogen or develop a bias, read on.

> **Back to Nature**
>
> Is "that time of the month" cramping your style? Consider hypnosis. Hypnosis, done by an accredited hypnotherapist, is a useful tool for helping you relax instead of tense when you feel menstrual cramps coming on. Some women do better with a posthypnotic suggestion to behave in certain ways, while learning self-hypnosis is more effective for others.

Back Pain and Your Menstrual Cycle

You probably don't need a calendar to know where you are in your menstrual cycle—your body does a pretty good job of telling you. Cramps, headache, and backache are all too familiar signals for many women that it's time for their periods. While stress can certainly aggravate menstrual discomfort, responsibility really rests with those hormones. (Not that we mean to give hormones a bad rap—they have many good and useful purposes. It's just that sometimes they get, well, annoying!)

Remember those hormonally softened connective tissues we just mentioned? They can sag a bit when it comes to supporting your muscles and bones. Your back, which bears most of the burden of keeping you in motion, can pick up the slack for only so long without complaining. The result—sore, aching muscles.

But wait—there's more. Your pelvis and lower back are part of the same structure. While it may seem like all the action takes place in your pelvic area, your lower back is just too close. The same sensory nerves serve them both. Instead of cramps in your lower abdomen, you may feel an achy, crampy discomfort in your lower back (referred pain). Sometimes you feel both.

> **Back Basics**
>
> **Dysmenorrhea** is the medical term for the pain and discomfort that can accompany a woman's menstrual period. In primary dysmenorrhea, symptoms start when bleeding starts and last a couple days. In secondary dysmenorrhea (dysmenorrhea from other causes), symptoms can start several days before your period.

Just because these events are an act of nature doesn't mean you have to grit your teeth and suffer through them. There are many approaches to relieving premenstrual and menstrual discomfort, which doctors call *dysmenorrhea*, from NSAIDs and other analgesics to hypnotism and visualization. If pelvic and lower-back pain make your periods miserable, first get a thorough gynecological exam from your primary care physician, women's health care professional, or gynecologist. If everything checks out, try these tips:

➤ Make exercise a part of your daily routine. Regular exercise lowers your body's progesterone and estrogen levels, reducing their influence on your body and your mood.

➤ Take an NSAID that works by blocking prostaglandins, such as naproxen. Prostaglandins are the chemical messengers that carry pain signals to the brain. Keep a journal so you know how far in advance of your period your symptoms start, and start taking an NSAID then. Take it at the first hint of discomfort (or even for a day ahead of time if you have severe cramps and your period is fairly predictable) and then regularly (don't wait until those prostaglandins build up in your system) for the next 24 to 48 hours (every six hours with food).

➤ Practice relaxation and stress-reduction techniques to help yourself feel more calm and in control. Remind yourself that your pain is time-limited. Stress and the sense of having no control over what's happening with your body magnify your pain.

➤ Do yoga postures that gently stretch your abdominal and lower-back muscles. This improves the flow of circulation to these areas, bringing the cells more oxygen and nutrition.

➤ Rest with a hot water bottle or heating pad against the area that hurts most (your lower back or your lower abdomen).

Back Off!

Keep the intensity of your exercise reasonable. Unless you're a competitive athlete in training for a specific event, stay within the recommendations of The American College of Sports Medicine—60 minutes of aerobic exercise three to five times a week. Very intense exercise can stop menstruation completely (as can low body weight). This becomes a risk factor for osteoporosis, since you don't have estrogen to maintain bone density.

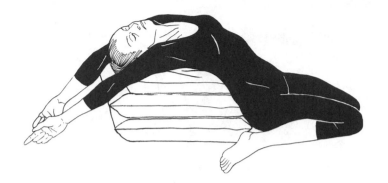

This yoga back stretch over a stack of pillows helps open the lower back and reduce the pain of menstrual cramps. It is also effective during pregnancy for reducing lower-back discomfort. After the stretch, bend forward to relax the back in the opposing direction.

Endometriosis and Lower-Back Pain

Endometriosis, says one woman who suffers its effects, is like going through labor every month—only there's no reward at the end. In this condition, bits of tissue similar to the lining of the uterus (called the *endometrium*) migrate to other parts of your body. Though most commonly found in the abdomen, these tissue fragments can appear just about anywhere within your body—researchers aren't entirely sure how they get to where they end up.

Acting like long-distance extensions of your uterus's endometrium, these misguided bits of tissue do what your endometrium does. When the lining of your uterus thickens in biological anticipation of pregnancy, these wayward orphans do the same. And when your uterus sloughs away the buildup when there is no pregnancy, these orphan fragments bleed, too.

While your uterus drains its surplus outside your body via your vagina, the endometrial tissues residing elsewhere have no outlets. The bleeding they produce pools around them, and your body responds to the resulting irritation by creating *cysts* to surround and contain it. These cysts get a little larger with each menstrual cycle, and begin to interfere with the regular functions of the tissues they've invaded. This causes pain.

Endometrial tissue often lodges itself in the connective tissues of your lower back and your pelvic cavity, becoming quite painful as the condition progresses. While in its early stages, endometriosis is hard to distinguish from dysmenorrhea, certain symptoms become prominent. Low-back pain, especially toward the end of your period, is a key symptom of endometriosis.

Back Basics

Endometrium means "within the uterus" and is the medical term for the blood-rich tissue that lines your uterus. A **cyst** is a swelling or growth that contains fluid or other material. It comes from the Greek word *kystis*, which means "sac."

291

Sites of endometriosis in the female reproductive system. Endometriosis can make menstrual cramps more painful, sometimes causing intense lower-back pain and discomfort.

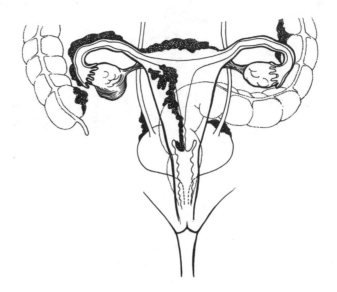

Back Talk

Do food cravings drive you crazy right before or during your period? Try giving in! In research studies, women who ate the carbohydrates (pasta, breads, desserts, potatoes, and cereals) they craved were less irritable and had less physical discomfort than those who denied their cravings. Carbohydrates appear to increase your levels of seratonin, a natural chemical substance that elevates mood. Beware, however, that some women experience the opposite effect—giving in to carb cravings worsens their menstrual discomfort.

Doctors generally use NSAIDs or other analgesics to relieve the symptoms of endometriosis, including back pain. Birth control pills or other hormone combinations can also control symptoms by preventing or limiting the hormone swings that go with menstruation. Some hormone treatments even prevent menstruation or cause "medical menopause." Severe endometriosis may require *laparoscopic* surgery to *cauterize* or remove the endometrial cysts. Many women report their endometriosis takes a dramatic turn for the better following pregnancy, though this doesn't hold true for all. While its symptoms are the biggest problem for most women, endometriosis causes infertility in some. Most women with endometriosis find relief after menopause, when the monthly cycles that trigger their symptoms cease.

Massage, especially in the low back and buttock muscles, often provides relief from endometrial (and menstrual) low-back pain. Deep massage can break up painful muscle contractions, allowing you to rest and sleep (which in itself is healing). To get a similar effect when you have no one to give you a massage, try lying on the floor with a soft rubber ball (such as a tennis ball) under your lower back. Use the pressure of your weight on the ball to relieve muscle tension, moving the ball to different points for maximum relief. Remember to stretch after such a self-massage—while lying on your back (not on the ball!), bring your knee to your chest and then across your body toward the opposite side.

> **Back Basics**
>
> In **laparoscopic** surgery, the surgeon makes a small incision and inserts a flexible, lighted tube called a laparoscope (a specialized endoscope). Through the laparoscope, the surgeon can view inside the pelvic and abdominal cavities. By passing special instruments or a laser through the laparoscope, the surgeon can remove or **cauterize** (burn away) the tissue.

Back Health During Pregnancy

When you're pregnant, your back does double duty. It supports the extra weight your little passenger generates (amazingly little of which actually belongs to him or her). It also tries to stabilize your increasingly out-of-balance body as your belly blooms to become your most prominent physical feature. Although minor low-back ache is very common (over half of all women during pregnancy), it usually goes away right after delivery. Very few women actually develop more than minor (until you've been through it) backache. The biggest risk for significant back problems when you're pregnant is having had them previously.

We once used to refer to pregnancy as "confinement"—the pregnant woman retreated to her private quarters and generally stayed still and out of action until her baby was born. We now know such inactivity sets the stage for a wide range of complications. Regular exercise and activity during pregnancy is an important part of your health and of your baby's.

How Your Body Changes

It might be easier to talk about the parts of your body that *don't* change with pregnancy—let's see, those would be…oh, never mind. Everything changes. The most obvious changes take place on the front side of your body, which gives your back plenty of work. Everyone notices your swelling belly. But your breasts are enlarging, too, preparing for their role in providing nutrition for your baby after birth.

Many of your body's changes are magical to experience (morning sickness excepted). By the time you feel your baby's first movements, in about your fifth or sixth month, you're starting to feel other changes, too. Your pelvis starts to feel heavy as the baby's weight stresses the ligaments. Your lumbar curve becomes more pronounced as your back looks for ways to more comfortably carry its growing load—which backfires, because you just end up with a backache.

The added weight of pregnancy throws the pelvic tilt off balance, causing a condition called "lordosis" or a swayback effect. To achieve the correct posture, try contracting your buttock muscles and consciously pushing the pelvis forward; place your hands under your belly at the joints where your thighs meet your hips and feel the pelvis as it moves forward into proper alignment.

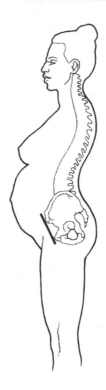

Back Off!

Ask your obstetrician before you take any medication to soothe your aching back, even if it's something you took all the time before you were pregnant. Anything you take also enters your baby's system, and many substances are not known to be safe for an unborn child. Aspirin affects your blood's clotting action, so don't take products containing aspirin during pregnancy. Aspirin and NSAIDs can actually close off the special circulation that the baby has and aren't recommended in pregnancy except in very special circumstances.

Toward the end of your pregnancy, you may feel pressure against your sacrum as your baby runs out of room and settles into the head-down position that will lead the way during delivery. And all those hormones coursing through your system have started softening your ligaments and pelvic joints (and your sacrum, too, which forms the back of your pelvis) in preparation for the Big Event. Resist this tendency toward swayback by practicing your posture exercises. Make a conscious effort to straighten your spine each time you stand up. If you feel like your tush sticks out, tuck it in by tilting your pelvis slightly.

Protecting Your Back and Your Baby

Back-healthy postures and movements are especially important to keep your back strong and healthy during pregnancy. This of all times is *not* when you want to take up armchair athletics! Your body's systems function far more effectively when you're in motion. Walking remains the ideal exercise—it's great for your back, and keeps your leg muscles in shape to help reduce the fluid retention and swelling that's a normal aspect of later pregnancy. Swimming is great, too, because it takes the weight off you and your back.

Discuss your regular exercise routine with your obstetrician or midwife. While many of your usual activities will be good for you during pregnancy, others might need some modification. Low-impact activities such as swimming and stationery cycling are gentler and kinder to your changing body. Vary your position frequently throughout the day. If you have to stand, put one foot on a small stool to relieve the pressure on your back.

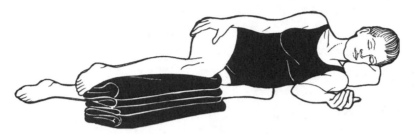

To take the strain off your back, lie on your left side with pillows to support your neck and your baby, and elevate your left leg as shown. This is a safe and comfortable position to get quick relief.

And don't forget that your center of gravity is out of kilter. Especially toward the end of your pregnancy, it's very easy to stumble and lose your balance. Your natural tendency to avoid falling forward onto your tummy puts tremendous stress on your back. Wear low-heeled shoes for both comfort and safety.

Five Back-Friendly Exercises for Pregnant Women

If there's ever a time when coworkers, friends, family members, and even complete strangers are especially accommodating, it's when you're pregnant. Take advantage of it by treating yourself to frequent relaxation breaks. These five exercises are great for your back and easy to do.

Tailor Sit and Stretch

Young children might recognize the tailor sit as the "crisscross applesauce" position. It's great for relieving pressure on your lower back. Some women like to do this exercise by sitting on the floor against a wall for added support.

1. Lower yourself to a sitting position on the floor. If it's later in your pregnancy, use a chair for support.

2. Fold your legs one over the other in the familiar cross-legged pose, with one foot under the opposite thigh and the other foot touching the opposite shin.

3. Outstretch your arms and rest your hands, palms facing up, on your knees.

4. Concentrate on feeling your lower back round out slightly. Be careful not to slouch, which puts strain on your shoulders and upper back.

5. Sit in this position as long as it's comfortable. Slouching or tingling in your legs or feet are signs that it's time to move.

The tailor stretch is similar to the tailor sit, and helps to loosen and relax the muscles of your upper back and shoulders.

1. Sit cross-legged as for the tailor sit.

2. Put your hands on your shoulders, then raise them together above your head. Stretch your right arm to reach as high as you can while still holding your left arm up.

3. Lower your right arm to the same height as the left, then relax both arms and put your hands on your shoulders again.

4. Repeat, this time stretching your left arm higher.

Pregnant Mountain Pose

This is the same yoga exercise from Chapter 5, "Posture Perfect," with a few alterations for pregnancy.

1. Stand with your feet together, toes pointing forward. Tilt your pelvis slightly forward so your baby doesn't press against your spine. Bend your knees slightly, and put your palms on top of your kneecaps.

2. Take in a deep, slow breath and let it out. Tighten your thigh muscles until your kneecaps pull up. Watch and feel them do this, then let your thigh muscles relax and your kneecaps return to their normal position.

3. Now stand up straight, with your hands at your sides (keep your pelvis slightly tilted). Try again to pull your kneecaps up with your thigh muscles. Hold for a few seconds, then relax. Take a slow, deep breath in and let it out.

Chair Stretch

You can do this easy and effective back stretch, adapted from yoga's downward facing dog pose, at home or at the office for a quick back release.

1. Perform this stretch with a strong and stable, straight-backed chair, or do it against a wall.

2. Stretch the back muscles forward from the hips and bend your knees if you need to, for a comfortable stretch. Don't strain.

3. Take in five deep breaths, holding for five counts on the inhale and 10 counts on the exhale.

4. Stand up and move into the pregnant mountain pose. Relax and center yourself.

5. Move on with your day with a refreshed, relaxed back.

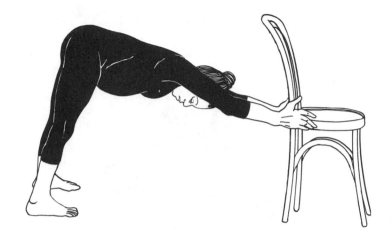

You can also try this stretch, a modified version of yoga's downward facing dog pose, against a wall. Bend your knees if you need to, and stretch only to a comfortable level. Feel your back really expand forward from the hips.

Pelvic Lift

For the first four months or so of your pregnancy, do this exercise lying on your back on the floor. After four months (or earlier if your obstetrician tells you not to lie on your back), do this exercise standing.

1. Lying version—Lie on your back on the floor and pull your knees up. Take in a slow breath. As you let your breath out, press the small of your back against the floor. Relax and take another breath in.

2. Standing version—Stand with your back against a wall. Take in a slow breath, pressing the small of your back against the wall as you do. Let your breath out, and relax your back.

Pregnant Squat

The pregnant squat helps to prepare you for labor by opening up the hip muscles and stretching out and strengthening the lower back.

1. Be sure to use the pillow, as shown in the following illustration, for support. Use as many pillows as you need to move into this pose. Stack them high, if need be!

2. Stretch your legs only as far as is comfortable, and hold the pose only as long as it remains easy. Once strain or discomfort sets in, move into the tailor sit position.

3. While holding the pose, take deep breaths, holding for five counts on the inhale and 10 counts on the exhale.

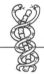

Back Care

Both pregnancy and breast-feeding put extra demands on your body to supply calcium. Most obstetricians keep women on prenatal vitamin supplements, which are high in calcium and other important nutrients, for as long as they're breast-feeding their babies. You need about 1,200 mg of calcium daily to meet this increased demand. Eat foods that are high in calcium, too—it's almost impossible to get too much calcium when you're pregnant or nursing.

297

If this pose is uncomfortable, move into the tailor sit and relax.

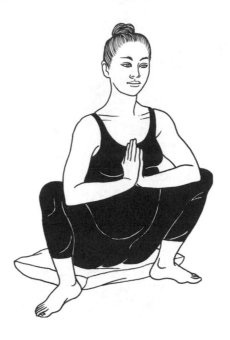

Just for New Moms

Perhaps the greatest letdown after the joy of giving birth is that first look in the mirror and the recognition that the body you've acquired over the past nine months didn't snap back to the old you as soon as its passenger disembarked. Don't worry, things will get back to normal. Just be patient with yourself, and take care of your body as it restores itself.

Few new moms get enough sleep, which makes most of them cranky and irritable. Even a routine pregnancy and delivery puts your body through a rigorous workout, and it wants its rest. Yet all too often, when you get a chance to nap or sleep, you're too keyed up to doze off.

When you have a few minutes to yourself (you will, we promise), dim the lights, put on some soothing music, and light an aromatherapy or scented candle. Retreat to the position that gave you such comfort during your pregnancy, the tailor sit. Close your eyes, let your body feel the music, and let the candle's fragrance swirl through your senses. Feel the tension drain from your head, down your neck and your arms, and out of your palms. Feel more tension travel down your back, into your legs, and out the bottoms of your feet. Slowly open your eyes. Isn't that better? Now see if you can catch a few winks before reality reclaims you (blow out the candle first).

Postpartum Hints and Tips

As you regain your strength and get to sleep for longer than 10 minutes at a time, remember to claim a few minutes here and there for a little exercise. Many of the exercises you did while you were pregnant will serve you well now—they're gentle, easy, and they help you feel better. Weather permitting, step outside for a short walk. Alone or with your baby, you'll find the fresh air invigorating.

Baby carriers with adjustable straps can really be back-savers, too, though your baby won't be ready for a backpack until she can sit up alone. If your back hurts, avoid slings or droopy carriers. And beware those handy car seats you can cart from car to everywhere else with baby in them! They're heavy and force you to carry your baby away from your body.

If You've Had a C-Section

You don't think much about how much your abdominal muscles support your back until you can't use them. When you have a *c-section*, the obstetrician cuts through your abdominal muscles to get to your uterus. Which direction that incision goes makes a major difference in how easily and quickly it heals.

The most common c-section incision runs horizontally across the lower part of your abdomen, under the bulge of your belly at the pubic hairline. This incision often is called a bikini cut; since it follows the grain of the underlying muscles, it heals smoothly. Rarely, the obstetrician may have to do a vertical incision, splitting you from your belly button to your pubic hairline, to get the baby out in a hurry. This incision can be slower to heal because it cuts across the grain of the muscles. Every contraction of the healing muscles hurts because it pulls against the sewn edges.

Without your abdominal muscles to help out, your back works overtime. Relieve the stress on your back by using your leg muscles to help you move between sitting, standing, and lying positions. Stretch frequently, to keep your back muscles from getting stiff and sore. And walk as much as you can tolerate. This gets your abdominal muscles involved in activity again (and helps you feel better in general).

Back Basics

A **c-section** is a surgical delivery. The phrase is short for cesarean section, said to be so named because the first person known to be born by this method was the ancient Roman ruler Julius Caesar.

Your Back and Breast-Feeding

Mothers and babies both enjoy the bonding that takes place during breast-feeding. It's such a wonderful chance for you both explore and enjoy each other in relative peace. Don't let a backache encroach on these touching times. Choose a comfortable place to sit that gives your back good support. Settle in before you begin. If you get uncomfortable while your baby is still nursing, pause for just a moment to get rearranged.

Here are some ways you can support your baby during breast-feeding without putting additional stress on your back:

➤ Use a special nursing pillow. These resemble swimming tubes except they're thinner in the back than the front and go around your waist to provide a comfortable cushion for your baby.

➤ Use the "football hold." Hold your baby's head in your hand and tuck her feet under your arm. Rest your arm on a regular or nursing pillow for additional support. Your baby nurses at the breast on the same side you're holding her. When you switch to the other breast, switch your baby to the other arm, too.

➤ Lie in bed on your side with your baby beside you and facing you. Let him nurse from the "down" breast. To switch to the other breast, lie on your other side.

Your breasts will be much larger and heavier than usual while you're breast-feeding. Without your baby's internal acrobatics to distract you, you're more likely to notice the strain this creates for your back. Remember to stretch often. A good nursing bra (get it professionally fitted, if you can) can provide additional support, giving your back a bit of a break.

Menopause Is More Than Hot Flashes

The Change, as we call it, hits women in their middle years. This transition couldn't be more aptly named. Only in pregnancy does a woman's body undergo a greater transition.

During menopause, your body alters much of the hormone production that has marked the cycles of its adult life. Literally translated, menopause means "end of monthly." It is the end of menstruation and the end of fertility. For many women, it is also a wonderful beginning, the start of a time when they regain control of their bodies and their lives.

Freedom from hormones doesn't come without a price, however. All those years your estrogen has been giving you monthly cramps, it's also been protecting the calcium reserves in your bones. Once your body stops producing estrogen, you lose this protective action and become vulnerable to osteoporosis.

Preventing Osteoporosis

Your bone strength and density reaches its peak when you're about 35 years old. By the time you reach age 45 (age 60 for men), you already have a condition (fortunately reversible) called osteopenia—which means you're losing about $1/2$ percent of bone mass every year. Further complicating matters, your body absorbs less calcium from your diet. And the less active you are, the more calcium your body pulls from your bones to meet its needs.

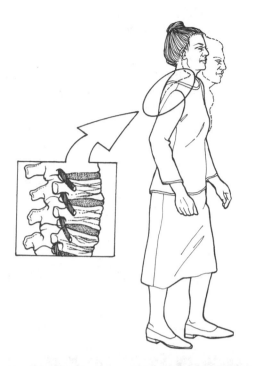

In osteoporosis, the vertebrae of the back can collapse as the bones weaken, causing fractures. Over time, these compression fractures produce a stooped posture.

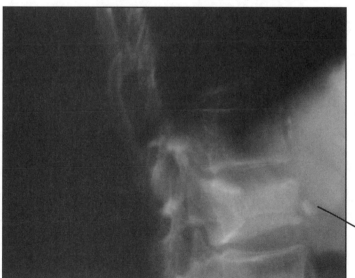

This patient has osteoporosis and a compression fracture. Notice the decrease in height of the fractured vertebra and the "thinness" (blackness) of the bones, showing loss of calcium. Reprinted by permission of Richard A. Deyo, M.D., M.P.H., University of Washington Medical Center.

vertebral compression fracture

Osteoporosis, which means "porous bones," is sometimes called the silent thief. You can't feel the calcium leeching from your bones, and can't see your bones getting thinner and lighter. One day you step off a curb wrong or take a minor fall, and a bone breaks. Fractures are the most serious consequence of osteoporosis. Each year 1.3 million people in the United States—8 in 10 of them women—suffer broken bones because of osteoporosis. Hip fractures are the most devastating because they often require surgical repair and months of rehabilitation. (Plus 50 percent of people who have a hip fracture never live independently again, and 20 percent die of a related problem.) Spine fractures can also be serious and painful.

A recent study reported in *USA Today* (conducted by Opinion Research for Mission Pharmacal) shows the interesting relationship between what women *know* about preventing or slowing osteoporosis and what they actually *do*. Check it out:

	Know	Do
Calcium supplement	88%	54%
Balanced diet	87%	77%
Healthy weight	80%	70%
Low body fat	66%	59%
Aerobic exercise	66%	38%
Weight training	65%	30%

Back to Nature

Calcium and fiber are both essential for health. They may not be so good together, however. Fiber appears to decrease your body's ability to absorb calcium. Take your fiber and your calcium separately. And watch the protein. High levels of protein take calcium from your body.

Calcium Supplements

Women going through and beyond menopause should take calcium supplements to keep their bones strong. It is possible, though difficult, to get the calcium you need—1,000 mg a day, or three to four servings—from your diet. Foods that are high in calcium include dairy products, broccoli, kale, collards, tuna, canned sardines and salmon with bones in, and spinach. Most calcium supplements also include small amounts of vitamin D, which your body needs to process calcium. Dairy products are also high in vitamin D, though most high-calcium vegetables are not. Supplements come in a wide range of formulas and sources; your doctor can help you identify the ones that are the best fit with your situation and lifestyle.

Hormone Replacement Therapy (HRT)

It's clear that taking estrogen supplements after menopause preserves your body's protection against calcium loss. It also reduces your cholesterol and long-term risk of heart attack. What's less clear is at what cost these protections come. HRT is controversial; it does appear to carry a slightly increased risk of breast cancer and blood clots, but protects against ovarian cancer, Alzheimer's dementia, hair and tooth loss, and skin wrinkling.

Replacement estrogen formulas range from synthetic (manufactured in a laboratory) to natural (cultivated from plant and animal sources). There's no clear evidence that one is better than the other. If you're approaching or past menopause, discuss HRT with your doctor to determine whether it's a good choice for you.

Other Medications

There are several medications available that help prevent bone loss or restore bone mass after menopause. They affect the way your bones rebuild their calcium stores after your body takes a withdrawal. The most powerful are estrogen (hormone replacement therapy after menopause), alendronate, and raloxifene. Doctors usually recommend a calcium supplement, vitamin D (in a multivitamin), and plenty of moderate weight-bearing exercise at the same time.

Exercise for Back Health

The most effective way to prevent osteoporosis is to stay active. Weight-bearing exercise (walking, jogging, dancing, jumping rope) has the greatest effect as far as encouraging your bones to build more mass. (If your doctor's already told you that you have osteoporosis, ask her what exercises are safe for you to do.) At a minimum, walk at least two miles at a time three or four times a week. Walking outside is refreshing but not always possible. Where there are shopping malls, there are usually mall walkers. The mall gives you a protected walking environment and company if you want it.

The Least You Need to Know

➤ The hormones that shape your female body also give your back some distinguishing features.

➤ Hypnosis and visualization are often effective methods for coping with menstrual discomfort.

➤ Pregnancy causes backache, but rarely causes serious back problems. Proper posture and frequent stretching help reduce your back's load.

➤ Calcium, vitamin D, and regular, gentle weight-bearing exercise are effective prevention tools for osteoporosis.

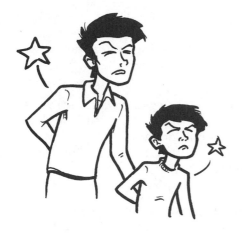

Chapter 26

It's All in the Family

In This Chapter

➤ Your baby and the soothing touch of massage

➤ Older children and back pain

➤ Saving your back when you're doing chores

➤ Back health for seniors

As an adult, you've earned certain rights through your struggles on the battlefield of life. But you don't have dibs on back problems. Children as young as 10 can have backaches and muscle strains.

Baby Backs

Baby bones get their start as soft cartilage. Within each is the core from which the calcification process begins and spreads. Though this process begins before birth, it's not complete until early adulthood.

A baby doesn't begin to develop control over the large muscles in her body until she's three or four months old. Her back muscles aren't strong enough to hold her in an unsupported sitting position for longer than a few minutes until she's eight or nine months old. Like every other part of your baby's body, her back grows and changes daily during her first year.

Infant Massage

Babies love massage. Of course, they don't know that's what it is. They just know you're touching and stroking them, and that feels good. A baby's other senses develop gradually, so touch is a key way of linking to the rest of the world during a baby's early months. Studies show that an infant appears able to distinguish her mother's touch from the touch of others within a few weeks following birth.

Even though they seem too young to have a care in the world, babies actually do feel stress. The entire transition from warm womb to the outside world is a bit harsh, despite your best efforts to soften it for your baby. Your touch tells your baby you're still there and you're still connected, even though the umbilical cord is gone.

Generally, doctors recommend that you avoid putting powders and oils on your baby's delicate skin for the first few months. Stroke your baby's bare skin with gentle pressure. Your touch should not be so firm that you indent the skin, but not so light that it tickles (which is an irritating sensation to an infant).

Back to Nature

Babies love being naked, as long as they stay warm. And they love to feel a caring caress against their tender skin. You don't have to get fancy to give your baby a back rub. Just use flowing, gentle strokes. If you're lying beside your baby, try to make eye contact while you're massaging him.

Massaging in gentle circles with your fingertips aids baby's digestion. The same stroke is used for baby's back. A light touch is all that's needed; avoid vigorous rubbing. Less is more for babies, who are easily overstimulated by harsh touch.

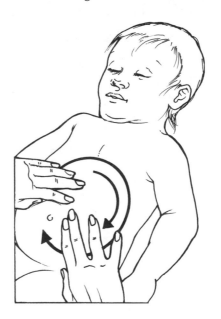

Use long, sweeping effleurage strokes, always moving toward the direction of your baby's heart (you don't want to fight the natural flow of blood back to the heart). Depending on your baby's age, he may watch you or may drift into sleep. Be sure he stays warm while his skin is exposed.

Take your cues from your baby to determine when she's had enough. She may start fidgeting or crying, or fall asleep. Or she may try to watch your face and to make eye contact. Your baby can react to massage in different ways depending on whether she's upset or this is a routine bonding activity between the two of you.

Toting That Toddler

Are you a parent with young children? Lifting your squirming, energetic offspring can give you a real pain in the back. Getting your child in and out of a car seat is a particular hazard. You're usually bent over, tugging at buckles and struggling with straps. Wouldn't it be nice if cars came with pop-up roofs just for parents?

Your awkward position means you're lifting 20 to 30 pounds of squirming child at a clear disadvantage. The usual rules of lifting are hard to apply—you can't pull the weight (your child) close to you, or use your leg and abdominal muscles to help your back. There's a strain just waiting to happen!

Keep that injury waiting. Take a look at where your child's car seat is installed in your car. Can you sit on the seat beside your child instead of leaning into the car from outside? Is your child old enough to climb down from the car seat and let you lift her at the door, where you can bend at the knees and pull her close to you? Experiment with different body positions to find ones that put less stress on your back.

Kids and Back Pain

Young children (under age six) don't often have back pain in the same way adults do. They may complain of soreness or aches after unusual physical activity, such as a day at the beach or an afternoon of roller skating. Occasionally a child falls on his tailbone, which can be a very painful experience. Though it's difficult for a child to break his soft bones, it's a possibility to consider if the pain doesn't start to go away in 48 hours.

If you're hearing your child complain of the same kind of back pain that plagues you, you might need to keep your discomforts more to yourself. Children are quite impressionable, and may unknowingly take on your pain. (It's amazing how kids pick up on

Back Off!

Don't put your young child in the hot tub or spa to ease her muscle aches! Children have more surface area (because of their height and weight ratio) exposed to warm water, which causes them to overheat and dehydrate much faster than adults might.

Back to Nature

Those special backpacks for carrying kids can be a great convenience. For your safety and your child's, be sure your child sits correctly in the seat and is securely belted in before you put the pack on your back. If you're wearing the pack correctly, your child's weight is fairly well balanced but still throws your center of gravity off. Always bend at the knees, not at the waist—both to protect your back and to keep your little one from tumbling out. Don't carry your child on your back while skiing, skating, bicycling, or similar activities—the risk of injury is very high for you both.

what we least expect them to notice.) Don't automatically disregard your child's, but try not saying anything about your back pain for a few days and see if your child stops complaining, too. Spend some time, too, asking your child about how he sees your pain and health (and his) to see how your problems are affecting him. Children may be afraid you're going to die, for example, if you make a comment like "this back pain is going to kill me!"

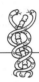

Back Care

Does your child have a noticeable sideways curve in his or her spine when you look at it from the back? If so, have your doctor check your child for scoliosis. Though not usually a serious problem, scoliosis typically progresses as your child grows. It can cause back pain, leg pain, and even spinal deformities if left untreated.

Back Off!

If your child complains of back or neck pain and has a fever or seems reluctant to move his or her head, see a doctor immediately. These can be early signs of infection affecting the spinal cord and brain. Though such infections (meningitis) are rare, they are serious and require urgent medical attention.

So Young, Yet So Much Sitting: Preteens

Between the ages of 6 and 12, back pain could become a problem. Today's children, as active as they are, spend more time sitting behind a desk or in front of a television or video game than they spend doing anything else. This creates the same problems for children as it does for adults. No one's back, no matter how young, likes to stay in the same position very long.

Encourage your child to take frequent breaks from whatever he's doing. Most schools break lessons into 20-minute segments for children under age 10, mostly because that's about the limit of their little attention spans but also because their bodies need to stretch and move.

Children also can have referred pain to the back, especially from urinary tract and kidney infections. As in adults, such infections can cause pain in the low to middle back and usually a fever. Suspected infections require immediate medical attention. Urinary tract infections are far more common in girls than in boys.

Growing Pains: Adolescents

Kids on the edge of adolescence live in bodies that are out of control. Hormones rage and growth spurts—your child can change literally overnight, with growth of several inches in a few months more the norm than the exception. Both hormones and growth can cause aches and pains in your child's back (and also legs and arms, if he's growing rapidly).

Adolescents are quite sensitive and uncertain about their changing bodies, and may not even confide in you about aches and pains unless they become intolerable.

You probably won't get too far trying to give your adolescent a backrub, unless you catch her when her defenses are down and she's willing to allow you near enough to touch her. Circular strokes and some gentle kneading might help her aching back feel better.

Low-back pain is a common companion to the menstrual cycle. Heat to the lower back or sometimes to the lower abdomen can help relieve this aching (moist heat often feels better). An anti-inflammatory drug such as ibuprofen taken regularly for the first day or two of the period can help.

Housework and Home Improvements

Here comes the weekend. What's on your "honey do" list? With our busy lifestyles today, probably more than you can accomplish. Though for a while it's nice to say, "Not this weekend, dear, I have a backache," eventually reality catches up with you and it's time to tackle chores.

It wouldn't hurt to treat your weekend's work as an athletic event. After all, you're going to be running here and climbing there—you might as well take exercise credit for your efforts.

Your spouse or other family members may disagree with us on this (and we respect their right to do so), but we suggest you quit when you're tired rather than trying to finish one more chore. A tired back is a more vulnerable back—and we've never known chores to do themselves when you weren't looking. What you don't do today will be waiting for you tomorrow...or next weekend.

Back Care

When your child watches television, works or plays at the computer, or plays video games, set a 20- or 30-minute timer. When the timer goes off, have your child take an activity break to do something physical. This stretches muscles that have been slumped and cramped, and gives your child a needed change of scenery.

Beware the Bends

Many tasks around the house and yard require you to bend. Gardening, washing floors, vacuuming carpets, even raking leaves and mowing the lawn (as long as you're pushing, not riding, the mower) all put your back in a less than ideal position.

If you're pulling weeds or planting flowers, get down on your knees on the ground rather than bending over at the waist. Try a gardening stool or kneeling pad. Straighten up every few minutes. Do a couple quick stretching exercises before you return to your duties. It might take you a little longer to finish, but you'll feel better when you're done.

When you have to pick something up from the ground, even if it's not heavy, bend with your knees instead of at the waist. This gives you better balance and also protects your back from possible muscle strain.

Steps and Ladders

Steps and ladders pose special hazards. First of all, you usually have stuff in your hands while you're trying to climb up. This alters your center of gravity and your sense of balance. A tumble is just a misstep away—and can cause serious injuries.

Second, once you get to your destination, the last thing you want to do is move. Whether you're painting, cleaning gutters, or handling some other chore, you stretch as far as you can to reach as much as you can. Not always the smart choice—it's easy to strain a back muscle or even fall from your pinnacle.

As a matter of safety, any time you're on a ladder or other high place, be sure someone is around to "spot" for you (to stand at the ready in case you lose your balance) or at least to hear you scream if you fall. If not tending to your medical needs, this person could hand you equipment and supplies so you don't have to keep climbing up and down.

It's also important to use the right ladder for the job. If you need to clean gutters, use a ladder tall enough to get you to the roof line, not a stepladder that puts you just a couple of feet off the ground. Be sure whatever ladder you use is properly positioned and stable before stepping onto it.

Back Care

Do you have high or second-story windows, or lots of windows all around your house? Consider hiring a window-cleaning service to take care of spring cleaning for you. The workers have all the right equipment—climbing and cleaning—and can get the job done in a fraction of the time it would take you, and rates are generally lower than you'd expect.

Your Turn to Do Windows

Cleaning windows, especially those on a second level, can combine both the best and the worst. You get a good workout—spray on, rub off, spray on, rub off. You also can get into some pretty peculiar postures, particularly if you're on a ladder or a roof. Watch your reach. With cleaning supplies in one hand and the other hand trying to keep you from the clutches of gravity, your perch can quickly become precarious.

Safe Sex for Your Back

As we've said throughout this book, there's no reason for life as you know it to end just because your back hurts. Sure, you might have to make some changes. But you should be able to continue enjoying a full and pleasurable life—including sex.

Experiment with different positions and even locations that allow you to get close and yet don't stress your back. Take things slow and easy. If you're resuming sexual activity following surgery, you'll probably want to avoid positions that put pressure on your back or cause your back to arch (or sag).

You Can Teach an Old Back New Tricks

Your back changes as you grow older, there's no way around it. Your intervertebral disks stiffen and lose their resilience. Your bones begin to show wear and tear. Is life as you know it over?

Good heavens, no! There are those who would argue it's just beginning, but that's another book. The fact is, you don't have to let your aging back change your life. With proper care and regular exercise, you can keep your back feeling young and strong for many years.

Three Exercises for an Aging Back

Though we might think of the 20s and 30s as the prime years for physical activity, the 40s, 50s, and 60s are even more important when it comes to bone and back health.

By the time you reach your mid to late 30s, your body has slowed its calcium processing way down. In your early adulthood, your forgiving body lets you get away with a lot. By the time you hit middle age, your body's stopped forgiving and started forgetting.

The older your back gets, the more important it is to reawaken it, to keep it flexible and mobile. You want to regularly stretch and relax your muscles, and extend your range of motion. In addition to the stretching exercises and yoga postures in other chapters of this book, the following three exercises can help you do this.

Forward Stretch

1. Sit in a chair with your feet flat on the floor and your knees apart.
2. Take in a slow, deep breath, hold it for a count of six, then let it out.
3. Slowly extend your hands toward your knees and drop your head to your chest.
4. Reach between your knees toward your toes, and let your body bend forward from the waist so your chest is between your thighs. (If you can't get that far down, don't worry—just go as far as is comfortable for you.)
5. Feel the muscles in your back stretch and your vertebrae extend. Hold for a count of six, then slowly return to your original position.
6. Take a slow, deep breath in and hold it for a count of six. Slowly release it. Repeat the entire cycle three or four times.

Shoulder Rolls

1. You can do this exercise sitting or standing, as long as you keep your spine straight.
2. Put your hands in your lap or at your sides. Face straight ahead. Take a slow, deep breath in, hold it for a count of six, and let it out.

311

3. Slowly rotate your left shoulder in a circular motion, moving your shoulder forward and then through the rotation and back to its original position.

4. Repeat with your right shoulder.

5. Repeat with both shoulders at the same time.

6. Take a slow, deep breath in, hold it for a count of six, then let it out. Repeat the entire sequence three or four times to relax and stretch the muscles in your neck, shoulders, and upper back.

Yoga Lightning-Bolt Posture for Seniors

1. Sit on the edge of a hard-seated chair with your feet tucked under and your knees forward.

2. Slowly lean forward so your torso is over your thighs.

3. Raise your arms over your head with your palms facing each other, as though you were getting ready to dive into a pool of water.

4. Slowly try to raise yourself from the chair. If you're steady, hold your posture for a count of six.

5. Reverse your movements to return to your starting position.

6. Repeat the sequence three or four times.

> **Back to Nature**
>
> Yoga postures are ideal for developing strength and balance. If either is a bit weak for you, have a chair handy for support. Many yoga postures can easily be adapted to meet your needs.

Back Health for the Oldest Old

The older you get, the more at risk you are for osteoporosis. Though we think of osteoporosis as a disease of postmenopausal women, by the time you reach your eighth decade, the odds even out. Men who are 80 and older are just as likely to have osteoporosis as are women of the same age.

This is partly because your body slowly loses its efficiency in absorbing and metabolizing calcium and phosphorus, two minerals essential for bone strength and density. It's also partly because you tend to eat less as you get older, and take in fewer minerals and vitamins in general.

Many doctors recommend that people over age 60 take a multiple vitamin and mineral supplement. Women should talk with their doctors about calcium supplementation, too. Weight-bearing exercise is helpful in maintaining muscle mass. Just walking for 30 to 45 minutes three or four times a week can make a world of difference for your back and for your attitude.

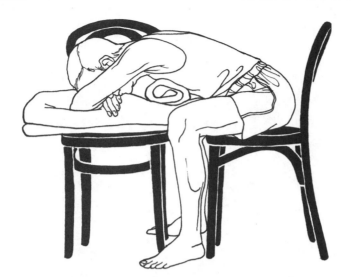

Seniors (or anyone!) can benefit from this pose. Place a folded blanket on the seat of one hard, straight-backed chair. Roll another towel and use it to cushion the chest as you bend forward to stretch out the lower back muscles. It's a wonderful supportive stretch that gives instant relief.

Aging muscles aren't as resilient as they once were, either. If you're over 70, you're more susceptible to muscle strains and pulls. Again, regular physical activity is the key to maintaining back health—it doesn't matter how old you are, your back still likes to be active. Treat your back with plenty of TLC. It's served you well so far, and it can keep doing so for many years to come if you take good care of it.

The Least You Need to Know

➤ Babies have very sensitive skin and respond well to gentle massage.

➤ Older children spend as much time as adults do sitting because they're invariably seated in front of computers, televisions, and video games. They need frequent stretch breaks to protect their backs.

➤ When housework and yard chores get you climbing around, be sure you use the right stepstool or ladder for the job, and have someone there to hand you supplies and equipment.

➤ Your "old" back can still have plenty of service left in it, if you treat it right.

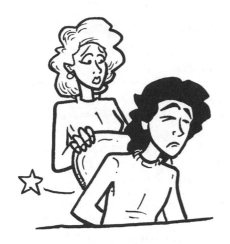

Chapter 27

Back Expectations

In This Chapter

➤ Dealing with a loved one's back problem

➤ Finding back-healthy activities you both can enjoy

➤ Watching out for your back's well-being

➤ How well do you treat your back? A self-quiz

Even with a bad back, life goes on. What you expect from your life has a lot to do with what you actually get. People who look on the bright side are more satisfied with what they see than those who focus on what's wrong.

When Someone You Love Has a Bad Back

It's not easy living with someone who has back pain, especially chronic. In fact, it can be downright challenging at times. Unless you have back pain, too, it's hard to understand what your loved one is going through. You can't see anything wrong, you can't feel anything wrong—all you know is your life has changed as a result.

Hang in there. Your support means more than you know. The very aspects of back problems that are hard for your loved one—pain that won't go away yet may have no apparent cause or cure, the limitations it imposes on his or her lifestyle—worry you, too. There are ways you can help, and things you can do for yourself to make it easier to "go with the flow."

How to Get Someone You Love to Go to the Doctor

Back pain can be an odd problem. Some people rush to the doctor with every little twinge, convinced that it's something either serious or that the doctor should be able to "fix" it. Now you know, because you've been paying attention as you've been reading this book, that doctors often can't fix back problems because they can't pin them down (and that most back pain improves on its own). So if your loved one is at the doctor's office so often there's a chair there with a nameplate, pass this book on when you're finished with it.

At the other end of the continuum is the person who won't go to the doctor under any circumstances. Fear is usually behind this resistance—what if the doctor finds something serious? With back problems, fortunately, that's very rare. Remember the "red flags" from Chapter 4 ,"Your Aching Back." If any of these are present, your loved one really needs to see a physician without delay.

But if your loved one's only complaint is pain and the limitations it places on life, you might suggest some of the self-treatments we discuss in this book. Unless your loved one is having leg pain, numbness, or other signs that there are nerve problems, the doctor probably can't do much more than your loved one can do on his or her own.

Back to Nature

If your loved one's back pain is taking all the joy out of life but he or she won't go to the doctor, see if a visit to a chiropractor might be a more agreeable option. A chiropractor can identify and treat a wide range of back problems, as well as alert you to anything an M.D. or D.O. should evaluate.

Back Off!

Anyone with back pain and a fever should see a doctor right away. This combination of symptoms can signal a serious infection that requires prompt medical attention.

Encouraging Back-Healthy Habits

Where is your loved one's aching back right now? Parked on the couch in front of the television? While lying around might be all he or she feels like doing, it's just about the worst possible thing for back health. Your back likes to be active. Even when you think it wants to rest, it needs exercise and activity for mobility and flexibility.

Suggest a short walk after dinner for starters. You might have to cajole and tease, but try to keep it light. Nagging and whining won't help anything (even you won't feel any better). But be gently persistent. Look for things to do together that involve some level of activity—shopping, or even going to the library (hey, you have to at least walk from the car to the building—just don't check out 20 books all at once). Just start getting out together as much as you can. An important first step in dealing with back pain is for your loved one to realize that he or she can hurt and still have a life.

Little Things You Can Do to Help

In reality, of course, only your loved one can do what needs to be done for his or her back health. You can make all the suggestions in the world, but that's the extent of your power. Sometimes the power of suggestion can be quite strong, especially when the promise of shared participation accompanies it.

What's Bad for Your Loved One Is Bad for You

Your loved one has back pain, and doesn't feel like doing much of anything. So what do you do? Probably the same! Doing nothing is no better for you than it is for your significant other.

A Sedentary Lifestyle Has Its Costs

Remember, an active back is a happy back. Your back wants you to stretch it and strengthen it so it stays flexible and mobile. When your lifestyle is so *sedentary* that you don't move much, you increase your risk of back problems. You also increase your risk of osteoporosis, particularly if you're a postmenopausal woman, and your risk of heart disease. Inactive people are also more likely to suffer from depression (a lack of joy in living).

Fortunately, the "cure" is simple—exercise! Regular, moderate physical activity, even just 20 or 30 minutes a day, works wonders for your back, your cardiovascular system (heart, lungs, and blood vessels), and your state of mind. It doesn't even have to be 20 or 30 minutes all at once—just five minutes here, 10 minutes there will do the trick. (Although sustained aerobic exercise at least three times a week is the very best way to keep your heart healthy, studies show even moderate activity increases life span.) Walking is the easiest way to get your body in shape, though activities such as swimming and bicycling are good, too.

Back Basics

A **sedentary** lifestyle has very little physical activity.

When Your Back Hurts, Too

If statistics could talk, they'd tell you that if your significant other has back problems, you're more likely to have them, too. With so many variables coming into play with back pain, it's hard to determine the reasons behind the probability. Of course, there's nothing contagious about back pain. Researchers believe there are numerous factors that put you at greater risk.

One of them might be that you pick up the slack—literally—in your household. Because your loved one can't lift, push, pull, or carry, you do. After all, someone still has to change the sheets on the bed, run the laundry, and wash the floors.

Other factors are more psychosocial—that is, they relate to the emotional and social aspects of your life. When your significant other has back problems that limit his or her activities, your life becomes limited, too. After a while, this limitation is all you know. You can begin behaving as though your back bothers you, too, and before you know it, it is.

Take Care of Yourself

It's hard, when someone you love hurts, to move forward with your life even if your loved one can't come along right now. But it's important for your health and well-being that you do just that. Develop a routine of relaxation and exercise to keep your life and your body balanced and healthy. You feel selfish, you say? Don't! How can you take care of someone else if you're not in good shape yourself?

Taking Good Care of Your Back: A Self-Quiz

How happy do you keep your back? See how you answer these questions now, then come back to them a month or so after finishing this book to see if your answers are different.

1. Your idea of time for yourself is…
   a) Being at work an hour before everyone else.
   b) No one's home but you, so you can stay in your jammies if you want.
   c) Planning an outing to a favorite location once a week.

2. Your meeting is out 20 minutes early. Now you have time to…
   a) Grab a latte and a bagel.
   b) Zip over to the bookstore to buy that book on yoga.
   c) Give yourself a neck massage.

3. Your favorite way to relax is…
   a) Fall asleep in front of the TV.
   b) Take a walk on the beach or in the park.
   c) Find a quiet place where you can close your eyes, do a few breathing exercises, and re-center yourself.

4. You need to burn off some energy. You decide to…
   a) Hit a few balls on the tennis court.
   b) Take your bicycle out for a spin.
   c) Go for a swim.

5. You're on the 14th hole and just hit a beautiful shot down the green. On your follow-through, you got a sharp, stabbing pain in your lower back. You…
   a) Finish the game—you can't quit when you have the best score for the year.

b) Send someone to the clubhouse for some ice, and do a few stretches to see if it goes away.

c) Call it a day. After all, it's only a game.

6. Your report is due this afternoon, and you've been working on it at your computer since you first got in. You suddenly realize it's near noon and you haven't taken a break. You...

a) Keep working—time's a-wasting.

b) Do a few shoulder shrugs and neck stretches, then get back to your computer.

c) Save your work, stand and do a few back stretches, then walk downstairs for a little fresh air.

7. There's a large box outside your door when you get home. No one else will be home for an hour or so. You...

a) Drag it in the house so you can open it.

b) Open it right where it stands so you can see what's inside.

c) Wait for your neighbor, who'll be home in about 10 minutes.

Give yourself five points for each A, three points for each B, and one point for each C. If you have 25 or more points, you haven't been paying attention. If you have 15 to 24 points, you think about your back sometimes but not often enough. If you have 14 or less points, treat yourself to a massage!

Prevention Is the Best Cure

You've heard the cliché hundreds of times: "An ounce of prevention is worth a pound of cure." We're repeating it one more time because it's so true. Reducing your risk of back trouble through exercise and activity is a much less painful route than working your way through an episode of back pain.

Keep Small Problems Small

Did you have a small ache in your lower back when you came home from work? Maybe you sat longer than usual today, twisted just wrong, or just happened to notice the discomfort in the car on the drive home. Keep it small. Do a few relaxation techniques as soon as you notice the first twinge. When you get home, ice the spot for 15 or 20 minutes, and then gently massage the area (if you can reach it; if not, have your significant other give you a hand). Take a relaxing, warm shower or bath, followed by a few back exercises or yoga postures, before you go to bed. In all likelihood, you'll wake up in the morning feeling refreshed and ready to face another day.

Have Patience

One of the most difficult aspects of back pain for most people is that it takes so long to go away. We're used to getting what we want, NOW. While we want to respect the natural healing process, we also want it to get going.

Take a deep breath, and have a little patience. You can't hurry healing. It just takes time. What you can do to help it along is take care of your back while it's healing. Pamper it, even, with massages and relaxing showers or baths. Take every opportunity to stretch and flex your back muscles. If it makes you feel better, see your chiropractor for a few adjustments. Just give your back the time it needs to heal.

It's All Relative

The good thing about back pain is that it changes often. Some days are worse than others, which isn't so good, but many more are better. Look forward to those days, and let that carry you through the others. Keep yourself busy, so your pain has less of your attention. You might be surprised at how effectively you can shut it down by shutting it out with activities and other interests.

Stay Informed

Learn everything you can about back pain and back problems. It won't make either go away, but it will give you a better understanding of how the back functions—and malfunctions. Knowledge also is empowering. When you know what the doctor means when she says "ankylosing spondylitis," you no longer fear strange words with too many syllables and too little meaning.

It's also possible your quest for information will lead you to solutions your loved one and his or her primary caregiver haven't considered or tried. Some approaches are likely to be holistic in nature, while others might involve new wonder drugs or miracle surgeries. New treatments are being developed, and the standard ones are being rigorously tested to find out whether or not they're effective, and for which back problems. The knowledge you've acquired in your search for answers is a good filter for separating the hype from the help.

Find Reliable Information Sources

There's an abundance of information available about back pain and back problems. Some might even say its overwhelming. Because the causes of back pain are often so difficult to pin down, and because most back problems eventually heal themselves, theories and ideas run wild. Someone tries something unconventional and is "cured," and suddenly the whole world knows because it's posted to a newsgroup on the *Internet*.

Never mind that no one else has tried the "cure," or that it's never been tested in any way, shape, or form. It worked for Dan, whose back pain kept him in bed for three years, so it could work for your loved one. This can be very, very scary stuff. Desperate people are often willing to try desperate measures. When those measures appear to work, they get all the credit. But no one has any idea whether there was a real relationship between Dan's miracle recovery and the alfalfa sprouts and raspberries he whirred in the blender with a handful of vitamin pills and drank every morning. (Ugh!) Was it the raspberries? Was it the alfalfa sprouts? Was it the vitamins? Who knows!

A good rule of thumb is to verify any information that you find interesting with at least two independent sources. If you locate the information on the *World Wide Web*, go to the library and try to find similar information in magazine articles or medical journals (not the same one sponsoring the Web site where you found the material in the first place). Beware of advertising ahead of scientific testing. "Promising" and "new" often mean "untested" and "experimental."

Back Basics

The **Internet** is a worldwide network of linked computers. It provides access to nearly endless information, from databases at research institutes to newsgroup discussions (people who write messages to other people with similar interests). The **World Wide Web** is a structure that organizes the material available through the Internet so it's easier to find and use.

Don't Be Afraid to Ask Questions

When you come across information that seems like it might help you or your loved one, don't be afraid to schedule an appointment with your doctor, chiropractor, or other primary health care provider. If it's a valid approach, there'll be something in a professional journal or your health care provider has already learned of it. If your doctor comes up empty, ask where to go next to find out more.

Sometimes you can check with a professional organization to get more information about a treatment or an approach that interests you. Your local medical society or association might be able to direct you to doctors who are studying or even using the approach.

Back Care

When you find information on the World Wide Web, check the address of the Web site or Web page that you're visiting. If it ends in ".com," it's a commercial site and odds are high its owner has something to sell. More reliable information sources are government agencies (".gov") and not-for-profit organizations (".org").

Think Positive

If an eight-ounce glass has four ounces of water in it, is it half full or half empty? If you see the glass as half full, you're excited and grateful to still have water. If you see it as half empty, however, you're bemoaning the loss of something you'll never get back. Sure, there'll be other water, but not the same water that's missing. How dreary! How you see life makes all the difference. Sure, you're going to have bad days. Everyone does, whether they have back problems or not. Look on the bright side.

The Power of Focus

Jon Kabat-Zinn, Ph.D., is known throughout the world for his writings and teachings in meditation and disease. He observes that disease and health co-exist as two parts of the same whole. Your back pain, and your back health, are simply different presentations of the same thing. If you focus on your pain, that's what you see and feel, and that's what drives your life. If you focus on health, however, you begin to perceive your back as healthy. Mind and matter begin working together.

Regain Control

People who believe they are in control of their lives are better able to cope with the variances life throws at them. The more control you believe you have, the more aspects of your life you begin to control. Studies show that how much control you feel you have—or don't have—may have a greater influence than the nature of the problem on whether your back problem becomes disabling. This is not to suggest your back problem isn't real. It's just yet another reminder of how connected your body and your mind are to each other.

Support Your Soul

What's good for your soul is good for your body. Studies show that people who go to church regularly and who feel a strong bond to their faith (it doesn't matter what religion or belief system) are more likely to survive serious illness or injury. They are also better able to handle the little things life throws at them because they have a clear sense of an existence that extends beyond them. This keeps them grounded in the reality that back pain doesn't define their lives; it's merely one aspect of living.

The Least You Need to Know

➤ It's okay to feel frustrated when a loved one has back problems.

➤ Treating small aches and pains with TLC (tender loving care) can keep them from getting big enough to interfere with your life.

➤ When you live with someone who has back pain, you're more likely to develop back problems yourself.

➤ You owe it to yourself to take care of your back.

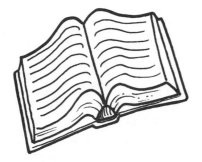

Glossary

Abduction   The action of moving your arms and legs away from your body.

Acupuncture   The ancient Chinese practice of stimulating certain points along the body's energy meridians.

Acute pain   *See* Pain, acute.

Adduction   The action of moving your arms and legs toward your body (laterally, or to the sides).

Adhesions   Abnormal growths of fibrous tissue that connect normally separate body parts.

Adjunctive therapies   Those that complement the chiropractic or other care that's the primary treatment.

Aerobic   "With oxygen."

Allopathic   Conventional Western medicine as practiced by an M.D.

Alternative medicine   In Western cultures, approaches to health care that are not allopathic. Also called complementary medicine.

Anaerobic   "Without oxygen."

Analgesic   A drug that relieves pain. Many anti-inflammatory drugs also work as analgesics.

Ankylosing spondylitis   A form of arthritis that affects the spine and sacroiliac joints (where the spine joins the pelvis).

Antibiotic   A drug that fights bacterial infections.

Anti-inflammatory   A medication that reduces swelling or inflammation.

Antiseptic   A chemical that cleans skin and other surfaces, destroying bacteria and microorganisms that could cause disease.

Arthroscope   Special lighted, flexible tube inserted into a small incision through which a surgeon performs a surgical procedure.

Biofeedback   A process of consciously affecting body activities that usually happen without conscious intervention, such as muscle tenseness and pain perception.

Biopsy   A procedure in which a small section of tissue is surgically removed for examination under a microscope.

Board certified   Means that a physician has completed extensive additional training and passed a series of rigorous tests in his or her chosen specialty.

Cauda equina   A branching nerve structure at the base of your spinal cord that resembles the tail of a horse.

Chemonucleolysis   Injecting an enzyme called chymopapain into the center of a herniated disk.

Chi   Energy, both physical and metaphysical. Eastern cultures view chi as an animated and nourishing force that sustains all life and existence, and sometimes refer to chi as "cosmic breath."

Chiropractic   The philosophy and practice of the healing method that uses spinal adjustments and manipulations to restore alignment to the spine and related structures.

Complementary medicine   *See* Alternative medicine.

Congenital   A condition or abnormality with which you are born.

CT scan   A process whereby a computer compiles multiple x-ray images into "slices" of images to give a dimensional perspective of body parts such as the spine.

Deqi   The tingling sensation you feel when an acupuncture needle is inserted.

Dermatomes   Areas of your body supplied by certain root nerves from your spine.

Diathermy   A form of heat treatment using high-frequency electrical currents directed into body tissues.

Disk prolapse   A bulge or tear in an intervertebral disk.

D.O.   Doctor of osteopathy.

Effleurage   Long, stroking movements that massage larger body areas.

Electromyography   A test that measures and records the electrical activity of your muscles, helping to determine whether there is any damage to the nerves or muscle tissue that affects a muscle's ability to contract and relax.

Epidural   An injection of an anesthetic agent into the epidural space (between the dura mater and the spinal cord) to numb the root nerves branching from the spinal cord.

Ergonomics   The science of "human engineering." Objects that are ergonomic are designed to interact with people in ways that make tasks easier and more efficient.

Extension   The action of straightening.

Failed Back Surgery Syndrome (FBSS)   The name for the collective symptoms some people experience when back surgery is not successful.

Fascia   The thin, membrane-like tissue that covers connective tissues.

Fiber optics   Bundles of hair-like glass threads that transmit light at its full strength from the light source to the end of an endoscope.

Fibromyalgia   Chronic pain syndrome involving the muscles and fibrous tissues.

Flexion   The action of bending.

Herniated disk   A disk in which its thick, fibrous wall weakens and stretches, allowing its jelly-like center to bulge through.

Internet   A worldwide network of linked computers.

Isokinetic contraction   An osteopathic technique that strengthens muscle fibers through contraction against resistance.

Isometric contraction   An osteopathic technique that encourages flexibility in connective tissue to restore a joint to its normal function.

Isometric exercise   Exercise that uses static resistance (pushing against a nonmoving force) to increase muscle strength.

Kyphosis   The outward curve of your thoracic spine. This often becomes more prominent and abnormal in people with osteoporosis.

Laminae   The bony arches of the vertebrae that you can feel when you run your fingers down your spine.

Ligaments   Tough bands of connective tissue that link bones together.

Lordosis   The inward curve in your lumbar spine.

Magnetic resonance imaging (MRI)   Computer technology that uses high-powered magnetic energy to "look" inside the body without surgery.

Mantra   Sanskrit word meaning "free from constant thought."

Mechanical injuries   Injuries that affect the way in which your back functions.

Metabolism   The process by which your cells use energy and clear waste.

Metaphysical   "Beyond the body."

Minimally invasive procedures   Surgeries that require very small incisions.

Motor nerves   Nerves that carry signals of action away from the brain.

Myelography   A process in which a dye is injected into the fluid around the spinal cord to highlight the structures of the spine. X-ray or CT scanning is then used to take pictures of the structures.

Myofascial   Involving both the muscle and fascia.

Myositis   Inflammation of the muscles.

Neuron   Nerve cell.

Neuropeptides   Biochemical substances found in brain cells as well as many other kinds of cells throughout the body.

NPO   Medical shorthand for "nothing by mouth."

NSAID   The abbreviation for "nonsteroidal anti-inflammatory drug."

Orthotics   Devices, usually custom-made for your feet, that fit into your shoes to alter the way you walk and stand.

Osteoarthritis   A condition in which the cartilage (tough, elastic tissue that keeps bone ends from rubbing against each other) in joints deteriorates, sometimes causing pain and instability.

Osteoarticular adjustment   Osteopathic manipulation of the relationship between bones at a joint to restore mobility.

Osteopathic manipulation therapy (OMT)   An osteopathic process of evaluation, diagnosis, and treatment.

Osteopathy   A form of medicine that views the human body as a unified organism, at the core of which is the musculoskeletal system.

Osteoporosis   A condition that results when the bones lose density and mass, becoming weak and susceptible to breaking.

Over-the-counter (OTC)   A medication you can buy without a prescription.

Pain, acute   Pain that comes on suddenly.

Pain, chronic   Pain that has been present for longer than six to eight weeks.

Pain, referred   The pain you feel in one place in your body that is caused by a problem somewhere else.

Petrissage   Small, kneading movements that massage a specific muscle or tendon.

Physiology   The study of how the human body works.

Placebo   A substance or device that looks like the real thing but actually has no therapeutic effect.

Podiatrist   Doctor of Podiatric Medicine (D.P.M.) who specializes in foot care.

Posthypnotic suggestion   An idea the hypnotherapist suggests to your mind when you're in a hypnotic state that will trigger a response or reaction when you're fully conscious.

Postoperative   After the surgery; often shortened to "postop."

Prolotherapy   Injecting an irritating substance into a spinal joint to encourage new connective tissue to grow.

Psychosomatic   "Mind and body."

Radionuclide   A radioactive substance that, when injected into the body, releases energy that some tissues absorb better than others, allowing this difference to make a picture (for example, bony tumors look darker than normal tissue).

Reflex   A body reaction over which you have no conscious control.

Rehabilitation   An integrated treatment approach that blends various methods and therapies to help people return to self-sufficiency.

Rheumatoid arthritis   A condition in which your body's immune system attacks your joints as though they were invaders.

Ruptured disk   *See* Disk prolapse.

Sciatica   Pain that follows the sciatic nerve down the buttock and back of your leg to below the knee.

Scoliosis   A side curvature of the spine.

Sedentary   A lifestyle that has very little physical activity.

Sensory nerves   Nerves that carry signals of sensation to the brain.

Soft tissues   Your muscles, tendons, and ligaments   body parts that are soft compared to bone.

Spasm   An involuntary muscle contraction that continues for a period of time.

Spina bifida   An abnormal gap that forms between the vertebrae in a developing unborn child, leaving part of the spinal cord outside the spine at birth.

Spinal stenosis   The narrowing of the opening in the vertebra through which nerves pass as they leave the spinal cord.

Spondylolisthesis   A painful condition in which one vertebra slips over the top of another, putting pressure on the spinal nerves and sometimes the spinal cord and causing pain.

Sterile   Germ free.

Subluxation   A situation in your spine where your facet joints are slightly out of alignment.

Survival of the fittest   A phrase for how traits within a species that are useful in helping that species survive are passed on to future generations.

Syndrome   A collection of symptoms that together describe a disorder. The cause is usually unknown.

Tendons   Tough bands of connective tissue that attach muscles to bones.

Ultrasound imaging   A technique that uses focused, high-frequency sound waves to generate images of internal body organs.

Ultrasound therapy   A form of heat treatment that uses high-frequency sound waves to relax muscles and increase their blood supply.

Vertebrae   The irregularly shaped bones that form your spine; just one is a vertebra.

World Wide Web   A structure that organizes the information available through the Internet so it's easier to find and use.

X-rays   A form of electromagnetic energy that, as it passes through an object, temporarily creates an electrically charged particle called an ion that shows up as an image on film.

Yin-Yang   In Traditional Chinese or Oriental Medicine, opposites that exist in pairs to form the whole (such as female/male, dark/light, cold/hot).

Yoga   A Sanskrit word meaning "union" or "to yoke together."

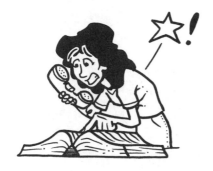

Who Treats Back Pain?

Many different practitioners treat back problems. This table summarizes who does what.

Practitioner	Scope of Practice
Acupuncturist	Many medical professionals can qualify to perform acupuncture. Scope of practice depends on profession.
Allopathic physician (M.D.)	Comprehensive primary and specialty health care. Can prescribe medications and perform surgery.
Chiropractor (D.C.)	Uses physical adjustments to treat conditions of the spine.
Family practitioner	M.D. or D.O. specializing in general health care needs.
Massage therapist (L.M.T.)	Performs therapeutic massage; may specialize in sports massage.
Neurosurgeon, neurologist	M.D. or D.O. specializing in conditions involving nerves.
Orthopedic surgeon	M.D. or D.O. specializing in conditions involving bones.
Physiatrist	M.D. or D.O. specializing in conditions involving mobility and physical rehabilitation.
Occupational therapist (O.T., L/O.T.)	Uses various therapies to restore physical functions necessary for activities of daily living (ADLs) and the return to work following serious injury.
Osteopathic physician (D.O.)	Functions the same as allopathic M.D. physician (primary or specialty care), with additional training in musculoskeletal manipulations. Philosophy of practice emphasizes holistic approach.
Physical therapist (P.T., R.P.T., M.P.T.)	Uses exercise and physical activities to relieve soft-tissue pain and restore function.
Traditional Chinese Medicine (TCM) doctor	Trained in TCM methods including acupuncture, energy therapies, and herbal treatments. (Sometimes called Traditional Oriental Medicine, or TOM.)

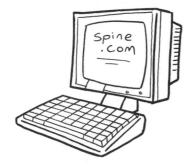

Resources for Back Pain

American Academy of Orthopedic Surgeons (AAOS)
6300 N. River Road
Rosemont, IL 60018-4262
Phone: 800-346-AAOS or 847-823-7186
Web site: www.aaos.org

The AAOS is the membership organization of physicians who specialize in orthopedics. It provides to patients information materials on a wide variety of orthopedic conditions and treatments.

American Physical Therapy Association (APTA)
111 North Fairfax Street
Alexandria, VA 22314
Phone: 800-999-2782
Web site: www.apta.org

The APTA is a national membership organization for the physical therapy profession. It provides continuing professional education for its members and general information for the public.

Associated Bodywork and Massage Professional (ABMP)
28677 Buffalo Park Road
Evergreen, CO 80439-7347
Phone: 800-458-ABMP (2267)
Fax: 303-674-0859
Web site: www.abmp.com

The ABMP is a national membership organization for practitioners in bodywork and massage. The organization provides information and educational materials for its members, information about massage and bodywork for the general public, and career information for those interested in working in bodywork or massage.

MedWeb

The Robert W. Woodruff Health Sciences Center Library of Emory University
Web site: www.medweb.emory.edu/MedWeb

This electronic reference source provides World Wide Web links to a vast number of medical and health care resources.

ChiroWeb.com

Web site: www.chiroweb.com

This electronic reference source provides comprehensive information about chiropractic care. It's a commercial Web site sponsored by chiropractors across America.

National Association for Chiropractic Medicine (NACM)

15427 Baybrook Drive
Houston, TX 77062
Phone: 281-280-8262
Fax: 281-280-8262
Web site: www.chiromed.org

From the Web site: "The National Association for Chiropractic Medicine (NACM) is a consumer advocacy association of chiropractors who confine their scope of practice to scientific parameters and seek to make legitimate the utilization of professional manipulative procedures in mainstream health-care delivery. The NACM offers consumer assistance in finding member practitioners."

American Chiropractic Association (ACA)

Phone: 800-368-3083
Web site: www.amerchiro.org

The ACA is a professional organization for chiropractors. The ACA provides information about back care, the philosophy and practice of chiropractic, and member chiropractors. It also sells related products and publications.

American Association of Acupuncture and Oriental Medicine (AAAOM)

433 Front Street
Catasauqua, PA 18032
Phone: 610-266-1433
Fax: 610-264-2768
Web site: www.aaom.org

Provides information about Traditional Oriental Medicine (TOM; also called Traditional Chinese Medicine, or TCM). The AAAOM is active in education, legislation, and professional standards.

American Osteopathic Association (AOA)

142 East Ontario Street
Chicago, IL 60611
Phone: 800-621-1773
Web site: www.am-osteo-assn.org

The AOA is the professional membership organization for osteopathic physicians. It can provide information about osteopathic care and physicians.

Endometriosis Association
8585 North 76th Place
Milwaukee, WI 53223
Phone: 800-992-3636 or 414-355-2200
Web site: www.endometriosisassn.org

The Endometriosis Association provides information about all aspects of endometriosis, from current research and treatment approaches to support groups and services.

National Health Information Center (NHIC)
P.O. Box 1133
Washington DC 20013-1133
Phone: 800-336-4797
Web site: www.nhic-nt.health.org

Sponsored by the Office of Disease Prevention and Health Promotion (ODPHP), U.S. Department of Health and Human Services, the NHIC is a health information referral service. It puts health professionals and consumers who have health questions in touch with those organizations that are best able to provide answers.

National Institutes of Health (NIH)
Bethesda, Maryland 20892
Phone: 301-496-4000
Web site: www.nih.gov

The National Institutes of Health are a collection of agencies and services within the U.S. federal government that conduct research and provide educational materials about health-related issues. NIH health resources are vast and diverse. Those available through the NIH Web site include CancerNet, AIDS information, Clinical Alerts, the Women's Health Initiative, and the NIH Information Index (a subject-word guide to diseases and conditions under investigation at NIH).

Occupational Safety and Health Administration (OSHA)
U.S. Department of Labor
Public Affairs Office - Room: 3647
200 Constitution Avenue
Washington, DC 20210
Phone: 800-321-6742 or 202-693-1999
Web site: www.osha.gov

OSHA is a division of the U.S. Department of Labor. Its mission "is to save lives, prevent injuries and protect the health of America's workers." OSHA is a good resource for information about workplace health and safety, regulations, and standards.

333

Scoliosis Association
P.O. Box 811705
Boca Raton, FL 33481-1705
Phone: 800-800-0669 or 561-994-0669

Founded by scoliosis patients and family members, the Scoliosis Association supports early detection, treatment, and research. There are numerous chapters throughout the United States.

Spondylitis Association of America
P.O. Box 5872
Sherman Oaks, CA 91413
Phone: 800-777-8189
Web site: www.spondylitis.org

The Spondylitis Association of America provides information about ankylosing spondylitis, spinal arthritis, and related conditions.

Texas Back Institute: Back Pain Hotline
6300 West Parker Road
Plano, TX 75093
Phone: 800-247-BACK (247-2225)
Web site: www.texasback.com

The Texas Back Institute claims to be the largest freestanding specialty clinic in the United States. Its practitioners include physicians, chiropractors, psychologists, and physical therapists (among others), and it treats patients from all across the United States. Through its Web site, the clinic offers information about back pain, back problems, and back treatments.

Index

A

abdominal exercises, 145
abdominal muscles, 20-23
  C-sections, 299
  functions, 21
abnormal results of
  diagnostic tools, 111
acetaminophen, 129, 132-133
activities
  avoiding back pain, 271
    planning ahead, 271
  resuming, 204-207
    driving, 205
    going back to work, 206
    household duties,
      205-206
    shoe choice, 207-208
    sitting and standing,
      204-205
    sleep positions, 206-207
acupuncture, 223-224
  acumassage, 225
  acupressure, 225
  choosing acupuncturists,
    231-232
    as caregiver, 232
    qualifications, 231-232
  acupuncturists
    scope of practice, 329
    selection of, 231-232
  heat treatments
    cupping, 225
    moxibustion, 225
  risks, 225
  Western medicine, electro-
    chemical interference,
    229-231
acupuncturists
  scope of practice, 329
  selection of, 231-232
    as caregiver, 232
    qualifications, 231-232
acute back pain, 42-44
adhesions, 215

adjunctive therapies,
  chiropractic care, 218
  nutrition and exercise, 218
  psychic health, 218-219
adjustments, chiropractic care
  lower-back pain, 216-217
  neck and shoulders,
    216-217
  treatment of back pain, 217
  treatment of nerve pain,
    217-218
adolescents and back pain,
  308-309
adrenaline, 230
adreno-cortico-trophic hormone. *See* ACTH
aerobic exercises, 153
aging
  as source of back pain, 34-37
    osteoporosis, 34-35
  back exercises, 311-313
    forward stretch, 311
    shoulder rolls, 311-312
    yoga lightning bolt
      posture, 312
  supplements, 312-313
aids and devices,
  ergonomics, 273
alcohol, effects on
  back pain, 281
alendronate, 303
alignment, yoga, 156
allopathic health care
  physicians (M.D.), 329
  versus alternative health
    care, 115-116
alternative health care
  medicine. *See* natural healing
    alternatives
  versus allopathic health care,
    115-116
anaerobic exercises, 153
  yoga, 153
analgesics, 10, 128
Anaprox, 131

anesthesiology, 190-193
  blocks and locals, 192-193
  general anesthesia, 192
  pain management after
    surgery, 193-194
ankle-jerk, 101
ankylosing spondylitis, 91-92
anti-inflammatory medicines,
  10-13, 128
  NSAIDs, 131-132
antibiotics, wound care, 202
anticoagulants, 43
antiseptic solution, 201
apitherapy. *See* bee and snake
  venom
arthroscope, 194
asanas, 151, 152
aspirin, 132-133
attitude, influence on back
  pain, 164-165

B

backpacks, as source of back
  pain, 37-38
backs
  bad habits, 10
  curves, 95-96
    kyphosis, 96-98
    lordosis, 96-98
    scoliosis, 95
  exercises, 146-147
    abdominal stretch, 146
    body curls, 147
    leg lifts, 147
    low back rotation,
      147-148
    stretches, 61, 146-147
  frequency of back pain, 5
  infants, 305-307
  physical structure, 15-21
    five sections, 23-25
    intervertebral disks, 17-18
    ligaments, 18
    muscles, 18-20